£80
'18
innere

Recent Results in Cancer Research

Volume 206

More information about this series at http://www.springer.com/series/392

Wojciech Golusiński · C. René Leemans
Andreas Dietz
Editors

HPV Infection in Head and Neck Cancer

Springer

Editors
Wojciech Golusiński
Department of Head and Neck Surgery
The Greater Poland Cancer Centre
Poznan University of Medical Sciences
Poznań
Poland

Andreas Dietz
Department of Head Medicine and Oral Health, Clinic of Otolaryngology
University of Leipzig
Leipzig
Germany

C. René Leemans
Department of Otolaryngology-Head and Neck Surgery
VU University Medical Center/Cancer Center Amsterdam
Amsterdam
The Netherlands

ISSN 0080-0015 ISSN 2197-6767 (electronic)
Recent Results in Cancer Research
ISBN 978-3-319-43578-7 ISBN 978-3-319-43580-0 (eBook)
DOI 10.1007/978-3-319-43580-0

Library of Congress Control Number: 2016947932

Printed on acid-free paper

This Springer imprint is published by Springer Nature
The registered company is Springer International Publishing AG Switzerland

Contents

Part I
Epidemiology and Molecular Biology of HPV Positive HNSCC

HPV in Head and Neck Cancer—30 Years of History

Stina Syrjänen, Jaana Rautava and Kari Syrjänen

Abstract

The interesting history of papillomavirus (PV) research has been reviewed before. The history of human papillomavirus (HPV) in head and neck region starts in 1901 when the contagious transmission of warty lesions into the mouth via oral sex was described, although the confirmation of their viral etiology had to wait until 1907. Ullman was the first to associate the human wart virus with laryngeal warts. Parsons and Kidd described the natural history of oral PV infections in rabbits already in 1942, but these findings were corroborated in humans only recently. Koilocytotic atypia described by Koss and Durfee in 1956 was recognized as a sign of HPV infection in cervical precancer lesions only in 1976–1977 (Meisels and Fortin; Purola and Savia). This prompted systematic surveys of head and neck lesions for the detection of koilocytosis since the late 1970s, and the authors of this communication were the first to propose the HPV involvement in a subgroup of head and neck cancers. Brandsma and Abramson demonstrated HPV16 DNA in tonsillar SCCs in 1989. Since the early 2000s, HPV research of head and neck squamous cell carcinomas (HNSCC) has made impressive progress, confirming that the specific anatomic site plays a key role in determining the susceptibility to HPV infection. The most likely cancer sites associated with HPV are the base of the tongue and palatine tonsils, followed by

S. Syrjänen (✉) · J. Rautava
Department of Oral Pathology, Faculty of Medicine, Institute of Dentistry, University of Turku, Lemminkäisenkatu 2, 20520 Turku, Finland
e-mail: stina.syrjanen@utu.fi

S. Syrjänen · J. Rautava
Department of Pathology, Turku University Hospital, University of Turku, Turku, Finland

K. Syrjänen
Department of Clinical Research, Biohit Oyj, Helsinki, Finland

W. Golusiński et al. (eds.), *HPV Infection in Head and Neck Cancer*,
Recent Results in Cancer Research 206, DOI 10.1007/978-3-319-43580-0_1

oral cavity, larynx, and sinonasal mucosa. There is substantial geographic variation in HPV association with HNSCC. Patients with HPV-associated HNSCC are younger, and survival is better than in the absence of HPV.

Keywords
History · Human papillomavirus (HPV) · Head and neck squamous cell carcinomas (HNSSC)

1 Introduction

The present-day understanding of papillomavirus (PV) research is a result of a long history of intense work consisting of important innovations and contributions of a countless number of past and present scientists. The past history of PV research is dual consisting of (1) basic virology research, and (2) an increasing awareness of human papillomaviruses (HPV) as a significant cause of human diseases emerging from the late 1970s. Several excellent reviews exist on the history of PV research (Syverton et al. 1950; Bäfverstedt 1967; Grodzicker and Hopkins, Oriel in 1989; Lancaster and Olson 1982; Gross 1983; Orth 1986; Oriel 1989; zur Hausen and de Villiers 1994; Lowy and Schiller 2006; Syrjänen and Syrjänen 2008; zur Hausen 2009). Since the early 2000s, the studies on HPV and head and neck cancer have increased overwhelmingly.

This chapter summarizes shortly the main milestones of the HPV research which have made an impact in the stepwise understanding of HPV as an etiological agent in a subgroup of head and neck squamous cell carcinomas (HNSCC). One has to note that this type of listing represents the personal preferences of the authors, and the missing of someone's name in the list by no means signifies the lack of importance of their work. The head and neck region discussed here comprises a number of distinct anatomic sites including oral cavity, nasal cavity, paranasal sinuses, nasopharynx; oropharynx, hypopharynx, and larynx. This historical review on the role of HPV in head and neck cancers is specifically acknowledging the early papers published during the next 10 years after the original observations and is summarized in the Tables 1, 2, 3, and 4.

Table 1 Detection of HPV in oral carcinomas during the first 10 years after the original report

Reference	Lesion	No. of cases	Method	HPV-positivity		Types detected
Syrjänen et al. (1983a, b, c, d)	SCC	40	ICH	8/40	20 %	
Syrjänen et al. (1983a, b, c, d)	SCC	1	ICH	0/1	0 %	
Syrjänen et al. (1983a, b, c, d)	SCC	6	ICH	0/6	0 %	

(continued)

Table 1 (continued)

Reference	Lesion	No. of cases	Method	HPV-positivity		Types detected
Jin and Toto (1984)	Verrucous Ca	7	ICH	0/7	0 %	
Löning et al. (1985)	SCC	6	SB	3/6	50 %	
de Villiers et al. (1985)	SCC	7	SB	3/7	43 %	2, 16
Adler-Storthz et al. (1986)	Verrucous Ca	9	ISH	1/9	11 %	2
Syrjänen et al. (1986)	SCC	2	ISH	1/2	100 %	16
de Villiers et al. (1986)	SCC	11	SB	4/11	36 %	2, 16
Löning et al. (1986)	SCC	6	ISH	3/6	50 %	11, 16
Milde and Löning (1986)	SCC	7	ISH	4/7	57 %	16
Maitland et al. (1987)	SCC	15	SB	7/15	47 %	16, unknown
Lookingbill et al. (1987)	SCC	1	DB	1/1	100 %	11, 16
Löning et al. (1987)	SCC	13	DB	5/13	38 %	6/11, 16/18
Ostrow et al. (1987)	SCC	3	SB	1/3	33 %	16
Dekmezian et al. (1987)	SCC	4	ISH	4/4	100 %	
Gassenmaier and Hornstein (1988)	SCC	68	ISH	16/68	23 %	2, 6, 11, 16
Lee et al. (1988)	SCC	2	SB	1/2	50 %	
Syrjänen et al. (1988)	SCC	51	ISH	6/51	12 %	16, 18
Brandsma and Abramson (1989)	SCC	39	SB	2/39	5 %	
Chang et al. (1989)	SCC	17	SB	13/17	76 %	
Maitland et al. (1989)	SCC	50	PCR	25/50	50 %	16
Demetric et al. (1990)	SCC	1	ISH, SB	1/1	100 %	16
Ishibashi et al. (1990)	SCC	6	SB	0/6	0 %	
Kashima et al. (1990)	SCC	29	SB,ISH	6/29	21 %	
Greer et al. (1990a, b)	SCC	2	DB	2/2	100 %	6/11, 16/18
Greer et al. (1990a, b)	Verrucous Ca	20	ISH	4/20	20 %	6/11, 16/18
Chang et al. (1990)	SCC	40	ISH, PCR		11/40 28 %	16(69 %), 6, 18
Kulski et al. 1990	SCC	5	SB	1/5	20 %	6/11, 16/18
Niedobitek et al. (1990)	SCC, tonsil	21	ISH	6/28	21 %	16
Arndt et al. (1991)	SCC	11	SB	7/11	64 %	6/11, 16/18
SCC, tonsil	9	SB	5/9	56 %	6/11, 16/18	
Tsuchiya et al. (1991)	SCC	23	ISH, SB	3/23	13 %	Unknown

(continued)

Table 1 (continued)

Reference	Lesion	No. of cases	Method	HPV-positivity		Types detected
Abdelsayed et al. (1991)	SCC	36	ISH	2/36	6 %	6/11, 16/18
Palefsky et al. (1991)	SCC	25	PCR	8/25	32 %	
Yeudall and Campo (1991)	SCC	39	SB		3/39 8 %	4, 16, 18
SCC	39	PCR	18/39	46 %		
Watts et al. (1991)	SCC	23	SB, PCR, E6	16/23	70 %	6/11, 16/18
Verrucous Ca	49	SB, PCR	27/49		55 %	16/18
Shroyer et al. (1993)	SCC	10	ISH, PCR	1/10	10 %	16/18
Verrucous Ca	3	ISH, PCR	0/3	0 %		
Zeuss et al. (1991)	SCC	15	ISH	0/15	0 %	
Young and Min (1991)	SCC, Verrucous Ca	27	ISH	0/27	0 %	
Adler-Storthz et al. (1992)	Verrucous Ca	9	ISH	3/9	33 %	2
Brachman et al. (1992)	SCC	11	PCR	1/11	9 %	
Howell and Gallant (1992)	SCC	8	SB	1/8	13 %	16
SCC, metastasis	2	SB	1/2	50 %	16	
Honig (1992)	SCC	12	ISH	7/12	60 %	6, 11, 16, 18
Shindoh et al. (1992)	SCC	24	SB	8/24	33 %	16, 18
Holladay and Gerald (1993)	SCC	37	DB	7/37	19 %	16, 18
Verrucous Ca	2	DB	0/2	0 %		
Noble-Topham et al. (1993)	Verrucous Ca	25	PCR	12/25	48 %	6/11, 16, 18
Woods et al. (1993)*	SCC	18	PCR, L1	14/18	78 %	6, 11, 16, 18
SCC metastasis	5	PCR	5/5 100 %	6, 11, 16, 18		
Cox et al. (1993)	SCC	8	SB	4/8	50 %	16
Guitart et al. (1993)	Verrucous Ca	1	ISH	1/1	100 %	6

Table 2 Detection of HPV DNA in palatine tonsil carcinomas during the first 10 years after the original report

Technique	No of positive cases/total	6/11	16	18	16/18	16/33	31	33	X	First author (year)
SB	2/7 (29 %)	1	1							Brandsma and Abramson (1989) [29]
SB	1/1 (100 %)		1[a]							Ishibashi et al. (1990) [30]
ISH	6/28 (21 %)		6							Niedobitek et al. (1990)[23]
SB	1/1 (100 %)		1							Bercovitch et al. (1991)[31]
ISH	5/14 (36 %)				5					Arndt et al. (1992)[24]
PCR	10/10 (100 %)		4			1		3	2	Snijders et al. (1992)[5]
PCR	12/14 (86 %)		7			1		2	2	Snijders et al. (1994)[25]
PCR	2/3 (67 %)									Brachman et al. (1992)[32]
PCR, SB, Virapap	3/6 (50 %)		3							Watanabe et al. (1993)
SB + PCR	1/4 (25 %)		1							Ogura et al. (1993)[33]
PCR	2/4 (50 %)		2							Lewensohn-Fuchs et al. (1994)
PCR	3/7 (43 %)								ND	Brandwein et al. (1994)[34]
PCR + SB	9/15 (60 %)		8						1	Paz et al. (1997)[9]
SB + PCR	1/1 (100 %)		1							Turazza et al. (1997)[35]
PCR + SB	11/21 (52 %)		8					1	2	Andl et al. (1998)[36]
PCR + SB	19/44 (43 %)	3	40							Schwarz (1998)[37]
PCR	14/22 (63 %)		11					1	2	Wilczyski (1998)[38]
PCR	2/2 (100 %)	1[a]			1[a]					Badaracco et al. (2000a, b)[39]
PCR	6/13? (46)?						6[b]			Lopez-Lizarraga et al. (2000)[40]
SB	1/1 (100 %)		1							Ishiji et al. (2000)[41]

(continued)

Table 2 (continued)

Technique	No of positive cases/total	6/11	16	18	16/18	16/33	31	33	X	First author (year)
PCR	2/4 (50 %)	1			1					Badaracco (2000)[1]
PCR	32/52 (62 %)									Gillison et al. (2000)[f7]
PCR	26/60 (43 %)		26		1					Mellin et al. (2000)[6]
PCR	12/22 (55 %)		11					1		
Total	221/432 (51 %)	7(3 %)	186 (84 %)	7(3 %)	3(1.4 %)	6(2.8 %)	9(4.6 %) 13(6 %)			

[a]Triple infection 6, 16, 18
[b]One infection with several HPV types 6, 18, 31, 35
[c]Double infections HPV 5/16, ADX1/16
[d]HPV 12, HPV 59
[e]One unidentified and HPV 59
[f]Includes also tumors of lingual tonsils

Table 3 Detection of HPV DNA in sinonasal carcinomas during the first 10 years after the original report

Type of technique			HPV genotypes detected						Total (%)		
Lesion		No.	6	6/11	11	16	16/18	18	Other	HPV+	Author and year
SCP	IH	1								100	Syrjänen et al. (1983a)
IP	ISH	14	1	5	5[c]					79	Syrjänen et al. (1987a)
SCC	ISH	3		3						100	
SCC	ISH	40		4		1		1		2.5	
SCC		2		1						50	Furuta et al. (1991)
SCC	PCR	8	1							12	Judd et al. (1991)
SCC	PCR	24				1				4	Kashima et al. (1992)
SCC	PCR	49		6		1				14	Furuta et al. (1992)
SCC	ISH[b]	35	1	1		3					Sarkar et al. (1992)
SCC	PCR	3		1					33		Tyan et al. (1993)
SCC	ISH[b]	22							57b[a]	86	Wu et al. (1993)

IP, inverted papilloma; SCC, squamous cell carcinoma; IH; immunohistochemistry; ISH, in situ hybridization; PCR, polymerase chain reaction; [a]19 cases HPV 57b-positive; [b]Double infection with HPV6/11 and 16 in 13 cases; [c]Double infection HPV 11&16 in 3 cases; ND, not clearly defined
SCC and papillomas
ISH+PCR

Table 4 Studies reporting on HPV detection in laryngeal squamous cell carcinomas during the first 10 years after the original report

Method/histological type		HPV-positive	Number/total	%	Authors and year
Detection method	Histological type	HPV types detected			
IHC	SCC	ND	13/36	36.1	Syrjänen et al. (1982)
SB	VCA	16	5/5	100	Abramson et al. (1985)
DB, SB	VCA	16	6/6	100	Brandsma et al. (1986)
SB	SCC	30	0/41	0	Kahn et al. (1986)
SB	SCC	16	1/36	3	Scheurlen et al. (1986)
SB	SCC	16	1/1	100	Stremlau et al. (1987)
DB	SCC	ND	0/4	0	Löning et al. (1987)
ISH	SCC	6, 11, 16	15/116	13	Syrjänen et al. (1987a, b)
SB, DB	SCC	6	1/1	100	Zarod et al. (1988)
IHC, SB	AOP, SCC	6	1/1	100	Kashima et al. (1988)
SB	SCC	11, 16	6/60	10	Brandsma and Abramson (1989)
PCR	SCC	16, 18	4/10	40	Kiyabu et al. (1989)
SB	JOP, SCC	6	4/4	100	Ward and Mounts (1989)
ISH	JOP, AOP, SCC	11	2/4	50	Lindeberg et al. (1989)

(continued)

Table 4 (continued)

Method/histological type		HPV-positive	Number/total	%	Authors and year
Detection method	Histological type	HPV types detected			
SB	SCC	NA	0/3	0	Ishibashi et al. (1990)
PCR	SCC	6, 16	7/34	20,5	Hoshikawa et al. (1990)
FISH	SCC	6, 11, 16, 18	5/50	10	Kulski et al. (1990)
PCR	SCC	16	26/48	54	Perez-Ayala et al. (1990)[a]
PCR	VCA	16	3 /3	100	Perez-Ayala et al. (1990)[a]
DB	SCC	6, 11, 16, 18	3/3	100	Vonka et al. (1990)
SB	SCC	16	3/6	50	Hong et al. (1991)
SB	SCC	16	1/1	100	McCullough and McNicol (1991)
PCR	SCC	6, 11, 16, 33	5/10	50	Morgan et al. (1991)
PCR	SCC	16, 18	4/28	14.3	Ogura et al. (1991)
SB	SCC	16	3/6	50	Wang et al. (1991)
PCR	SCC	16	3/4	75	Watts et al. (1991)
ISH	SCC	16, 18	12/27	44	Arndt et al. (1992)
PCR, SB	SCC	16	11/16	68.8	Yao et al. (1992)
DB, PCR	SCC	11, 16, 18	16/43	37.0	Anwar et al. (1993)
PCR	SCC	16	3/40	8	Brandwein et al. (1993)
PCR	VCA	ND	17/20	85	Kasperbauer et al. (1993)
ISH	SCC	16, 18	1/1	100	Makowska et al. (1993)
PCR, SB	SCC	16, 18	2/16	13.2	Ogura et al. (1993)
PCR	SCC	11, 16, 18	2/10	20	Tyan et al. (1993)
IHC, ISH	SCC	7	1/10	10	Van Rensburg et al. (1993)

2 Milestones

Warts were known since the classical Greek era, but the infectious nature of cutaneous warts was not understood until the studies by Payne (1891) and Jadasson (1896). This contagious mode of transmission was confirmed also for genital condylomas some 10 years later, when Heidingsfield described a prostitute, who had acquired condyloma lesions in her tongue as a result of oral sex (Heidingsfield, 1901). Only a few years later, the viral etiology of these lesions was demonstrated by Ciuffo (1907), who used a cell filtrate of a common wart to transfer the infection. Human wart virus was later associated with laryngeal warts (Ullman 1923). In 1942, Parsons and Kidd published their milestone study where they showed that oral papillomatosis of rabbits is a viral disease. They also described the most likely sites in oral mucosa to be infected with PV. In addition, they showed that even irritation/trauma could activate a latent PV infection and the virus could be transmitted via saliva. The data of that pioneering study are still timely, while no similar natural history studies on oral papillomas in the humans exist even today.

In 1949, Ayre and Ayre (1949) described the morphology of “halo cells” in Pap smears and cervical biopsies, originally calling them as a precancer cell complex. One of their patients subsequently developed a carcinoma in situ (CIS) lesion, and the authors renamed this cytological abnormality as a “nearocarcinoma” in 1951. While studying the cytological smears collected during a screening program from cervical precancer lesions, Koss and Durfee could confirm Ayre’s discovery. They published their classical paper in 1956 and renamed this cellular abnormality as koilocytotic atypia (Koss and Durfee 1956). Later, Koss admitted, however, that the viral etiology of the koilocytotic atypia was not suspected in 1956, although the wart-like epithelial changes pointed to that direction (Koss 1987).

From a clinical point of view, a major breakthrough was made by two research groups, unaware of each other, who both described koilocytotic cells in Pap smears derived from flat epithelial lesions, frequently associated with cervical precancer lesions (dysplasia) (Meisels and Fortin 1976; Purola and Savia 1977). These two reports prompted the interest of many cytopathologists in these lesions from a completely new perspective, while realizing that by observing the cytopathic effects of a virus on light microscopy, one could probably “see” the etiological agent of cervical cancer precursors. This leads also us to start a systematic survey of head and neck lesions for the presence of koilocytosis as a sign of viral infection. From the very beginning, the concept of HPV only as a sexually transmitted disease was also questioned by us, because oral and laryngeal papillomas were frequently found in young children.

HPV research today owes much to one of the pioneers in the field, to Dr. Harald zur Hausen, who turned his interest on HPV in the early 1970s. The first of his classical series of four works from 1974 to 1976 attempted to detect virus-specific DNA in human tumors, he completed nucleic acid hybridization experiments with complementary RNA of human wart virus (zur Hausen et al. 1975). In 1980, Gissmann and zur Hausen isolated and characterized a new virus, which proved to be the etiological agent of classical genital warts, and designated this new virus as HPV6 (Gissmann and zur Hausen 1980). Characterization of the first of these genital HPV types led to the isolation of its closest relative from a laryngeal papilloma receiving the label HPV11 (Gissmann et al. 1982). At that time, all attempts to detect homologous DNA in laryngeal squamous cell carcinomas failed, however (Gissmann et al. 1982). One of the absolute highlights of the early 1980s was the isolation and characterization of a new HPV type from cervical cancer, which subsequently has proved to be the single most important HPV type of them all, namely HPV16, by Dürst and his colleagues in 1983 (Dürst et al. 1983). In 1984, HPV18 was isolated and characterized from cervical carcinoma (Boshart et al. 1984).

Currently, more than 200 PVs have been sequenced and numbered according to the order of the characterization of the genome. PVs are classified as a taxonomic family of their own since 2004 (de Villiers et al. 2004). Alpha papillomaviruses contain most of the mucosal HPV genotypes. It became evident that different genotypes are responsible for cutaneous common warts and genital warts. During the same period, zur Hausen formulated his hypothesis of HPV as an etiological agent of cervical cancer (zur Hausen et al. 1975, 1976) which was later acknowledged by nomination as the Nobel Laureate in Medicine and Physics in 2008.

In parallel with the impelled interest in HPV lesions of the genital tract and skin, the suspected HPV origin of two additional lesions was confirmed: first the juvenile-onset laryngeal papillomas and later the adult-onset papillomas. Quick and coworkers described epithelial atypia in these lesions, with possible implications in their known risk for malignant transformation (Quick et al. 1978, 1979, 1980). Soon, conclusive clinical and virological evidence on the similarities between genital condylomas and laryngeal papillomas was provided (Quick et al. 1980). Within the next two years, HPV involvement in laryngeal squamous cell carcinomas was suggested by us, based on their morphological characteristics and detection of HPV antigens by immunohistochemistry (IHC) (Syrjänen and Syrjänen 1981; Syrjänen et al. 1982).

The HPV etiology of inverted papilloma of the nasal cavity/paranasal sinuses was suggested by us in 1983 (Syrjänen et al. 1983a, b, c, d). Even if these lesions are relatively rare, this concept is clinically important, due to the high tendency of inverted papillomas to recurrence (known well before any evidence on HPV) and an increased risk for malignant transformation.

The same period witnessed the extension of HPV research into yet another group of squamous cell lesions, subsequently gained a substantial clinical importance, i.e., the first evidence on HPV involvement in benign (Jenson et al. 1982) and malignant (Syrjänen et al. 1983a, b, c, d) squamous cell tumors of the oral mucosa. Evidence was also provided, for the first time, that HPV may be the etiological agent of a subgroup of oral squamous cell carcinomas as well.

Finally, the description of the technique how to make virus-like particles (VLP) in vitro, by Kirnbauer et al. (1992), opened completely new visions into at least two important areas of HPV research: (1) HPV serology and (2) HPV vaccination. The authors succeeded in expressing the L1 major capsid proteins of BPV1 and HPV16 in insect cells using a Baculovirus vector and analyzed their conformation and immunogenicity. The L1 proteins were expressed at high levels and, surprisingly, assembled into structures that closely resembled native PV virions (Kirnbauer et al. 1992). These self-assembled BPV L1 VLPs mimicked intact bovine PV (BPV) virions, and induced neutralizing antisera in rabbits, with similar immunogenicity as the real viral particles. It became immediately evident that VLPs were good candidates for testing the levels of antibodies and potentially also the antigen to be used for preventing HPV infections (Kirnbauer et al. 1992). Subsequent studies resulted in the development of the first-generation prophylactic vaccines against HPV6, 11, 16, 18 (Gardasil®, Merck) or against HPV16 and HPV18 (Cervarix®, GSK).

3 HPV and Oral Cavity Cancer

As early as in 1983, we presented an original observation and hypothesis that HPV is present in a subset of oral cancers and accordingly also an etiological factor of these cancers (Syrjänen et al. 1983a, b, c, d). In that pioneering study including 40 lesions, 16/40 (40 %) showed HPV-suggestive changes on light microscopy, and of those, 8/16 (50 %) expressed HPV structural proteins upon immunohistochemical staining (IHC) (Syrjänen et al. 1983b). This non-commercial HPV common antiserum was made against HPVs present in pooled HPV lesions (Pyrhönen 1978). A few years later, the same biopsy samples were re-examined for the presence of HPV DNA using ISH and PCR, and 12/40 disclosed the presence of HPV11, 16, or 18 DNA (Chang et al. 1990). Prompted by our original reports, also other groups became interested in the association of HPV and oral cancer. The studies published during the subsequent 10 years since our original report are summarized in Table 1. In 1985, HPV DNA was found in oral cancer samples by two research groups; Löning et al. reported HPV11 and 16 DNA in 3/6 oral carcinomas, and de Villiers et al. HPV2 in one and HPV16 in 2/7 tongue carcinomas. With in situ hybridization (ISH), we were able to localize HPV DNA in the tumor cells. HPV6, 11, 16, and 18 DNA was found in 6/51 oral SCCs and in 6/21 oral precancer lesions (Syrjänen et al. 1988).

Snijders et al. (1996) analyzed 221 SCCs of the aerodigestive tract. With the HPV GP5+/6+ general primer-mediated PCR, 32 % of the samples scored positive. The HPV prevalence ranged from 70 % in tonsillar SSC down to 10 % in hypopharyngeal SCC (Snijders et al. 1996). Approximately 60 % of oral carcinomas proved to be HPV-positive, with HPV16 by far the most frequent type in all sites. In addition, HPV6, 7, 33, 35, and 59 were detected, albeit infrequently. Later, it has been shown that HPV prevalence is higher in oral cancer patients younger than 60 years (Syrjänen et al. 1988; Balaram et al. 1995; Cruz et al. 1996).

Miller and Johnstone (2001) were the first to present a meta-analysis based on pooled data from non-controlled studies between 1982 and 1997 to estimate HPV prevalence in precancer lesions, oral cancer, and normal oral mucosa. They found that the frequency of HPV detection in normal oral mucosa [10.0 %; 95 % confidence interval (CI), 6.1–14.6 %] was significantly less than in leukoplakia (22.2 %; 95 % CI, 15.7–29.9 %), intra-epithelial neoplasia (26.2 %; 95 % CI, 19.6–33.6 %), verrucous carcinoma (29.5 %; 95 % CI, 23–36.8 %), and OSCC (46.5 %; 95 % CI, 3 7.6–55.5 %). The pooled odds ratio (OR) for the subset of studies directly comparing the prevalence of HPV in normal mucosa and OSCC was 5.4, confirming the trend observed in the overall sample (Miller and Johnstone 2001). However, this analysis was not based on case–control studies. In the review of Kreimer et al. (2005), HPV prevalence in OSCC was 23.5 % (Kreimer et al. 2005). HPV16 was the most common type present, being detected in 16.0 % of OSCC and accounting for almost 70 % of the HPV-positive cases. HPV18 was the next most common oncogenic HPV type, detected in 8 % of OSCC (Kreimer et al. 2005; Adelstein et al. 2009). The wide variations in HPV detection rates have been explained by differences in sampling (e.g., oral scrapings, cells acquired with mouthwash, or biopsies), as well as by the different sensitivity and specificity of HPV testing methods.

Because the earlier meta-analyses lacked the design of case–control studies, a meta-analysis was performed including only case–control studies assessing HPV in oral cancer, with healthy oral mucosa as controls (Syrjänen et al. 2011). Collectively, 1885 cases and 2248 controls of OSCC and 956 cases and 675 controls of oral potentially malignant disorders (OPMD) were available for analysis. Significant association was found between pooled HPV DNA detection and OSCC (OR = 3.98; 95 % CI: 2.6–6.02) and even for HPV16 only (OR = 3.86; 95 % CI: 2.16–6.86). HPV was also associated with OPMD (OR = 3.87; 95 % CI: 2.87–5.21). In a subgroup analysis of OPMD, HPV was also associated with oral leukoplakia (OR = 4.03; 95 % CI: 2.34–6.92), oral lichen planus (OR = 5.12; 95 % CI: 2.40–10.93), and epithelial dysplasia (OR = 5.10; 95 % CI: 2.03–12.80).

To conclude, the evidence emerged through different lines of research during the past 30 years supporting the view that a subgroup oral cancers are linked with HPV, exactly as suggested by us already in 1983. The recognition of HPV in etiology has raised two questions: (1) Is HPV testing needed in routine diagnostics? (2) the role of HPV vaccination in prevention of oral HPV infection?

4 HPV and Palatine Tonsil Cancer

Brandsma and Abramson (1989) were the first to report on the presence of HPV16 DNA in 2 of 7 tonsillar SCCs among the 100 HNSCC samples analyzed with Southern blot hybridization. They also suggested that the anatomic site in the head and neck region plays a role in determining the susceptibility to HPV infection, the most likely infection sites being the tongue (18 %), tonsils (29 %), and pharynx (13 %). In their study, they also analyzed the matched control samples (n = 116) from the same anatomic region and could confirm the presence of subclinical HPV in subjects with no history of papilloma or oral malignancy. The subsequent studies on the HPV detection in palate tonsil carcinoma are summarized in Table 2.

A year after the original report, Ishibashi et al. (1990) described an additional tonsillar SCC infected with episomal form of HPV16. The same HPV type was also detected in two lymph node metastasis, suggesting the direct role of HPV infection in the development of SCC. In 1992, Snijders et al. had described two HPV16-positive tonsillar carcinomas, where HPV16 was episomal. They also found two HPV33-positive carcinomas where HPV was either integrated or both in episomal and integrated state (Snijders et al. 1992). Importantly, Snijders and coworkers were the first to show that E6/E7 mRNAs were present exclusively in the neoplastic cells, providing further evidence for viral etiology of tonsillar carcinomas (Snijders et al. 1992).

Niedobitek et al. in 1990 localized HPV16 DNA in the tumor cells in 6/28 carcinomas, of which 5 were poorly and 1 was moderately differentiated, while the two highly differentiated carcinomas and one in situ carcinoma were HPV-negative. Subsequently, several studies have later confirmed that the HPV association is related to tumor histology, as originally suggested by Niedobitek et al. (1990).

Bercovitch et al. (1991) described the presence of integrated HPV6 in a tonsillar carcinoma. Arndt et al. (1992) used in situ hybridization for HPV detection and found that 65.5 % of the 61 HNSCC cases were HPV16/18-positive, with the following anatomic subsites: 12 laryngeal carcinomas (44 %), five tonsillar tumors (35.7 %), eight tumors of the hypopharynx (66.6 %), and three tongue carcinomas (37.5 %). The largest series of tonsillar carcinomas analyzed until 2002 was reported by Mellin and coworkers. Of the 84 tonsillar carcinomas, 46 % tested HPV DNA-positive, which was in episomal state in most cases (Mellin et al. 2000, 2002). They also reported that patients with HPV-positive tonsillar cancer and especially with episomal form had the best survival (Mellin et al. 2002). In 2000, Gillison and coworkers analyzed 52 tonsillar cancers among the 253 newly diagnosed HNSCC. Totally 62 % of the tonsillar cancers were positive with ISH. HPV-positive oropharyngeal cancers were less likely to occur among moderate to heavy drinkers (OR = 0.17; 95 % CI = 0.05–0.61) and smokers (OR = 0.16; 95 % CI = 0.02–1.4), had a characteristic basaloid morphology (OR = 18.7; 95 % CI = 2.1–167), were less likely to have TP53 mutations (OR = 0.06; 95 % CI = 0.01–0. 36), and had improved disease-specific survival (hazard ratio [HR] = 0.26; 95 % CI = 0.07–0.98). Table 2 summarizes the studies reported during the first 10 years following the original report on the HPV presence in tonsillar carcinomas.

Since the early days, several meta-analyses have been completed and they confirm HPV as a main etiological agent of oropharyngeal cancer, mainly palatine tonsils and base of the tongue (Ndiaye et al. 2014). The highest HPV prevalence rates have been reported from the USA and Sweden, reaching 70–90 %. As with the other HNSCCs, a wide geographic variation in HPV prevalence is evident and HPV16 is the main genotype involved in these cancers.

5 HPV and Sinonasal Cancer

The coexistence of two different epithelia (columnar cells and stratified squamous epithelium) creates squamo-columnar junctions at multiple sites in the respiratory tract, entities that are thought to be a prerequisite for the spread of HPV infections in this region (Syrjänen 1997; Syrjänen and Syrjänen 2000).The increased interest in sinonasal cancer parallels the research activity focused on their benign counterparts, sinonasal papillomas since the 1980s, when the evidence on possible causal role of HPV was first provided (Syrjänen et al. 1983a, b, c, d, 1987a, b; Siivonen and Virolainen 1989).

Papillomas of the sinonasal mucosa have been recognized since 1854, when first described with the name inverted papilloma (Ward 1854). Based on a meta-analysis of the reports covered until 1992, the overall recurrence rate is substantial (32 %), varying from 0 to 100 % (Syrjänen 2003). Similarly, the reported prevalence of metachronous and synchronous malignancy varies within a wide range, 3–16 % and 0–100 %, respectively (Bielamowicz et al. 1993; Lawson et al. 1995). It was not until 1983, however, that HPV was first suggested as a potential etiological agent of sinonasal papillomas and their malignant counterparts by us (Syrjänen 1983). This hypothesis was based on the immunohistochemical detection of HPV antigen expression in a single papilloma, soon confirmed by in situ hybridization (ISH) demonstrating HPV DNA both in benign and malignant sinonasal lesions (Syrjänen 1993; Syrjänen et al. 1987a, b; Siivonen and Virolainen 1989).

Following these primary reports, a slowly expanding research interest in HPV and sinonasal cancer has been noted (MacKay et al. 2005; Hpoffman et al. 2006). HPV as a possible etiological agent in sinonasal cancer has gathered from either reports on malignant transformation of HPV-associated papillomas and/or HPV DNA detection in sinonasal carcinomas. Table 3 summarizes the early papers on HPV detection in sinonasal carcinomas. By 2002, a literature survey found that 21 % of the 322 sinonasal carcinomas analyzed so far were HPV-positive (Syränen 2003). In a more recent meta-analysis (Syrjänen and Syrjänen 2013), 35 studies were eligible, covering 492 sinonasal SCCs from different geographic regions. Altogether, 133 (27.0 %) cases tested HPV-positive. The results also showed that it seems to be too premature to conclude that sinonasal carcinomas in different geographic regions have a different etiology, as hypothesized in some studies

To conclude, it seems that approximately 20–30 % of the sinonasal carcinomas are associated with HPV similarly as other head and neck cancers, except oropharyngeal cancers.

6 HPV and Nasopharyngeal Cancer

Nasopharynx is the region of the respiratory tract connecting the nasal cavity to the pharynx. At birth, the nasopharynx is lined by a typical respiratory epithelium. However, this pseudostratified columnar ciliated epithelium is gradually replaced by stratified, non-ciliated epithelium, and with advancing age, by mature squamous epithelium. Nasopharyngeal cancer (NPC) is among the few human malignancies where viral etiology has been firmly established. The evidence is compelling to implicate the important causal role of Epstein–Barr virus (EBV) in the development of NPC (Hyams 1971; Giannoudis et al. 1995). These data have recently stimulated a few studies looking for the evidence on possible HPV involvement in NPCs, the well-differentiated SCCs in particular (Dickens et al. 1992; Huang et al. 1993; Tyan et al. 1993; Hörding et al. 1994; Giannoudis et al. 1995; Shen et al. 1996).

Using PCR, Dickens et al. (1992) found evidence for HPV 16/18 DNA in NPC samples. Huang et al. (1993) established two cell lines from well-differentiated EBV-negative NPCs and could demonstrate HPV 16-related sequences in both of these (Huang et al. 1993). In a series of 30 NPCs analyzed for EBV and HPV sequences using PCR, EBV was present in all (100 %), and interestingly, HPV DNA was found in 14/30 (46.7 %) of the cases. All 14 cases contained HPV16 (Tyan et al. 1993). In another study, a series of 15 well-differentiated NPCs of the squamous type were analyzed for HPV DNA using PCR (Hörding et al. 1994). HPV DNA was present in 4/15 (26.7 %) of the tumors. Giannoudis et al. (1995) analyzed 63 NPCs from Greece for EBV and HPV sequences and found HPV DNA in 12/63 (19 %) of the cases Giannoudis et al. 1995).

Taken together, there seems to be emerging evidence that HPV16 might be involved in the development of a subset of NPC, the well-differentiated squamous cell type, whereas the two other types of NPC are closely linked with EBV. So far, little evidence has been provided suggesting the synergistic action of these two tumor viruses in this anatomic region.

7 HPV and Laryngeal Cancer

Laryngeal carcinoma (LSCC) may arise as a late complication of preexisting squamous cell papilloma (SCP), but the vast majority of these malignant lesions do develop without any antedating papilloma, through cancer precursor lesions (dysplasia, intraepithelial neoplasia, carcinoma in situ). So far, too little attention has been paid to these precancer lesions with regard to the evidence for HPV involvement (Lindeberg and Krogdahl 1997; Poljak et al. 1997; Sugar et al. 1997).

The association of HPV with laryngeal carcinoma was first suggested by detecting typical cytopathic effects of HPV in these lesions (Syrjänen and Syrjänen 1981). The presence of HPV was confirmed by IHC staining to demonstrate the expression of HPV structural proteins (Syrjänen et al. 1982). The most convincing evidence to implicate HPV in laryngeal cancer is derived from the studies demonstrating HPV DNA in the cancer lesions by different hybridization techniques and PCR (Syrjänen 1997; Syrjänen et al. 1987b; Syrjänen and Syrjänen 2000; Kashima et al. 1997; Herrero et al. 2003).

The published literature was subjected to systematic review and meta-analysis just recently (Gama et al. 2016). One hundred seventy-nine studies were eligible, comprising 7347 LSCCs from different geographic regions. Altogether, 1830 (25 %) cases tested HPV-positive considering all methods, with effect size of 0.269 (95 % CI: 0.242–0.297; random-effects model). In meta-analysis stratified by the (1) HPV detection technique and (2) geographic study origin, the between-study heterogeneity was significant only for geographic origin ($P = 0.0001$). In meta-regression, the HPV detection method ($P = 0.876$) or geographic origin ($P = 0.234$) was not significant study-level covariates.

Taken together, benign laryngeal papilloma is among the first lesions that were confirmed to be associated with HPV. The role of HPV in laryngeal cancer has been long disputed, but now convincingly demonstrated by extensive meta-analysis (Gama et al. 2016). Not unlike in the other head and neck malignancies, the prevalence of HPV in laryngeal cancer also levels off at around 25 %, thus reflecting the HPV-attributable fraction in these malignancies.

References

Abramson AL, Brandsma J, Steinberg B, Winkler B (1985) Verrucous carcinoma of the larynx. Possible human papillomavirus etiology. Arch Otolaryngol 111:709–715

Adelstein DJ, Ridge JA, Gillison ML, Chaturvedi AK, D'Souza G, Gravitt PE, Westra W, Psyrri A, Kast WM, Koutsky LA, Giuliano A, Krosnick S, Trotti A, Schuller DE, Forastiere A, Ullmann CD (2009) Head and neck squamous cell cancer and the human papillomavirus: summary of a National Cancer Institute State of the Science Meeting, November 9–10, 2008, Washington, D.C. Head Neck 31:1393–1422

Adler-Storthz K, Newland JR, Tessin BA, Yeudall WA, Shillitoe EJ (1986) Human papillomavirus type 2 DNA in oral verrucous carcinoma. J Oral Pathol 15:472–475

Adler-Storthz K, Ficarra G, Woods KV, Gaglioti D, DiPietro M, Shillitoe EJ (1992) Prevalence of Epstein-Barr virus and human papillomavirus in oral mucosa of HIV-infected patients. J Oral Pathol Med 21:164–170

Andl T, Kahn T, Pfuhl A, Nicola T, Erber R, Conradt C, Klein W, Helbig M, Dietz A, Weidauer H et al (1998) Etiological involvement of oncogenic human papillomavirus in tonsillar squamous cell carcinomas lacking retinoblastoma cell cycle control. Cancer Res 58:5–13

Anwar K, Nakahuki K, Imai H, Naiki H, Inuzuka M (1993) Over-expression of pS3 protein in human laryngeal carcinoma. Int J Cancer 53:952–956

Arndt O, Bauer I, Brock J (1991) Use of the Dot-Blot technique in the detection of human papillomavirus(HPV) deoxyribonucleic acid (DNA) in malignant tumors of the oropharynx. Laryngorhinootologie 70:441–444

Arndt O, Zeise K, Bauer I, Brock J (1992) Detection of human papillomaviruses (HPV) in laryngeal papilloma. An in situ hybridization study. Laryngorhinootologie 71:132–136

Atula S, Grenman R, Syrjänen S (1997) Fibroblasts can modulate the phenotype of malignant epithelial cells in vitro. Exp Cell Res 235:180–187

Ayre JE (1962) Is·carcinoma in situ reversible? In: Wied GL (ed) Proceedings of the first international congress of exfoliative cytology. Vienna, pp 94–102

Ayre JE, Ayre WB (1949) Progression of precancer stage to early carcinoma of the cervix within 1 year; combined cytologic and histologic study with report of a case. Am J Clin Pathol 19:770–778

Badaracco G, Venuti A, Morello R et al (2000a) Human papillomavirus in head and neck carcinomas; prevalence, physical status and relationship with clinical/pathological parameters. Anticancer Res 20:1301–1306

Badaracco G, Venut A, Bartolazzi A et al (2000b) Overexpression of p53 and bcl-2 proteins and the presence of HPV infection are independent events in head and neck cancer. J Oral Pathol Med 29:173–179

Bäfverstedt B (1967) Condylomata acuminata- past and present. Acta Derm Venereol (Stockh) 47:376–381

Balaram P, Nalinakumari KR, Abraham E, Balan A, Hareendran NK, Bernard HU, Chan SY (1995) Human papillomaviruses in 91 oral cancers from Indian betel quid chewers–high prevalence and multiplicity of infections. Int J Cancer 61:450–454

Bercovich JA, Centeno CR, Aguilar OG, Grinstein S, Kahn T (1991) Presence and integration of human papillomavirus type 6 in a tonsillar carcinoma. J Gen Virol 72:2569–2572
Bielamowicz S, Calcaterra TC, Watson D (1993) Inverting papilloma of the head and neck: the UCLA update. Otolaryngol Head Neck Surg 109:71–76
Boshart M, Gissmann L, Ikenberg H, Kleinheinz A, Scheurlen W, zur-Hausen H (1984) A new type of papillomavirus DNA, its presence in genital cancer biopsies and in cell lines derived from cervical cancer. EMBO J 3:1151–1157
Brachman DG, Graves D, Vokes E, Beckett M, Haraf D, Montag A, Dunphy E, Mick R, Yandell D, Weichselbaum RR (1992) Occurrence of p53 gene deletions and human papilloma virus infection in human head and neck cancer. Cancer Res 52:4832–4836
Brandsma JL, Abramson AL (1989) Association of papillomavirus with cancers of the head and neck. Arch Otolaryngol Head Neck Surg 115:621–625
Brandsma JL, Steinberg BM, Abramson AL, Winkler B (1986) Presence of human papillomavirus type 16 related sequences in verrucous carcinoma of the larynx. Cancer Res 46:2185–2188
Brandwein MS, Nuovo GJ, Biller H (1993) Analysis of prevalence of human papillomavirus in laryngeal carcinomas. Ann Otol Rhinol Laryngol 102:309–313
Brandwein M, Zeitlin J, Nuovo GJ, MacConnell P, Bodian C, Urken M, Biller H (1994) HPV detection using "hot start" polymerase chain reaction in patients with oral cancer: a clinicopathological study of 64 patients. Mod Pathol 7:720–727
Chang KW, Chang CS, Lai KS, Chou MJ, Choo KB (1989) High prevalence of human papillomavirus infection and possible association with betel quid chewing and smoking in oral epidermoid carcinomas in Taiwan. J Med Virol 28:57–61
Chang F, Syrjänen S, Nuutinen J, Kärja J, Syrjänen K (1990) Detection of human papillomavirus (HPV) DNA in oral squamous cell carcinomas by in situ hybridization and polymerase chain reaction. Arch Dermatol Res 282:493–497
Ciuffo G (1907) Innesto postiveo con filtrado di verrucae volgare. Gior Ital D Mal Ven 48:12–17
Cox M, Maitland N, Scully C (1993) Human herpes simplex-1 and papillomavirus type 16 homologous DNA sequences in normal, potentially malignant and malignant oral mucosa. Eur J Cancer B Oral Oncol 29B(3):215–219
Cruz IB, Snijders PJ, Steenbergen RD, Meijer CJ, Snow GB, Walboomers JM, Van-der-Waal I (1996) Age-dependence of human papillomavirus DNA presence in oral squamous cell carcinomas. Eur J Cancer B Oral Oncol 32B:55–62
de Villiers EM (2013) Cross-roads in the classification of papillomaviruses. Virology 445:2–10
de Villiers EM, Weidauer H, Otto H, zur Hausen H (1985) Papillomavirus DNA in human tongue carcinomas. Int J Cancer 36(5):575–578
de Villiers E-M, Fauquet C, Broker TR, Bernard H-U, zur Hausen H (2004) Classification of papillomaviruses. Virology 324:17–27
Dekmezian RH, Batsakis JG, Goepfert H (1987) In situ hybridization of papillomavirus DNA in head and neck squamous cell carcinomas. Arch Otolaryngol Head Neck Surg 113:819–821
Demetrick DJ, Inoue M, Lester WM, Kingma I, Duggan MA, Paul LC (1990) Human papillomavirus type 16 associated with oral squamous carcinoma in a cardiac transplant recipient. Cancer 15(66):1726–1731
Dickens P, Srivastava G, Liu YT (1992) Human papillomavirus 16/18 and nasopharyngeal carcinoma. J Clin Pathol 45:81–87
Dürst M, Gissmann L, Ikenberg H, zur Hausen HA (1983) papillomavirus DNA from a cervical carcinoma and its prevalence in cancer biopsy samples from different geographic regions. Proc Natl Acad Sci USA 80:3812–3815
Furuta Y, Shinohara T, Sano K, Nagashima K, Inoue K, Tanaka K, Inuyama Y (1991) Molecular pathologic study of human papillomavirus infection in inverted papilloma and squamous cell carcinoma of the nasal cavities and paranasal sinuses. Laryngoscope 101:79–85
Gama RR, Carvalho AL, Filho AL, Scorsato AP, López RV, Rautava J, Syrjänen S, Syrjänen K (2016) Detection of human papillomavirus in laryngeal squamous cell carcinoma: systematic review and meta-analysis. Laryngoscope. 126:885–893

Gassenmaier A, Hornstein OP (1988) Presence of human papillomavirus DNA in benign and precancerous oral leukoplakias and squamous cell carcinomas. Dermatologica 176:224–233
Giannoudis A, Ergazaki M, Segas J, Goitakis J, Adamopoulos G, Gorgoulis V, Spandidos DA (1995) Detection of Epstein-Barr virus and human papillomavirus in nasopharyngeal carcinoma by the polymerase chain reaction technique. Cancer Lett 89:177–181
Gillison ML, Koch WM, Capone RB, Spafford M, Westra WH, Wu L, Zahurak ML, Daniel RW, Viglione M, Symer DE, Shah KV, Sidransky D (2000) Evidence for a causal association between human papillomavirus and a subset of head and neck cancers. J Natl Cancer Inst 92:709–720
Gissmann L, zur Hausen H (1980) Partial characterization of viral DNA from human genital warts (Condylomata acuminata). Int J Cancer 25:605–609
Gissmann L, Diehl V, Schultz-Coulon HJ, zur Hausen H (1982) Molecular cloning and characterization of human papilloma virus DNA derived from a laryngeal papilloma. J Virol 44:393–400
Greer RO, Douglas JM, Breese P, Crosby LK (1990a) Evaluation of oral and laryngeal specimens for human papillomavirus (HPV) DNA by dot blot hybridization. J Oral Pathol Med 19:35–38
Greer RO, Eversole LR, Crosby LK (1990b) Detection of human papillomavirus-genomic DNA in oral epithelial dysplasias, oral smokeless tobacco-associated leukoplakias, and epithelial malignancies. J Oral Maxillofac Surg 48:1201–1205
Guitart J, McGillis ST, Bailin PL, Bergfeld WF, Rogers RS (1993) Human papillomavirus-induced verrucous carcinoma of the mouth-case report of an aggressive tumor. J Dermatol Surg Oncol 19:875–877
Hayes RB, Kardaum JWPF, de Bruyn A (1987) Tobacco use and sinonasal cancer: a case-control study. Br J Cancer 56:843–846
Heidingsfield ML (1901) Condylomata acuminata linguata. J Cutan Genitourin Dis 19:226–234
Herrero R, Castellsagué X, Pawlita M et al (2003) Human papillomavirus and oral cancer: the International Agency for Research on Cancer Multicenter study. J Natl Cancer Inst 95:1772–1783
Hoffmann M, Klose N, Gottschlich S et al (2006) Detection of human papillomavirus DNA in benign and malignant sinonasal neoplasms. Cancer Lett 239:64–70
Honig JF (1992) Non radioactive in situ hybridization for detection of human papilloma virus DNA in squamous cell carcinoma of tongue. Bull Group Int Rech Sci Stomatol Odontol 35:107–115
Howell RE, Gallant L (1992) Human papillomavirus type 16 in an oral squamous carcinoma and its metastasis. Oral Surg Oral Med Oral Pathol 74:620–626
Huang E-S, Gutsch D, Tzung K-W, Lin C-T (1993) Detection of low-level of Human papilloma virus type 16 DNA·sequences in cancer cell lines derived from two well-differentiated nasopharyngeal cancers. J Med Virol 40:244–250
Hyams VJ (1971) Papillomas of the nasal cavity and paranasal sinuses. A clinicopathological study of 315 cases. Ann Otol Rhinol Laryngol 80:192–206
Ishibashi T, Matsushima S, Tsunokawa Y, Asai M, Nomura Y, Sugimura T, Terada M (1990) Human papillomavirus DNA in squamous cell carcinoma of the upper aerodigestive tract. Arch Otolaryngol Head Neck Surg 116:294–301
Ishiji T, Kawase M, Honda M et al (2000) Distinctive distribution of human papillomavirus type 16 and type 20 DNA in the tonsillar and the skin carcinomas of a patient with epídermodysplasia verruciformis. Br J Dermatol 143:1005–1010
Jadassohn (1896) Sind die verrucae vulgares ubertragbar? Vehandel D Deutsch Dem Gesellsch 5:497–512
Jenson AB, Lancaster WD, Hartmann DP, Shaffer EL Jr (1982) Frequency and distribution of papillomavirus structural antigens in verrucae, multiple papillomas, and condylomata of the oral cavity. Am J Pathol 107:212–218
Jin Y-T, Toto PD (1984) Detection of human papovavirus antigens in oral papillary lesions. Oral Surg 58:702–705

Judd R, Zaki SR, Coffield LM, Evatt BL (1991) Sinonasal papillomas and human papillomavirus. Hum Pathol 22:550–556

Kahn T, Schwarz E, zur Hausen H (1986) Molecular cloning and characterization of the DNA of a new Human papillomavirus (HPV30) from a laryngeal carcinoma. Int J Cancer 37:61–65

Kashima H, Wu TC, Mounts P, Heffner D, Cachay A, Hyams V (1988) Carcinoma ex-papilloma: histologic and virologic studies in whole-organ sections of the larynx. Laryngoscope 98:619–624

Kashima HK, Kutcher M, Kessis T, Levin LS, de Villiers EM, Shah K (1990) Human papillomavirus in squamous cell carcinoma, leukoplakia, lichen planus, and clinically normal epithelium of the oral cavity. Ann Otol Rhinol Laryngol 99:55–61

Kashima HK, Kessis T, Hruban RH, Wu TC, Zinreich SJ, Shah KV (1992) Human papillomavirus in sinonasal papillomas and squamous cell carcinoma. Laryngoscope 102:973–976

Kasperbauer JL, O'Halloran GL, Espy MJ, Smith TF, Lewis JE (1993) Polymerase chain reaction (PCR) identification of human papillomavirus (HPV) DNA in verrucous carcinoma of the larynx. Laryngoscope 103:416–420

Kirnbauer R, Booy F, Cheng N, Lowy DR, Schiller JT (1992) Papillomavirus L1 major capsid protein self-assembles into virus-like particles that are highly immunogenic. Proc Natl Acad Sci USA 89:12180–12184

Koss LG (1987) Carcinogenesis in the uterine cervix and human papillomavirus infection. In: Syrjänen K, Gissmann L, Koss LG (eds) Papillomaviruses and human disease. Springer, Heidelberg, pp 235–267

Koss LG, Durfee GR (1956) Unusual patterns of squamous epithelium of the uterine cervix and pathologic study of koilocytotic atypia. Ann NY Acad Sci 63:1245–1261

Kreimer AR, Clifford GM, Boyle P, Franceschi S (2005) Human papillomavirus types in head and neck squamous cell carcinomas worldwide: a systematic review. Cancer Epidemiol Biomarkers Prev. 14:467–75 (Review)

Kulski JK, Demeter T, Mutavdzic S, Sterrett GF, Mitchell KM, Pixley EC (1990) Survey of histologic specimens of human cancer for human papillomavirus types 6/11/16/18 by filter in situ hybridization. Am J Clin Pathol 94:566–570

Lancaster WD, Olson C (1982) Animal papillomaviruses. Microbiol Rev 46:191–207

Lawson W, Ho BT, Shaari CM et al (1995) Inverted papilloma: a report of 112 cases. Laryngoscope 105:282–288

Lee NK, Ritter DB, Gross AE, Myssiorek DJ, Kadish AS, Burk RD (1988) Head and neck squamous cell carcinomas associated with human papillomaviruses and an increased incidence of cervical pathology. Otolaryngol Head Neck Surg 99:296–301

Lewensohn-Fuchs I, Munck-Wikland E, Berke Z, Magnusson KP, Pallesen G, Auer G, Lindholm J, Linde A, Aberg B, Rubio C et al (1994) Involvement of aberrant p53 expression and human papillomavirus in carcinoma of the head, neck and esophagus. Anticancer Res 14:1281–1285

Lindeberg H, Krogdahl A (1997) Laryngeal dysplasia and the human papillomavirus. Clin Otolaryngol 22:382–386

Lindeberg H, Syrjänen S, Kärjä J, Syrjänen K (1989) Human papillomavirus (HPV) type 11 DNA in squamous cell carcinomas and pre-existing multiple laryngeal papillomas. Acta Otolaryngol (Stockh) 107:141–149

Löning T, Ikenberg H, Becker J, Gissmann L, Hoepfner I, zur Hausen H (1985) Analysis of oral papillomas, leukoplakias, and invasive carcinomas for human papillomavirus type related DNA. J Invest Dermatol 84:417–420

Löning T, Hoepfner I, Milde K (1986) Characterization of mucosal papillomas and carcinomas. Pathologe. 7(4):187–191

Löning T, Meichsner M, Milde-Langosch K, Hinze H, Orlt I, Hormann K, Sesterhenn K, Becker J, Reichart P (1987) HPV DNA detection in tumours of the head and neck: a comparative light microscopy and DNA hybridization study. ORL 49:259–269

Lookingbill DP, Kreider JW, Howett MK, Olmstead PM, Conner GH (1987) Human papillomavirus type 16 in Bowenoid papulosis, intraoral papillomas, and squamous cell carcinoma of the tongue. Arch Dermatol 123:363–368
Lopez-Lizarraga E, Sanchez-Corona J, Montoya-Fuentes H, Bravo-Cuellar A, Campollo-Rivas O, Lopez-Demerutis E, Morgan-Villela G, Arcaute-Velazquez F, Monreal-Martinez JA, Troyo R (2000) Human papillomavirus in tonsillar and nasopharyngeal carcinoma: isolation of HPV subtype 31. Ear Nose Throat J 79:942–944
Lowy DR, Schiller JT (1994) A virus-like particle enzyme-linked immunosorbent assay detects serum antibodies in a majority of women infected with human papillomavirus type 16. J Natl Cancer Inst 86:494–499
Lowy DR, Schiller JT (2006) Prophylactic human papillomavirus vaccines. J Clin Invest 116:1167–1173
Maitland NJ, Cox MF, Lynas C, Prime SS, Meanwell CA, Scully C (1987) Detection of human papillomavirus DNA in biopsies of human oral tissue. Br J Cancer 56:245–250
Maitland NJ, Bromidge T, Cox MF, Crane IJ, Prime SS, Scully C (1989) Detection of human papillomavirus genes in human oral tissue biopsies and cultures by polymerase chain reaction. Br J Cancer 59:698–703
Makowska W, Rogozinski T, Zawadowski J, Waloryszak B (1993) Human papilloma virus infection in the case of larynx carcinoma. Otolaryngol Pol 47:23–25
McCullough DW, McNicol PJ (1991) Laryngeal carcinoma associated with human papillomavirus type 16. J Otolaryngol 20:97–99
McKay SP, Gregoire L, Lonardo F, Reidy P, Mathog RH, Lancaster WD (2005) Human papillomavirus (HPV) transcripts in malignant inverted papilloma are from integrated HPV DNA. Laryngoscope 115:1428–1431
Meisels A, Fortin R (1976) Condylomatous lesions of the cervix and vagina. I. Cytologic patterns. Acta Cytol 20:505–509
Mellin H, Friesland S, Lewensohn R, Dalianis T, Munck-Wikland E (2000) Human papillomavirus (HPV) DNA in tonsillar cancer: clinical correlates, risk of relapse, and survival. Int J Cancer 89:300–304
Mellin H, Dahlgren L, Munck-Wikland E et al (2002) Human papillomavirus type 16 is episomal and a high viral load may be correlated to better prognosis in tonsillar cancer. Int J Cancer
Milde K, Löning T (1986) Detection of papillomavirus DNA in oral papillomas and carcinomas: application of in situ hybridization with biotinylated HPV 16 probes. J Oral Pathol 15:292–296
Miller CS, Johnstone BM (2001) Human papillomavirus as a risk factor for oral squamous cell carcinoma: a meta-analysis, 1982–1997. Oral Surg Oral Med Oral Pathol Oral Radiol Endod 91:622–635
Morgan DW, Abdullan V, Quiney R, Myint S (1991) Human papilloma virus and carcinoma of the laryngo-pharyngx. J Laryngol Otol 105:288–292
Ndiaye C, Mena M, Alemany L, Arbyn M, Castellsagué X, Laporte L, Bosch FX, de Sanjosé S (2014) Trottier H.HPV DNA, E6/E7 mRNA, and p16INK4a detection in head and neck cancers: a systematic review and meta-analysis. Lancet Oncol. 15:1319–1331
Niedobitek G, Pitteroff S, Herbst H, Shepherd P, Finn T, Anagnostopoulos I, Stein H (1990) Detection of human papillomavirus type 16 DNA in carcinomas of the palatine tonsil. J Clin Pathol 43:918–921
Noble-Topham SE, Fliss DM, Hartwick RWJ, McLachlin CM, Freeman JL, Noyek AM, Andrulis IL (1993) Detection and typing of human papillomavirus in verrucous carcinoma of the oral cavity using the polymerase chain reaction. Arch Otolaryngol Head Neck Surg 119:1299–1304
Ogura H, Watanabe S, Fukushima K, Masuda Y, Fujiwara T, Yabe Y (1991) Presence of human papillomavirus type 18 DNA in a pharyngeal and laryngeal carcinoma. Jap. J Cancer Res 82:1184–1187

Ogura H, Watanabe S, Fukushima K, Masuda Y, Fujiwara T, Yabe Y (1993) Human papillomavirus DNA in squamous cell carcinomas of the respiratory and upper digestive tracts. Jpn J Clin Oncol 23:221–225

Oriel JD (1989) Human papillomaviruses and anal cancer. Genitourin Med 65:213–215

Orth G (1986) Epidermodysplasia verruciformis: a model for understanding the oncogenicity of human papillomaviruses. Ciba Found Symp 120:157–174

Ostrow RS, Manias DA, Fong WJ, Zachow KR (1987) Faras AJ.A survey of human cancers for human papillomavirus DNA by filter hybridization. Cancer 59:429–430

Parsons RJ, Kidd JG (1943) Oral papillomatosis of rabbis: a virus disease. J Exp Med 77:233–250

Payne A (1891) On the contagious rise of common warts. Br J Dermatol 3:185

Paz IB, Cook N, OdomMaryon T, Xie Y, Wilczynski SP (1997) Human papillomavirus (HPV) in head and neck cancer: an association of HPV 16 with squamous cell carcinoma of Waldeyer's tonsillar ring. Cancer 79:595–604

Poljak M, Gale N, Kambic V (1997) Human papillomaviruses: a study of their prevalence in the epithelial hyperplastic lesions of the larynx. Acta Otolaryngol Suppl 527:66–69

Purola E, Savia E (1977) Cytology of gynaecologic condyloma acuminata. Acta Cytol 21:26–31

Pyrhönen S (1978) Human wart-virus antibodies in patients with genital and skin warts. Acta Derm Venereol Stockh 58:427–432

Quick CA, Faras A, Krzysek R (1978) The etiology of laryngeal papillomatosis. Laryngoscope 88:1789–1795

Quick CA, Foucar E, Deliver LP (1979) Frequency and significance of epithelial atypia in laryngeal papillomatosis. Laryngoscope 89:550–560

Quick CA, Watts SL, Krzyzek RA, Faras AJ (1980) Relationship between condylomata and laryngeal papillomata. Clinical and molecular virological evidence. Ann Otol Rhinol Laryngol 89:467–471

Schwartz SM, Daling JR, Doody DR, Wipf GC, Carter JJ, Madeleine MM, Mao EJ, Fitzgibbons ED, Huang S, Beckmann AM, McDougall JK, Galloway DA (1998) Oral cancer risk in relation to sexual history and evidence of human papillomavirus infection. J Natl Cancer Inst 90:1626–1636

Shen J, Tate JE, Crum CP, Goodman ML (1996) Prevalence of human papillomaviruses (HPV) in benign and malignant tumors of the upper respiratory tract. Mod Pathol 9:15–20

Shindoh M, Chiba I, Yasuda M, Saito T, Funaoka K, Kohgo T, Amemiya A, Sawada Y, Fujinaga K (1995) Detection of human papillomavirus DNA sequences in oral squamous cell carcinomas and their relation to p53 and proliferating cell nuclear antigen expression. Cancer 76:1513–1521

Shroyer KR, Greer RO, Fankhouser CA, McGuirt WF, Marshall R (1993) Detection of human papillomavirus DNA in oral verrucous carcinoma by polymerase chain reaction. Mod Pathol 6:669–672

Snijders PJF, Cromme FV, van den Brule AJC et al (1992) Prevalence and expression of human papillomavirus in tonsillar carcinomas, indicating a possible viral etiology. Int J Cancer 52:845–850

Snijders PJ, Steenbergen RD, Top B, Scott SD, Meijer CJ, Walboomers JM (1994) Analysis of p53 status in tonsillar carcinomas associated with human papillomavirus. J Gen Virol 75:2769–2775

Snijders PJ, Scholes AG, Hart CA, Jones AS, Vaughan ED, Woolgar JA, Meijer CJ, Walboomers JM, Field JK (1996) Prevalence of mucosotropic human papillomaviruses in squamous-cell carcinoma of the head and neck. Int J Cancer 66:464–469

Snijders PJ, Steenbergen RD, Meijer CJ, Walboomers JM (1997) Role of human papillomaviruses in cancer of the respiratory and upper digestive tract. Clin Dermatol 15:415–425

Stremlau A, Zenner HP, Gissmann L, zur Hausen H (1987) Demonstration and organizational structure of the DNA of human papillomaviruses in laryngeal and hypopharyngeal carcinomas. Laryngol Rhinol Otol Stuttg 66:311–315

Sugar J, Vereczkey I, Toth J, Peter I, Banhidy F (1997) New aspects in the pathology of the preneoplastic lesions of the larynx. Acta Oto Laryngol 52–56
Syrjänen K (2003) HPV infections in benign and malignant sinonasal lesions. J Clin Pathol 56:174–181
Syrjänen KJ, Syrjänen SM (1981) Histological evidence for the presence of condylomatous epithelial lesions in association with laryngeal squamous cell carcinoma. ORL 43:181–194
Syrjänen K, Syrjänen S (2000) Papillomavirus infections in human pathology. Wiley, London-Paris, pp 1–615
Syrjänen S, Syrjänen K (2008) The history of papillomavirus research. Cent Eur J Public Health 16 (Suppl):S7–13
Syrjänen K, Syrjänen S (2013) Detection of human papillomavirus in sinonasal carcinoma: systematic review and meta-analysis. Hum Pathol 44(6):983–991
Syrjänen KJ, Syrjänen SM, Pyrhönen S (1982) Human papilloma virus (HPV) antigens in lesions of laryngeal squamous cell carcinomas. ORL 44:323–334
Syrjänen KJ, Pyrhönen S, Syrjänen SM (1983a) Evidence suggesting human papillomavirus (HPV) etiology for the squamous cell papilloma of the paranasal sinus. Arch Geschwulstforsch 53:77–82
Syrjänen K, Syrjänen S, Lamberg M, Pyrhönen S, Nuutinen J (1983b) Morphological and immunohistochemical evidence suggesting human papillomavirus (HPV) involvement in oral squamous cell carcinogenesis. Int J Oral Surg 12:418–424
Syrjänen KJ, Syrjänen SM, Lamberg MA, Pyrhönen S (1983c) Human papillomavirus (HPV) involvement in squamous cell lesions of the oral cavity. Proc Finn Dent Soc 79:1–8
Syrjänen KJ, Syrjänen SM, Lamberg MA, Happonen RP (1983d) Local immunological reactivity in oral squamous cell lesions of possible HPV (human papillomavirus) origin. Arch Geschwulstforsch 53:537–546
Syrjänen SM, Syrjänen KJ, Lamberg MA (1986) Detection of human papillomavirus DNA in oral mucosal lesions using in situ DNA-hybridization applied on paraffin sections. Oral Surg Oral Med Oral Pathol 62:660–667
Syrjänen S, Happonen RP, Virolainen E, Siivonen L, Syrjänen K (1987a) Detection of human papillomavirus (HPV) structural antigens and DNA types in inverted papillomas and squamous cell carcinomas of the nasal cavities and paranasal sinuses. Acta Otolaryngol Stockh 104:334–341
Syrjänen S, Syrjänen K, Mäntyjärvi R, Collan Y, Kärjä J (1987b) Human papillomavirus DNA in squamous cell carcinomas of the larynx demonstrated by in situ DNA hybridization. ORL J Otorhinolaryngol Relat Spec 49:175–186
Syrjänen SM, Syrjänen KJ, Happonen RP (1988) Human papillomavirus (HPV) DNA sequences in oral precancerous lesions and squamous cell carcinoma demonstrated by in situ hybridization. J Oral Pathol 17:273–278
Syrjänen S, Lodi G, von Bültzingslöwen I, Aliko A, Arduino P, Campisi G, Challacombe S, Ficarra G, Flaitz C, Zhou HM, Maeda H, Miller C, Jontell M (2011) Human papillomaviruses in oral carcinoma and oral potentially malignant disorders: a systematic review. Oral Dis 17 (Suppl 1):58–72
Syverton JT, Dascomb HE, Wells EB, Kooman J, Berry GP (1950) The virus induced papilloma to carcinoma sequence. Carcinomas in the natural host, the cottontail rabbit. Cancer Res 10:440–444
Tsuchiya H, Tomita Y, Shirasawa H, Tanzawa H, Sato K, Simizu B (1991) Detection of human papillomavirus in head and neck tumors with DNA hybridization and immunohistochemical analysis. Oral Surg Oral Med Oral Pathol. 71:721–725
Turazza E, Lapeña A, Sprovieri O et al (1997) Low-risk human papillomavirus types 6 and 11 associated with carcinomas of the genital and upper aero-digestive tract. Acta Ostet Gynecol 76:271–276
Tyan Y-S, Liu S-T, Ong W-R, Chen M-L, Shu C-H, Chang Y-S (1993) Detection of Epstein-Barr virus and Human papillomavirus in head and neck tumors. J Clin Microbiol 31:53–56

Ullman EV (1923) On the etiology of the laryngeal papilloma. Acta Otolaryngol 5:317–338
van Rensburg EJV, Venter EH, Simson IW (1993) Human papillomavirus DNA in aerodigestive squamous carcinomas demonstrated by means of in situ hybridization. S Afr Med J 83:516–518
Vonka R, Vesely J, Sibl O, Brichacek B (1990) The presence of human papillomavirus deoxyribonucleic acid in tumors in the otorhinolaryngologic area. Cas Lek Cesk 129:334–336
Wang AC, Hsu JJ, Hsueh S, Sun CF, Tsao KC (1991) Evidence of human papillomavirus deoxyribonucleic acid in vulvar squamous papillomatosis. Int J Gynecol Pathol 10:44–50
Ward N (1854) A mirror of the practice of medicine and surgery in the hospitals of London: London Hospital. Lancet 2:480–482
Ward P, Mounts P (1989) Heterogeneity in mRNA of human papillomavirus type-6 subtypes in respiratory tract lesions. Virol 168:1–11
Watanabe S, Ogura H, Fukushima K et al (1993) Comparison of Virapap filter hybridization with polymerase chain reaction and Southern blot hybridization methods for detection of human papillomavirus in tonsillar and pharyngeal cancers. Eur Arch Otorhinolaryngol 250:115–119
Watts SL, Brewer EE, Fry TL (1991) Human papillomavirus DNA types in squamous cell carcinomas of the head and neck. Oral Surg Oral Med Oral Pathol 71:701–707
Wilczynski SP, Lin BTY, Xie Y, Paz IB (1998) Detection of human papillomavirus DNA and oncoprotein overexpression are associated with distinct morphological patterns of tonsillar squamous cell carcinoma. Am J Pathol 152:145–156
Woods KV, Shillitoe EJ, Spitz MR, Schantz SP, Adler-Storthz K (1993) Analysis of human papillomavirus DNA in oral squamous cell carcinomas. J Oral Pathol Med 22:101–108
Wu TC, Trujillo JM, Kashima HK, Mounts P (1993) Association of human papillomavirus with nasal neoplasia. Lancet 341:522–524
Yeudall WA, Campo MS (1991) Human papillomavirus DNA in biopsies of oral tissues. J Gen Virol 72:173–176
Young SK, Min KW (1991) In situ DNA hybridization analysis of oral papillomas, leukoplakias, and carcinomas for human papillomavirus. Oral Surg Oral Med Oral Pathol 71:726–729
Zarod AP, Rutherford JD, Corbitt G (1988) Malignant progression of laryngeal papilloma associated with human papilloma virus type 6 (HPV-6) DNA. J Clin Pathol 41:280–283
Zeuss MS, Miller CS, White DK (1991) In situ hybridization analysis of human papillomavirus DNA in oral mucosal lesions. Oral Surg Oral Med Oral Pathol 71:714–720
zur Hausen H (1976) Condylomata acuminata and human genital cancer. Cancer Res 36:794
zur Hausen H (2009) Papillomaviruses in the causation of human cancers—a brief historical account. Virology 384(2):260–265 (Review)
zur Hausen H, de Villiers EM (1994) Human papillomaviruses. Annu Rev Microbiol 48:427–447
zur Hausen H, Gissmann L, Steiner W, Dippold W, Dregger I (1975) Human papilloma virus and cancer. Bibl Haematologica 43:569–571

Epidemiology of HPV-Positive Tumors in Europe and in the World

Xavier Castellsagué, Marisa Mena and Laia Alemany

Abstract

Strong evidence has accumulated in the last 15 years showing that infection by certain human papillomaviruses (HPVs) is etiologically involved in a subset of head and neck cancers (HNCs). In this chapter, epidemiologic-related topics on HNCs are reviewed: (i) HPV-attributable fractions and HPV-type distributions by different anatomical HNC sites, using not only HPV DNA but other more specific markers of causality; (ii) an update of the HPV-related HNCs burden worldwide and by regions; and finally, (iii) the determinants for HPV positivity in HNCs, focussing on gender, age, smoking habits, sexual behavior, and other related factors such as tonsillectomy performance. This information is essential in order to understand the burden of the disease and its dynamics and changing patterns, as well as for planning and assessment of the potential impact of HPV-based preventive strategies for HNCs.

Keywords

Epidemiology · HPV · Head and neck cancer · Burden of disease

1 The Contribution of HPV in the Etiology of HNCs

Strong evidence has accumulated in the last 15 years showing that infection by certain human papillomaviruses (HPVs) is etiologically involved in a subset of head and neck cancers (HNCs) (A Review of Human Carcinogens 2009). While virtually

X. Castellsagué (✉) · M. Mena · L. Alemany
Institut Catala d'Oncologia (ICO) L'Hospitalet de Llobregat, Catalonia, Spain
e-mail: xcastellsague@iconcologia.net

W. Golusiński et al. (eds.), *HPV Infection in Head and Neck Cancer*,
Recent Results in Cancer Research 206, DOI 10.1007/978-3-319-43580-0_2

all cervical cancers are considered HPV-driven (Walboomers et al. 1999), the quantitative assessment of the etiological involvement of HPVs in HNCs is challenged by their multifactorial etiology largely attributed to tobacco and alcohol use (IARC 1988, 2004; Gillison et al. 2012). Consequently, the unequivocal fraction of HPV-DNA-positive HNCs for which HPV infection is indeed the truly triggering carcinogenic event is unknown and its estimation remains a challenge (Herrero et al. 2003). Further, the mere presence of HPV DNA in HNCs is not sufficient to prove viral causation as it might just reflect a transient infection unrelated to the carcinogenic process (Holzinger et al. 2012; Ndiaye et al. 2014; Castellsagué et al. 2016).

Most previous studies and meta-analyses assessing the quantitative contribution of HPV in HNCs have used the presence and detection of HPV-DNA in the tumor as the sole criterion to classify the tumor as HPV-driven, probably resulting in an overestimation of the true impact of HPV in head and neck carcinogenesis. To accurately classify a tumor as HPV-driven, it is crucial to use in addition to HPV-DNA detection other markers related to HPV-induced carcinogenesis and thus assess the biological and oncogenic activity of the HPVs identified in HNCs.

1.1 The ICO Study on HPV in HNCs

The Catalan Institute of Oncology (ICO) conducted a large international study explicitly designed to generate robust estimates of HPV-attributable fractions (AFs) in HNCs by quantifying the expression of a selection of markers of HPV-induced carcinogenesis and using a strict single protocol that standardized the entire processing and testing of all tumor samples (Castellsagué et al. 2016).

The methods used in this study have been already published (de Sanjosé et al. 2010). In brief, formalin-fixed, paraffin-embedded cancer tissues of the oral cavity, pharynx and larynx were collected from pathology archives in 29 countries worldwide. All samples were subjected to central histopathological evaluation, DNA quality control, and HPV-DNA detection. Samples containing HPV-DNA were further tested for HPV E6*I mRNA detection and expression of p16^{INK4a}, pRb, p53, and Cyclin D1 by immunohistochemistry.

A total of 3,680 samples yielded valid results: 1,374 pharyngeal, 1,264 oral cavity, and 1,042 laryngeal cancers.

Figure 1 presents by major HNC site, estimated range of HPV-AFs using different combinations of markers of HPV carcinogenesis: HPV-DNA detection, HPV E6*I mRNA detection, and p16 over-expression. Ranges of AFs when considering HPV DNA plus E6*I mRNA and/or p16^{INK4a} were: 18.5–22.4 % for the oropharynx, 3.0–4.4 % for the oral cavity, and 1.5–3.5 % for the larynx. Corresponding estimates for pharynx unspecified subsite, nasopharynx, and hypopharynx were, respectively, 7.5–16.1, 1.1–5.9 and 2.4 % (Castellsagué et al. 2016). We observed that within both the oral cavity and the larynx, those subsites that were more proximal to the oropharynx showed higher HPV-AFs than those that were more distal to the oropharynx. Thus, HPV-AFs in combined oral cavity subsites that were

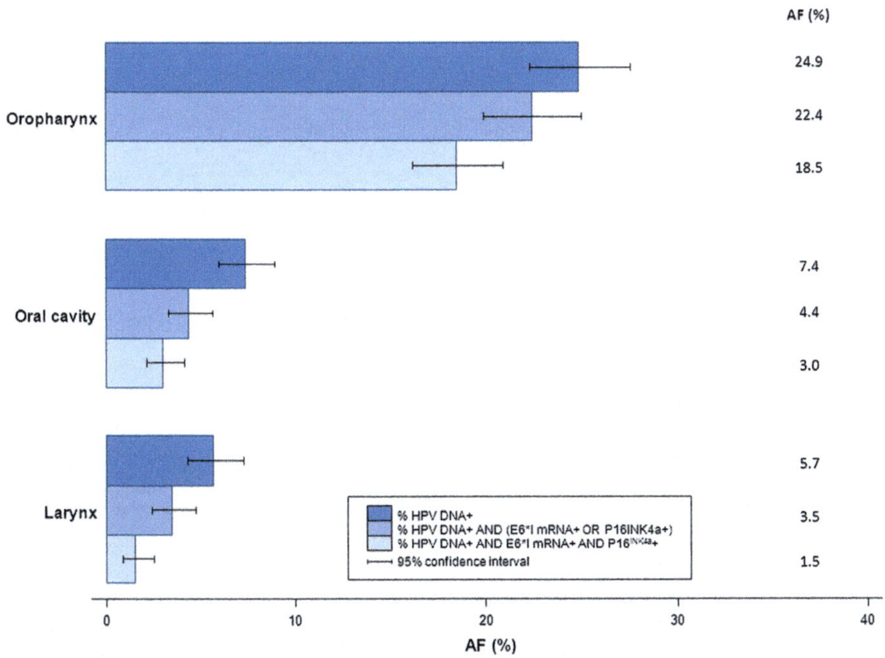

Fig. 1 HPV-attributable fractions for head and neck cancers according to positivity and/or over-expression of selected biomarkers of HPV-induced carcinogenesis

proximal to the oropharynx ranged (when considering HPV DNA plus E6*I mRNA and/or $p16^{INK4a}$) from 4.9 to 6.7 %, as opposed to 1.4–2.3 % in subsites that were distal to the oropharynx ($p < 0.001$ for both comparisons). Corresponding values in the larynx were 4.2 % versus 1.4–3.4 % in combined subsites that were proximal versus distal to the oropharynx, but these differences in the larynx were not statistically significant (Castellsagué et al. 2016).

Figure 2 shows oropharyngeal HPV-AFs by geography, gender, age group, and year of diagnosis. Estimates of HPV-AF in the oropharynx were highest in South America, Central and Eastern Europe and Northern Europe, and lowest in Southern Europe. Women showed higher HPV-AFs than men for cancers of the oropharynx. Globally, younger patients showed higher HPV-AFs than older patients and AFs tended to be higher in more recent decades with a statistically significant increasing trend in AFs with increasing recency.

1.2 HPV-Type Distribution in HNCs

Among HPV-DNA-positive cancer cases, the distribution of individual HPV types is different in HNCs when compared with cervical cancers, as HPV16 is systematically found in a much higher percentage of HNCs than of cervical cancer.

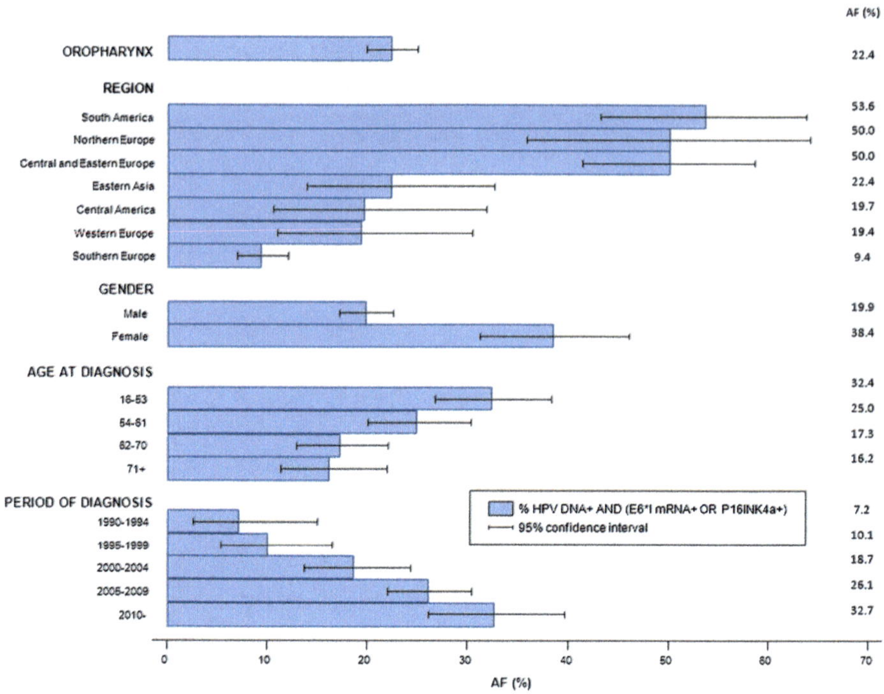

Fig. 2 HPV-attributable fractions for oropharyngeal cancer according to world region, gender, age, and period of diagnosis

Confirming results from several other studies, the ICO study found that HPV16 is the most frequently detected genotype among HPV-DNA-positive cases (75.2 %), but again with a wide range according to cancer site: 83 % in the oropharynx, 68.8 % in the oral cavity, and 50.8 % in the larynx (Castellsagué et al. 2016). The corresponding percentages for combined HPV types included in the nonavalent HPV vaccine (types 6, 11, 16, 18, 31, 33, 45, 52, and 58) were 89.7, 76.3, and 81.4 %, indicating that most HPV-positive HNCs could eventually be prevented through HPV immunization programs.

2 Burden of HPV-Related HNCs

HNC is the seventh cause of incident cancer cases worldwide, with an estimated 686,328 new cases and 375,622 deaths every year (Ferlay et al. 2013). These estimations include the oral cavity, larynx, and pharynx (nasopharynx, oropharynx, and hypopharynx). Among HNCs, oral cavity (including lips) is the most common, representing more than 40 % of the cases. HNC shows a wide worldwide geographical heterogeneity in terms of incidence rates (Ferlay et al. 2013), likely reflecting a wide variability in the prevalence of established risk behaviors. Moreover, 75 % of the HNC burden occurs in men. As mentioned in the previous section, the association of HPV with HNC is also very heterogeneous with dramatic variations across anatomical sub-sites and geographical regions. The oropharynx is the sub-site with strongest associations with HPV. In some regions of the world such as USA or Northern Europe, more than 70 % of oropharyngeal cancer cases are estimated to be HPV-related (Chaturvedi et al. 2011), as compared with only 17 % in Southern Europe (De Martel et al. 2012).

However, as explained before, the mere use of HPV-DNA detection is not appropriate to classify a HNC as HPV-driven. Thus, the precise estimation of the burden of HPV-related HNCs requires the use of accurate HPV-AFs that include not only HPV-DNA detection but also at least one additional marker of HPV-induced carcinogenesis such as mRNA and/or p16 over-expression. The ICO survey is currently the largest and most robust study that used these markers in the definition of HPV-AFs in 3,680 HNC cases from Europe, Central and South America, Africa and Asia (Castellsagué et al. 2016). Based on sex- and region-specific HPV-AFs (as defined by HPV-DNA positivity and at least positivity by one additional marker, either mRNA or p16), we were able to estimate more accurately the burden of HPV-driven HNC in most world regions (Table 1). For regions not appropriately covered by the ICO study, global HPV-AFs from the ICO study or from other studies that tested for at least two HPV-related markers were used as indicated in the table footnotes. As shown in the table, we estimate that every year about 45,000 new HNC cases can be attributed to HPV infection worldwide. That table details the estimated burden by world region and sex for each major HNC site. It is important to mention that the HPV-AFs used in the ICO study might slightly underestimate the real number of HPV-driven HNCs because most HPV-DNA-negative samples were not tested for the additional markers and also because the assignment of HPV-driven cancers required positivity for at least two HPV-related markers.

In terms of trends, during the last years it has been evidenced that the annual number of new oropharyngeal cancer cases is increasing in some parts of the world (Chaturvedi et al. 2013), as well as the fraction of oropharyngeal cancer associated with HPV infection (Mehanna et al. 2013). The increased incidences have been observed particularly among young men (<60 years old) in several economically developed countries despite concomitant declines in incidence for oral cavity and lung squamous cell carcinomas. These contrasts suggest a role of HPV infection in increasing oropharyngeal cancer incidence rates among men. However, among women, incidence increased for all three HNCs, supporting a dominant effect of smoking on increasing incidence rates (Gillison et al. 2015).

Table 1 HPV-attributable fractions and estimated annual number of incident HNC cases attributable to HPV (requiring positivity for both HPV DNA and at least one additional HPV-related marker) by region, sex, and anatomical site

	Oral cavity[a]				Oropharynx[b]				Larynx[c]				ALL SITES		
	Male		Female		Male		Female		Male		Female		Male	Female	All
	AFs (%)	HPV-driven N	AFs (%)	HPV-driven N	AFs (%)	HPV-driven N	AFs (%)	HPV-driven N	AFs (%)	HPV-driven N	AFs (%)	HPV-driven N	HPV-driven N	HPV-driven N	HPV-driven N
Europe	4.4[d]	1,873	2.6[d]	490	16.9[d]	3,753	40.2[d]	1,792	2.2[d]	792	4.3[d]	169	6,418	2,451	8,869
Asia	4.7[e]	5,264	3.8[e]	2,161	18.8[d]	6,619	17.6[d]	1,429	2.8[e]	1,925	9.2[e]	805	13,808	4,395	18,203
North America	8.9[f]	1,683	1.7[f]	164	71.2 [g]	6,551	55.2 [g]	1,334	2.8[e]	300	9.2[e]	254	8,534	1,752	10,286
Central-South America	6.4[d]	831	6.8[d]	520	37.8[d]	1,919	51.6[d]	629	4.8[d]	686	15.6[d]	343	3,436	1,492	4,928
Africa	4.7[e]	281	3.8[e]	268	19.9[e]	511	38.4[e]	564	2.8[e]	213	9.2[e]	97	1,005	929	1,934
Oceania	4.7[e]	107	3.8[e]	51	19.9[e]	215	38.4[e]	93	2.8[e]	20	9.2[e]	9	342	153	495
World		10,039		3,654		19,568		5,841		3,936		1,677	33,543	11,172	44,715

AFs HPV-attributable fractions; *N* Number of incident cases attributable to HPV infection

[a]The total number of cases in 2012 has been obtained from GLOBOCAN 2012. Oral cavity includes lip, base of tongue, mobile tongue, gum, floor of the mouth, palate, other and unspecified parts of mouth, and salivary glands

[b]The total number of cases in 2012 has been extrapolated from initial estimates reported in Forman et al. (2012), which were only reported for both sexes combined using old GLOBOCAN 2008 and cancer registry data. To estimate corresponding updated 2012 figures, we assumed: (1) the same geographical distribution of oropharyngeal cases across European regions as the corresponding distribution of "other pharynx" cases available in GLOBOCAN 2012; (2) the same increment of oropharyngeal cases from GLOBOCAN 2008 to GLOBOCAN 2012 as that of "other pharynx" cases; and (3) the same gender distribution of oropharyngeal cases by region as that of "other pharynx" cases in GLOBOCAN 2012. Oropharynx includes oropharyngeal parts as well as tonsil and base of tongue

[c]The total number of cases in 2012 has been obtained from GLOBOCAN 2012. Larynx includes glottis, laryngeal cartilage, and unspecified and overlapping lesions of larynx

[d]AFs derived from the ICO study (Castellsagué et al. 2016) in which a case was classified as HPV-related if it was positive for both HPV DNA and either $p16^{INK4a}$ or E6*I mRNA

[e]Since this region was not appropriately represented in the ICO study, site-and sex-specific global HPV-AFs from the ICO study were used

[f]AFs derived from Lingen et al. (2013) in which a case was classified as HPV-related if it was positive for HPV E6/7

[g]AFs derived from Jordan et al. (2012) in which a case was classified as HPV-related if it was positive for HPV E6/7

3 Determinants for HPV-Positive Head and Neck Cancers

As mentioned before, HPV-AFs in HNCs are highly heterogeneous across geographical regions, particularly in oropharyngeal cancers (Castellsagué et al. 2016). Distinct trends in tobacco and alcohol consumption, sexual behavior, and sociodemographic variables may lead among others to these observed heterogeneous patterns.

Besides HPV infection, tobacco and alcohol are the classic and well-established risk factors for HNCs. Tobacco prevalence estimates exhibit substantial variation across age groups, sex, and countries (Ng et al. 2014). Prevalence estimates by country can vary from below 5 % for women in some African countries to more than 55 % for men in Timor-Leste and Indonesia. Gender differences are also important, with an estimated age-standardized prevalence of 31 % for men and 6 % for women, in 2012 (Ng et al. 2014). Differences in smoking prevalence trends are also observed with highest declining rates observed in Canada, USA, and European Nordic countries, and increased prevalence rates in other countries (Ng et al. 2014). Moreover, and beyond prevalence variations, it is still unclear whether tobacco and/or alcohol use can act as co-factors and/or effect modifiers in risk of developing HPV-positive HNCs. A review of case-control studies addressing this issue showed inconsistent results, with two studies reporting positive interactions between HPV infection and tobacco, two showing no interaction, and finally three reporting a negative joint effect (Gillison et al. 2012).

Some studies indicate that the most likely explanation for the origin of HPV-related HNCs is a sexually acquired oral HPV infection that is not cleared, persists, and evolves into a neoplastic lesion. Sexual behavior is a clear risk factor for oral HPV acquisition and HPV-related HNCs (Gillison et al. 2008). Like for tobacco and alcohol consumption, sexual behavior greatly varies across regions with proportions of ever having oral sex in USA higher than 65 % compared to lower than 20 % in countries from Southern Europe such as Spain (Heck et al. 2010).

Gender and age are also factors that can affect HNCs HPV positivity. HPV-positive HNCs patients show younger ages at diagnosis than HPV-negative ones (Castellsagué et al. 2016), probably linked to differential sexual behavior of younger versus older cohorts. Regarding gender, a recent systematic review on differences in the proportion of HPV-AF in oropharyngeal cancers between men and women revealed heterogeneous HPV-related HNCs patterns with the highest men-to-women ratio found in USA (1.5) and lowest found in Asia and some European countries (0.7) (Combes et al. 2014). This last observation is in agreement with our recently published results of higher oropharyngeal cancer HPV-AFs in women from some European countries (Castellsagué et al. 2016). Combes and colleagues also evaluated the sex-specific lung cancer rates in order to assess whether the observed gender differences in HNC could be explained by differences in tobacco consumption and found that HPV prevalence in oropharyngeal cancers differs by gender and country mainly as a consequence of the vast international variation in male smoking habits (Combes et al. 2014). However, there are still unclear reasons for these gender findings besides gender differences in tobacco consumption. A recent work by D'Souza and colleagues showed differences in the natural history of oral HPV infections between men and women, such as a higher risk of acquiring an oral HPV infection with recent number of oral sexual partners among men and less HPV infection clearance in men (D'Souza et al. 2016)

Other factors may be contributing to this observed geographical heterogeneity in HPV-AFs in HNCs, for example trends in tonsillectomy rates. Tonsillectomy consists on the removal of the tonsils, the most susceptible head and neck site for HPV infection. Some countries have reported a decrease in tonsillectomies rates over time (Koshy et al. 2014; Fakhry et al. 2015), and a recent study reported both a decrease of this surgical procedure with a simultaneous increase in the risk of oropharyngeal cancer (Fakhry et al. 2015). Tonsillectomy likely reduces the palatine lymphoid tissue susceptible to carcinogenic factors and subsequent potential malignization.

References

A review of human carcinogens (2009) Part B: Biological agents/ IARC Working Group on the Evaluation of Carcinogenic Risks to Humans. Lyon, France: International Agency for Research on Cancer Monographs

Castellsagué X, Alemany L, Quer M et al (2016) HPV involvement in head and neck cancers: comprehensive assessment of biomarkers in 3680 patients. J Natl Cancer Inst 108(6):djv403

Chaturvedi AK, Engels EA, Pfeiffer RM et al (2011) Human papillomavirus and rising oropharyngeal cancer incidence in the United States. J Clin Oncol 29:4294–4301

Chaturvedi AK, Anderson WF, Lortet-Tieulent J et al (2013) Worldwide trends in incidence rates for oral cavity and oropharyngeal cancers. J Clin Oncol 31:4550–4559

Combes JD, Chen AA, Franceschi S (2014) Prevalence of human papillomavirus in cancer of the oropharynx by gender. Cancer Epidemiol Biomarkers Prev 23(12):2954–2958

De Martel C, Ferlay J, Franceschi S et al (2012) The global burden of cancers attributable to infections in the year 2008: a review and synthetic analysis. Lancet Oncol 13:607–615

de Sanjosé S, Quint WG, Alemany L et al (2010) Retrospective International Survey and HPV Time Trends Study Group. Human papillomavirus genotype attribution in invasive cervical cancer: a retrospective cross-sectional worldwide study. Lancet Oncol 11(11):1048–1056

D'Souza G, Wentz A, Kluz N et al (2016) Gender differences in risk factors and natural history of oral human papillomavirus (HPV) infection. J Infect Dis 10(pii):jiw063

Fakhry C, Andersen KK, Christensen J et al (2015) The Impact of Tonsillectomy upon the Risk of Oropharyngeal Carcinoma Diagnosis and Prognosis in the Danish Cancer Registry. Cancer Prev Res (Phila) 8(7):583–589

Ferlay J, Soerjomataram I, Ervik M et al (2013) GLOBOCAN 2012 v1.0, Cancer Incidence and Mortality Worldwide: IARC Cancer Base No. 11. Lyon, France: International Agency for Research on Cancer. http://globocan.iarc.fr. Accessed 09 Mar 2016

Forman D, de Martel C, Lacey CJ et al (2012) Global burden of human papillomavirus and related diseases. Vaccine 30(Suppl 5):F12–F23

Gillison ML, D'Souza G, Westra W et al (2008) Distinct risk factor profiles for human papillomavirus type 16-positive and human papillomavirus type 16-negative head and neck cancers. J Natl Cancer Inst 100(6):407–420

Gillison ML, Alemany L, Snijders PJ et al (2012) Human papillomavirus and diseases of the upper airway: head and neck cancer and respiratory papillomatosis. Vaccine. 30(Suppl 5):F34–F54

Gillison ML, Chaturvedi AK, Anderson WF et al (2015) Epidemiology of Human Papillomavirus-Positive Head and Neck Squamous Cell Carcinoma. J Clin Oncol 33 (29):3235–3242

Heck JE, Berthiller J, Vaccarella S et al (2010) Sexual behaviours and the risk of head and neck cancers: a pooled analysis in the International Head and Neck Cancer Epidemiology (INHANCE) consortium. Int J Epidemiol 39(1):166–181

Herrero R, Castellsagué X, Pawlita M et al (2003) IARC Multicenter Oral Cancer Study Group. Human papillomavirus and oral cancer: the International Agency for Research on Cancer multicenter study. J Natl Cancer Inst 95(23):1772–1783

Holzinger D, Schmitt M, Dyckhoff G et al (2012) Viral RNA patterns and high viral load reliably define oropharynx carcinomas with active HPV16 involvement. Cancer Res 72(19):4993–5003

IARC (1988) Monographs on the evaluation of carcinogenic risks to humans, vol. 44. Alcohol drinking. Lyon, France: International Agency for Research on Cancer Monographs

IARC (2004) Monographs on the evaluation of carcinogenic risks to humans, vol. 83. Tobacco Smoke and Involuntary Smoking. Lyon, France: International Agency for Research on Cancer Monographs

Jordan RC, Lingen MW, Perez-Ordonez B et al (2012) Validation of methods for oropharyngeal cancer HPV status determination in US cooperative group trials. Am J Surg Pathol 36(7):945–954

Koshy E, Bottle A, Murray J et al (2014) Changing indications and socio-demographic determinants of (adeno)tonsillectomy among children in England–are they linked? A retrospective analysis of hospital data. PLoS ONE 9(8):e103600

Lingen MW, Xiao W, Schmitt A et al (2013) Low etiologic fraction for high-risk human papillomavirus in oral cavity squamous cell carcinomas. Oral Oncol 49(1):1–8

Mehanna H, Beech T, Nicholson T et al (2013) The prevalence of human papillomavirus in oropharyngeal and non-oropharyngeal head and neck cancer—a systematic review and metaanalysis of trends by time and region. Head Neck 35:747–755

Ndiaye C, Mena M, Alemany L et al (2014) HPV DNA, E6/E7 mRNA, and p16INK4a detection in head and neck cancers: a systematic review and meta-analysis. Lancet Oncol. 15(12):1319–1331

Ng M, Freeman MK, Fleming TD et al (2014) Smoking prevalence and cigarette consumption in 187 countries, 1980-2012. JAMA 311(2):183–192

Walboomers JM, Jacobs MV, Manos MM et al (1999) Human papillomavirus is a necessary cause of invasive cervical cancer worldwide. J Pathol 189(1):12–19

Molecular Patterns and Biology of HPV-Associated HNSCC

Ruud H. Brakenhoff, Steffen Wagner and Jens P. Klussmann

Abstract

Head and neck cancer is the sixth most common cancer worldwide. The large majority are squamous cell carcinomas (HNSCC) that develop in the mucosal linings of the upper aerodigestive tract. These tumors develop either by exogenous carcinogen exposure (smoking, alcohol drinking) or by human papillomavirus (HPV) infection, particularly those in the oropharynx (OPSCC). HPV-positive (HPV+ve) and HPV-negative (HPV-ve) OPSCC are considered different disease entities. HPV+ve tumors are different at the molecular level and likely as a consequence have a much more favorable prognosis than HPV-ve tumors, despite their generally advanced stage at presentation. In general, HNSCCs develop in precancerous mucosal changes, and the apparent lack of precancerous HPV+ve mucosal changes is therefore remarkable. In this Chapter, head and neck carcinogenesis is discussed and the molecular differences between HPV+ve and HPV-ve tumors are outlined.

Keywords

Head and neck cancer · Human papillomavirus (HPV) · Molecular carcinogenesis · Genetic alteration · Expression profile · Epigenetics · MicroRNA (miRNA) · Oropharynx

R.H. Brakenhoff (✉)
Department of Otolaryngology-Head and Neck Surgery,
VU University Medical Center, Amsterdam, The Netherlands
e-mail: rh.brakenhoff@vumc.nl

S. Wagner · J.P. Klussmann
Department of Otorhinolaryngology, Head and Neck Surgery,
University of Giessen, Giessen, Germany
e-mail: jens.p.klussmann@hno.med.uni-giessen.de

W. Golusiński et al. (eds.), *HPV Infection in Head and Neck Cancer*,
Recent Results in Cancer Research 206, DOI 10.1007/978-3-319-43580-0_3

1 Introduction

1.1 Genetic Progression Model of Head and Neck Cancer

1.1.1 Precursor Lesions in the Mucosal Linings

By far most knowledge on the pathogenesis of squamous cell carcinomas in the upper aerodigestive tract has been obtained from oral cancers, the likely reason being that oral precancerous changes are most frequently diagnosed and the specimens are available for research. Leukoplakia, a white lesion in the mucosa of the oral cavity, is the most common precursor lesion of oral squamous carcinomas and its prevalence varies between 0.1 and 0.5 % (Napier and Speight 2008; van der Waal 2009). The common policy is to treat the lesion when possible and analyze the specimen or a biopsy by microscopic examination for dysplasia, graded as mild, moderate, or severe. Although criteria have been defined by the WHO, it is difficult to make an objective categorization of dysplasia due to a high inter- and intra-observer variation in assessment. After diagnosis and treatment when possible, patients are subsequently monitored by watchful waiting.

The percentage of oral leukoplakia that develops into cancer depends on various factors such as the study population, the used definition of leukoplakia, and the length of the observation time, but an annual transformation rate of 1–2 % per year is a reasonable assumption (van der Waal 2009; Napier and Speight 2008). Risk factors for progression are female gender, size, and the presence and grade of dysplasia. Most recent studies have identified genetic changes as the best predictors of malignant transformation (Zhang et al. 2012). HPV presence has been analyzed in leukoplakia lesions, but results are discordant, most likely due to false-positive results by the applied sensitive HPV-DNA assays. Most reliable studies suggest a very low prevalence of less than 1 % (reviewed in Ha and Califano 2004).

1.1.2 Field Cancerization

Oral leukoplakias are visible manifestations of precursor lesions that are macroscopically recognized. However, there are several histological and clinical indications that many precursor changes in the oral mucosa are not visible to the naked eye. Already in 1953, the term “field cancerization” was proposed to explain the high propensity to develop local recurrences after treatment of HNSCC and the high likelihood that multiple independent tumors develop in the head and neck mucosa. Slaughter et al. carefully studied oral cancer specimens and linked the frequent observation of dysplastic changes surrounding these tumors with the occurrence of local recurrences and multiple primary tumors (Slaughter et al. 1953). Thanks to the developments in molecular research during the last two decades, the process of field cancerization can now be defined in molecular terms. In 1996, the first genetic multistep progression model for HNSCC was postulated, based on the genetic characterization of morphological changes in the squamous epithelium (Califano et al. 1996). Loss of heterozygosity at chromosomes 3p, 9p, and 17p appeared to occur in dysplasia, apparently reflecting early carcinogenesis, while other alterations at 11q, 4q, and 8 were typically present in carcinomas, likely corresponding to a relatively late phase in carcinogenesis.

Using these genetic markers combined with *TP53* mutations, it was shown that in at least 35 % of the oral and oropharyngeal tumors, the carcinomas are surrounded by mucosal epithelium with such genetic changes (Tabor et al. 2001). This epithelium has a macroscopically normal appearance, but may be histologically dysplastic. This tumor-adjacent mucosal epithelium characterized by genetic changes has also been coined "field," in line with the earlier studies. Importantly, these fields often extend into the surgical margins and are an important source of local recurrences and second primary tumors that are so often seen in treated HNSCC patients.

There is some information on what seems to precede the development of fields. Van Houten et al. reported small p53-positive focal patches in tumor-adjacent mucosal epithelium (van Houten et al. 2002). These mutated p53-positive patches were considered equivalent to the "clones" or "clonal units" defined as a family of daughter cells from a common progenitor cell or adult stem cell which makes up the squamous epithelium and that has now become detectable by the mutation in p53. These p53-mutated clonal units were considered to represent the first oncogenic changes in the mucosa and formed together with the genetically defined fields on the basis of the hypothetical patch-field-tumor-metastasis progression model for HNSCC development (Leemans et al. 2011). Recent data support this model. By Axin2 lineage tracing experiments, the stem cells and the patches they form have been shown recently, at least in mouse skin (Lim et al. 2013).

The studies described above relate to HNSCC in general and were carried out before the distinction between HPV+ve and HPV-ve tumors had become apparent. Recently, it was studied whether HPV+ve tumors in the oropharynx are also surrounded by these large fields of altered cells. It was reasoned that HPV infection is likely the first carcinogenic event in HPV+ve tumors as is seen in the cervix and that HPV or better viral E6 transcripts could be used to study field cancerization surrounding HPV+ve tumors. Remarkably, in none of the tested surgical margins, E6 transcripts could be detected, strongly suggesting that HPV-induced field cancerization seems not to occur in the upper aerodigestive tract or, alternatively, that HPV infection is not the first carcinogenic event (Rietbergen et al. 2014). Hence, in contrast to HPV-mediated carcinogenesis in the cervix that can be followed by inspection and biopsies of acetowhite lesions, there are no indications for HPV-related precancerous changes in the upper aerodigestive tract. The molecular pathogenesis of HPV-induced squamous cancers in the upper aerodigestive tract remains an enigma and relies on the extrapolation of data collected in the invasive carcinomas.

1.2 Cancer-Associated Changes in Head and Neck Carcinogenesis

It has been well established that cancer arises by the accumulation of genetic and epigenetic changes in genes acting in cancer-associated signaling pathways, causing the acquired cancer-related phenotypes that have so elegantly been summarized by Hanahan and Weinberg (2000, 2011) and include limitless replicative potential, self-sufficiency in growth signals, insensitivity to antigrowth signals, evading apoptosis, invasion and metastasis, and angiogenesis. HPV+ve and HPV-ve tumors have been studied very well for their respective molecular changes, and the findings are summarized below.

1.2.1 Different Genetics in HPV+ve and HPV-ve Tumors

HPV cannot be cultured and most assays to test for HPV in tumor specimen are therefore based on particularly the detection of viral DNA. As these DNA-based assays are borrowed from the cervical cancer screening research field, they are very sensitive and easily overestimate the HPV-attributable fraction. In 2001, Van Houten et al. convincingly indicated that only a subgroup of the HPV+ve tumors assessed by DNA PCR actually shows expression of the viral oncogenes E6 and E7 (van Houten et al. 2001), and since then, presence of these transcripts is considered as the gold standard that HPV is actively involved in a tumor. In 2004, Braakhuis et al. showed for the first time that tumors stratified for the presence or absence of oncogenic HPV16 E6 transcripts show a different genetic pattern when analyzed by loss of heterozygosity analysis (Braakhuis et al. 2004) and later by microarray comparative genomic hybridization (Smeets et al. 2006). Most prominent in HPV+ve tumors is the absence of *TP53* mutations as well as the absence of loss of chromosome arms 3p, 9p and the amplification of 11q13, while these changes are very common in HPV-ve tumors. The gene on 3p is still unknown, but on the other chromosome arms, the relevant cancer genes have been identified, *CDKN2A* ($p16^{Ink4A}$) on 9p, *CCND1* (CyclinD1) on 11q13 and *TP53* on 17p. *TP53* is an established cancer gene in HNSCC. Somatic mutations are found in 60–80 % of the tumors (van Houten et al. 2002; Balz et al. 2003; Poeta et al. 2007; Cancer Genome Atlas 2015), and overexpression of a dominant-negative mutant of p53, in conjunction with ectopic expression of TERT (the catalytic subunit of telomerase) as well as overexpression of cyclinD1 or a $p16^{Ink4A}$-insensitive CDK4 mutant, causes cellular immortalization of in vitro cultured mucosal keratinocytes (Opitz et al. 2001; Rheinwald et al. 2002). In HPV+ve tumors, the p53 protein is not mutated, but bound and targeted for degradation by the HPV viral oncoprotein E6.

The identified tumor suppressor gene on chromosome arm 9p is *CDKN2A* encoding the $p16^{Ink4A}$ protein, while the oncogene on the amplified region 11q13 is *CCND1* encoding cyclinD1. Both proteins act in the Rb signaling pathway controlling the G1–S transition of the cell cycle. The cyclinD1/CDK4-6 complex phosphorylates the pRb proteins, inhibitors of the G1–S restriction point.

The *CDKN2A* gene encodes the cell cycle-inhibiting protein p16^{Ink4A}, which binds and disrupts the cyclinD/CDK4-6 complex. The p16^{Ink4A} cell cycle-inhibiting protein is frequently inactivated in HNSCC by mutation or methylation in combination with chromosomal loss or, in the majority of cases, by homozygous deletion (Reed et al. 1996; Cancer Genome Atlas 2015). *CCND1*, the gene encoding cyclinD1, is located at 11q13 and amplified or gained in >80 % of HPV-ve HNSCC (Smeets et al. 2006). Together with abrogation of p53, these changes cause cellular immortalization (Smeets et al. 2011). Hence, *TP53*, *CCND1*, and *CDKN2A* are established cancer genes in HPV-ve HNSCC. In HPV+ve tumors, the viral oncoprotein E7 abrogates this same pathway by binding and targeting the pRb proteins for degradation.

In functional studies using a conditionally immortalized in vitro model of oropharyngeal keratinocytes (Smeets et al. 2011), the consequences of p53 and pRb abrogation by the various viral and host cancer genes were investigated. Both, inactivation of p53 in oropharyngeal keratinocytes by knockdown with short hairpin RNA and expression of dominant-negative mutant p53R172H or expression of the HPV16 oncoprotein E6: all caused an extended lifespan. When combined with p16^{Ink4A} knockdown, ectopic cyclinD1 expression, or HPV16 E7 expression, the cells became immortal albeit in the context of ectopic TERT expression. Summarized, p53 is frequently inactivated in HNSCC: either by somatic mutation in HPV-ve tumors or by HPV E6 in HPV+ve tumors. The Rb genes (encoding pRb and the other pocket proteins p107 and p130) are targeted in HPV+ve HNSCC by HPV E7 protein, while in HPV-ve HNSCC, the genes encoding p16^{Ink4A} and cyclinD1 acting in the same pathway are inactivated or overexpressed, respectively. This is reflected in the differential losses and gains of the chromosomal regions that contain these genes and explains at least in part the genetic differences between HPV+ve and HPV-ve tumors.

The cancer-associated phenotype caused by inactivation of the p53 and pRb pathways in oropharyngeal keratinocytes is at least cellular immortalization. This phenotype also fits with the timing of the genetic events early in the progression of HPV-ve HNSCC in patients. Loss of 9p21 and the location of *CDKN2A* as well as *TP53* mutations are frequently found in precursor fields (Califano et al. 1996; Tabor et al. 2001; Leemans et al. 2011) and are considered as the earliest genetic changes. In HPV+ve HNSCC, these same pathways are likely also the first to be inactivated by the viral E6 and E7 oncoproteins, assuming that HPV infection is the initial carcinogenic event.

Although it has been postulated that abrogation of p53 is one of the first causative genetic hits by either somatic mutation or expression of HPV-E6, not all HPV-ve tumors do contain mutant p53. Approximately 60 % of HNSCC harbour a mutation in *TP53* and 20 % contain transcriptionally active HPV (Braakhuis et al. 2004). In the remaining 20 % of cases, p53 seems not to be inactivated (Smeets et al. 2009). There is the unlikely possibility that mutations have been missed, but it is more plausible that other genes in the p53 pathway are targeted (Berns et al. 2004) or that these tumors follow p53-independent routes of malignant progression. In most recent molecular profiling studies, it was shown that this subgroup of

HPV-ve and *TP53* wild-type tumors typically show *HRAS* and *CASP8* mutations (Cancer Genome Atlas 2015) and form a separate subgroup.

Besides abrogation of cell cycle regulation by the inactivation of the p53 and pRb pathways, likely also telomere shortening needs to be overcome in order to achieve limitless replicative potential. The activity of telomerase or TERT, the enzyme that is able to increase telomere length, is detectable in 80 % of the HNSCC (Califano et al. 1996). Moreover, in most in vitro models, TERT seemed a factor of importance (Rheinwald et al. 2002; Dickson et al. 2000) although the data are not consistent. It has been proposed that keratinocytes may follow alternative lengthening of telomeres (ALT), which is TERT independent (Opitz et al. 2001). The chromosomal location of TERT (5p15.33) is not known as frequently gained or amplified in HNSCC. In HPV+ve tumors, the role of increased TERT expression seems more important, at least in the cervix (Snijders et al. 1998).

The molecular catalog of head and neck cancer was recently published by The Cancer Genome Atlas consortium and is the largest overview of genetic and epigenetic changes in head and neck cancer at present (Cancer Genome Atlas 2015). In this study, 279 tumors were characterized by next-generation sequencing and array analysis for their molecular changes. In total, 36 cases were HPV+ve by the mapping of at least 1000 sequence reads to the HPV genome. The data confirmed the differential genetic patterns described above, but further noted frequent structural changes in HPV+ve tumors in *TRAF3*, a gene at chromosomal region 14q32, and frequently involved in anti-viral immune responses. With respect to the somatic mutations, more frequent TpC mutations were found in HPV+ve tumors, but the number of somatic mutations was not different between HPV+ve and HPV-ve tumors. Besides frequent deletions of *TRAF3*, frequent missense mutations in *PIK3CA* were identified in HPV+ve tumors and amplifications of *E2F1*. PIK3CA protein is the catalytical subunit of PI3-kinase, a lipid kinase that phosphorylates the phospholipid PIP2 to PIP3 and thereby activates the AKT proteins. Most recently, Sewell et al. reported 8 PIK3CA mutations in 33 HPV+ve tumors, but also showed that the HPV proteins interfered with AKT signaling (Sewell et al. 2014).

1.2.2 Different Expression Profiles HPV+ve and HPV-ve

Expression profiles based on the detection of mRNA can be generated by different methods such as Northern blotting, DNA microarrays, or qRT-PCR. Nowadays next-generation sequencing allows analysis of the transcriptome with high sample throughput and this method will likely replace DNA microarrays in future, which are still widely used in genome wide mRNA expression analysis.

Gene expression profiling has been used for more than one decade for the classification of HNSCC (Table 1). For instance in 2001, Hanna et al. utilized a cDNA array to analyze the expression profile of 1,187 tumor-related genes to predict the radiation response in tissue resistant and sensitive to radiation. Sixty tumor-related, differentially expressed genes were identified and used to generate a predicting model with cluster analysis (Hanna et al. 2001). In 2004, Chung and coworkers performed cDNA microarrays for 60 HNSCC samples covering

12,814 human genes. Four distinct subtypes could be identified with an EGFR pathway signature, a mesenchymal-enriched subtype, a normal epithelium-like subtype, and a subtype with high levels of antioxidant enzymes (Chung et al. 2004).

However, similar to genetic alterations, a therapeutically relevant molecular classification cannot be drawn from the results of these and other earlier gene expression studies due to lack of information about HPV status and/or absence of significant numbers of HPV+ve cases, small sample size and/or inhomogeneity of samples regarding tumor characteristics (e.g., primary localization) and treatment modalities.

Among the first studies with differentiation of HPV+ve and HPV-ve HNSCC, thirty-six HNSCC tumors were analyzed using Affymetrix Human 133U Plus 2.0 GeneChip (Slebos et al. 2006). This cohort contains 8 (22 %) HPV16-DNA+ve samples, all except one (larynx) derived from the oropharynx, while the majority of HPV-ve tumors (15 of 28) were derived from the oral cavity. HPV-DNA detection was confirmed by RT-PCR of HPV16-E6 RNA expression. The microarray revealed 91 genes that were differentially expressed between HPV+ve and HPV-ve HNSCC with statistical significance, which was confirmed (for a subset of genes) by RT-PCR. Among the highly expressed genes for HPV+ve samples, cell cycle regulators ($p16^{INK4A}$, p18, and CDC7) and transcription factors (TAF7L, RFC4, RPA2, and TFDP2) were found, while only two genes were significantly down-regulated in HPV+ve tumors (NAP1L2, a member of the nucleosome assembly protein (but not confirmed by RT-PCR) and KIRREL (NEPH1) a member of the immunoglobulin superfamily involved in cell–cell interactions). In addition to the microarray data, mapping of genes by chromosomal location revealed high levels of expression in HPV+ve tumors on chromosome 3q24-qter.

In 2007, Schlecht and coworkers reported a subset of 123 differentially expressed genes in HPV16+ve HNSCC by using a 27,323 gene containing cDNA microarray chip. Their cohort comprises 42 HNSCC patients from an inner city area of New York with 29 % of samples being positive for HPV16 (determined by MY09/11-PCR and RT-PCR of the HPV16-E6 oncogene). Differentially expressed genes were found in cell cycle control, DNA replication, carcinogen metabolism, immune response, and inflammation by gene ontology analyses. The retinoblastoma-binding protein (p18), replication factor-C gene, and an E2F-dimerization partner transcription factor (TFDP2) were among the most significantly overexpressed genes in HPV+ve HNSCC tumors which are consistent with cervical cancer. Specifically, downregulation of genes related to viral defense and immune response was found in HPV+ve tumors (including interleukins and interferon-induced proteins), indicating an immune modulating influence of HPV (Schlecht et al. 2007).

In the same year of the study above, 68 patients with primary HNSCC were analyzed using Affymetrix U133plus2 GeneChips covering over 47,000 transcripts (Winter et al. 2007). By clustering of genes whose in vivo expression correlated with the expression of 10 well-known hypoxia-regulated genes (e.g., CA9, GLUT1, and VEGF), a signature comprising 99 genes was obtained, of which 27 % were known previously to be hypoxia related. Median RNA expression of the genes of this signature was an independent prognostic factor for recurrence-free survival in a publicly available head and neck cancer data set and a significant prognostic factor for overall survival in a published breast cancer series. However, HPV status was not considered in this study.

In HPV-related and HPV-ve HNSCC, differentially expressed genes have been found in several cellular processes such as cell cycle regulation and apoptosis, transcription regulation, DNA replication and repair, keratinocytes differentiation, and immune response.

By immunohistochemical studies, $p16^{INK4a}$ was among the first proteins identified to be differentially expressed between HPV+ve and HPV-ve HNSCC (Klussmann et al. 2003). $p16^{INK4a}$ positivity has turned out to be a reliable surrogate marker for HPV-associated cancers in the clinical setting (Mooren et al. 2014; Prigge et al. 2015). As $p16^{INK4a}$, p21 is another tumor suppressor protein involved in cell cycle regulation and its expression has been shown to be strongly associated with favorable prognosis in HPV+ve tonsillar cancers (Hafkamp et al. 2009). In contrast, the expression of proteins associated with tumor cell survival (e.g., survivin) was less in HPV+ve OPSCC (Preuss et al. 2008a, b). Furthermore, expression of growth factor receptors (e.g., EGFR) is negatively correlated with positive HPV status (Reimers et al. 2007).

Using an integrated genomic analysis and validation technique, a limited number of HPV+ve tumor samples have been analyzed (Walter et al. 2013). Four gene expression subtypes, basal, mesenchymal, atypical, and classical, were identified for HNSCC. Interestingly, 10 of the 14 HPV+ve samples were classified as atypical ($n = 8$) or classical type ($n = 2$) and SOX2 and ALDH1 were highly expressed in both of these types. SOX2 and ALDH1 are thought to be involved in the acquisition of stem cell properties of tumor cells.

ALDH1 (aldehyde dehydrogenase 1) expression was significantly increased in metastasis of OSCC and with reduced survival, but ALDH1 expression did not correlate with positive HPV status (Qian et al. 2013b; 2014). SOX2 (sex-determining region Y-box 2) is known to be a lineage-survival oncogene in squamous cell carcinoma (Brcic et al. 2012). It was shown that SOX2 is involved in EMT (epithelial-to-mesenchymal transition) which is one of the first steps in metastasizing. Reduced SOX2 expression was associated with enhanced tumor cell motility and upregulation of genes related to cell motility like VIM (vimentin), which is a mesenchymal marker protein. Low SOX2 expression was also shown to be prognostic relevant to HNSCC patients at high risk of treatment failure (Bayo et al. 2015).

In gene expression profiles of 15 HPV-ve and 15 transcriptionally active HPV +ve tumors from the oropharynx only, 224 differentially expressed genes have been found by using a 135,000 probe containing Whole-Genome Tiling Array

(Roche NimbleGen 12x135K CGH array) (Mirghani et al. 2014). These genes were used to generate a predictive transcriptomic signature which may be used for case-by-case identification of OPSCC etiology as suggested by the authors. Interestingly, CDKN2A, PI3K, and PDCD1 were overexpressed in HPV16+ve OPSCC, consistently with other studies. But they were not included in the final signature because of their highly variable expressions level from one tumor to another.

Recently, Keck et al. identified five subtypes in HNSCCs based on gene expression consensus clustering (using an Agilent 4x44K v2 Microarray targeting 27,958 gene RNAs), copy number profiling, and HPV status (Keck et al. 2015). Among them, two biologically distinct subtypes were identified for HPV+ve tumors. One of them showed an immune and mesenchymal phenotype and was also represented by HPV-ve tumors. This subtype is characterized by expression of immune response genes (CD8, ICOS, LAG3, and HLA-DRA) and mesenchymal genes (vimentin, matrix metalloproteinases). Corresponding to a potential epithelial-to-mesenchymal transition, epithelial markers (P-cadherin and cytokeratins) are downregulated, also. Compared to HPV-ve tumors of this subtype, HPV +ve tumors of the immune/mesenchymal subtype display elevated activities in cell cycle pathway genes related to HPV, show a higher proliferation rate comparable to an already published signature (Whitfield et al. 2006) and are morphologically nonkeratinizing and poorly differentiated. Another subtype termed classical subtype was identified for HPV+ve as well as HPV-ve tumors. This subtype is characterized by a higher proliferation rate compared to the other groups and significant enrichment of altered gene expression for putrescine (polyamine) degradation pathway. Polyamines are required for eukaryotic cell growth, differentiation, and survival. The metabolic pathway of polyamines is frequently dysregulated in cancer, and elevated polyamine levels have been shown to correlate with increased cell proliferation (Gerner and Meyskens 2004). In particular, catabolic pathways seem to be important in epithelial cancers by producing reactive aldehydes and H_2O_2 that are capable of damaging critical cellular molecules including DNA. HPV+ve tumors of the classical subtype showed overexpression of cell cycle and cell division or related genes like CDKN2A and E2F2, whereas in HPV-ve tumors of the classical subtype altered expression of AKR1C1, AKR1C3, and ALDH3A1 were found. Those genes belong to xenobiotic metabolism pathway and are known to be associated with smoking, which also was different between HPV+ve and HPV-ve tumors of the classical subtype (74 % vs. 42 % heavy smokers in HPV-ve compared to HPV+ve tumors). Interestingly, loss of AKR1C3 expression was found in the transition of a laryngeal papillomatosis to a cancer of the larynx (Huebbers et al. 2013).

For HPV-ve tumors only, a basal subtype with significant enrichment for hypoxia signaling genes expression (e.g., HIF1A, CA9, and VEGF) was defined. Also, neuregulin signaling (including EGFR and NRG1 (neuregulin1/heregulin)) and overexpression of epithelial markers are characteristic features of this basal subtype. Opposed to the HPV+ve tumors of the immune/mesenchymal subtype, a highly keratinizing and well-differentiated morphology is common for the basal subtype.

In this study Keck et al. identified five HNSCC subtypes in an unsupervised way (Keck et al. 2015), strongly correlating with previously identified HNSCC subtypes (Chung et al. 2004) and resembling those found in squamous cell carcinoma of the lung (Wilkerson et al. 2010). Importantly, two distinct HPV+ve tumor subtypes were identified, providing a biologic basis for clinical heterogeneity also observed in HPV+ve HNSCC. This strongly suggests that beyond HPV, further biomarkers are required for HNSCC and also, that differential treatment approaches might be required for subgroups within the HPV+ve HNSCC (Table 1).

1.2.3 Regulation of Gene Expression by Epigenetics and MicroRNAs

Gene expression can be regulated at different levels. Here, we focus on differential epigenetic mechanisms in HPV+ve and HPV-ve HNSCC relevant to corresponding gene expression profiles. Epigenetic mechanisms are divided into three main groups: DNA methylation, histone modifications, and noncoding RNAs (ncRNAs).

As indicated by their name, ncRNAs are not translated into proteins. Highly abundant and functionally important RNAs belong to ncRNAs like tRNAs and ribosomal RNAs. Recently, many ncRNAs have been identified, but functional validations are often missing and some ncRNAs are considered to be non-functional (also referred to as Junk RNA). However, many ncRNAs are implicated in biological functions related to gene expression. Here, we focus on microRNAs, a group of trans-acting ncRNAs involved in regulation of gene expression.

MicroRNAs have been discovered in 1993 (Lee et al. 1993) and play a key role in posttranscriptional gene regulation in many cellular processes including cell division, development, cell death, and cell migration. They are transcribed by RNA polymerase II in the nucleus as primary microRNA (pri-miRNA) of 500–3,000 bases which are processed in a complex called Microprocessor by RNAse III (DROSHA) to generate 60–70 nucleotide precursor miRNAs (pre-miRNAs). This hairpin-like pre-miRNA contains the mature miRNA sequence in the double-stranded part of the stem loop. The pre-miRNAs are exported to the cytoplasm and further processed by DICER1 to produce the mature miRNAs, which are incorporated together with DICER1 and Argonaute (AGO) proteins in the miRNA-induced silencing complex (miRISC) (Fig. 1). Here, the miRNA directs the miRISC by sequence complementary to its target mRNAs and mediates gene suppression by targeted mRNA degradation and translational repression in so-called P bodies (processing bodies).

Recently, it was shown that HPV genomes encode their own miRNAs (Gu et al. 2011; Qian et al. 2013a). The role of these miRNAs is still rather unclear, but target predictions mapped potential miRNA-binding sites to the HPV genome (within HPV genes E5, E1, L1 and in the LCR region) as well as to host target sequences and suggest multiple functions in cell cycle regulation, immune functions, cell adhesion/migration, and carcinogenesis (Qian et al. 2013a).

Table 1 Expression profiles of HPV+ve compared to HPV-ve HNSCC

First author	Year	Anatomical site						HPV-	HPV+	Differently expressed genes (probes)	Analyzed genes (probes)
		Oropharynx	Oral cavity	Tonsils	Base of tongue/tongue	Larynx	Hypopharynx				
Keck	2014	X	X			X		75	55	1386	27,958
Mirghani	2014	X						15	15	224	(135,000)
Jung	2010	X	X		X		X	30	11 + 7	1498(2152)	>38,500
Lohavanichbutr	2009	X	X					78	41	(446)	>38,500
Martinez	2007			X	X			4	3	166	14,820
Pyeon	2007	X	X					26	16	92	>38,500
Schlecht	2007	X	X			X	X	30	12	149	(27,323)
Slebos	2006	X	X			X	X	28	8	91	>38,500

Numbers of differential expressed genes (or probes) are listed in relation to the anatomical site of the tumor sample, sample size (HPV−, HPV+), and quantity of analyzed probes in following studies: Keck 2014 (Keck et al. 2015), Mirghani 2014 (Mirghani et al. 2014), Jung 2010 (Jung et al. 2010), Lohavanichbutr 2009 (Lohavanichbutr et al. 2009), Martinez 2007 (Martinez et al. 2007), Pyeon 2007 (Pyeon et al. 2007), Schlecht 2007 (Schlecht et al. 2007), and Slebos 2006 (Slebos et al. 2006)

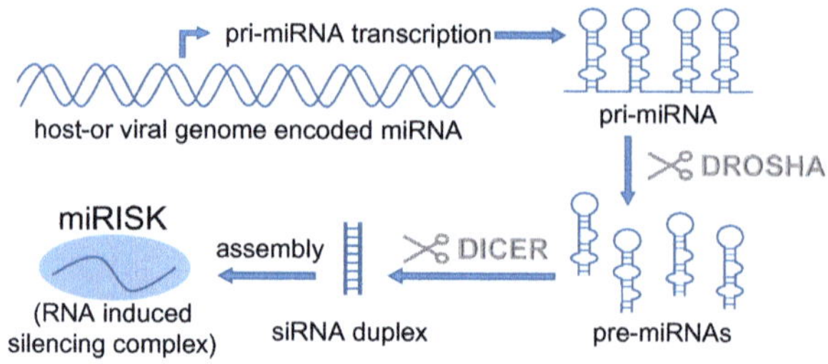

Fig. 1 Transcription and processing steps required for miRNA-induced silencing complex (miRISC) formation

Altered miRNA expression has been implicated in various diseases including cancer, and overexpression of "oncogenic" miRNAs and downregulation of tumor suppressor miRNAs are related to carcinogenic processes like tumor formation, invasion, and metastasis. The biogenesis of miRNAs can be influenced at different steps during miRNA maturation. Pri-miRNA transcription can be positively or negatively influenced by genetic alterations, epigenetic modifications or tumor suppressors, and oncogenes. Further on, pri-miRNA processing, nucleolar export and final maturation steps can also be affected. Finally, miRNA function can be biased by competing endogenous RNA (ceRNA) or by mutations of miRNA-binding sites.

A PubMed literature search for "mirna & expression & cancer" results in more than 16.000 hits. However, this number drops to 26 by adding "head&neck&HPV" to the search term, and only few studies have analyzed differential miRNA signatures in HPV+ve compared to HPV-ve cancers. As in "classical molecular biology," one cannot stick to the simplification that one miRNA has one target and therefore one function. Based on their rather small size, miRNAs may bind to several, often more than hundreds of more or less conserved target sequences. In addition, target genes can have numerous binding sites for different miRNA species, which makes gene regulation via miRNAs to a rather complex network of molecular interactions. Emerging techniques enlarge the knowledge on differential expressed miRNAs in HPV+ve compared to HPV-ve head and neck cancers; however, until now, data are rather inconsistent. Table 2 specifies miRNAs that were differentially expressed in HPV+ve compared to HPV-ve HNSCC in at least two publications. Given that one-third of the miRNAs are either upregulated in one study but downregulated in another study, shows that interpretation of miRNA data should be handled with care and experimental results highly depend on several factors like sample type, storage/processing, and analyzing techniques. Until now, no distinct picture of the role of miRNAs in HPV-associated HNSCC can be drawn, but their importance is obvious by considering the diverse and important functions of miRNA target genes in HNSCC (Table 2).

Besides ncRNAs, DNA methylation and histone modifications are two other important epigenetic processes affecting gene expression. In eukaryotes, methylation of cytosine typically occurs in a CpG dinucleotide and is associated with a

Table 2 Differential expressed miRNAs in HPV+ve compared to HPV-ve HNSCC

Reference	miRNA	Regulated in HPV+ compared to HPV-	Top-scoring targets (selected) based on number of validation methods (mirtarbase)	Target function
Lajer et al. (2011, 2012), Wald et al. (2011)	hsa-miR-363	Up	BCL2L11, CDKN1A, HI VEP1, CASP3, CD274	Apoptosis, cell cycle, transcriptional regulation, immunology
Lajer et al. (2011), Wald et al. (2011)	hsa-miR-26b	Up and down	PTGS2, EPHA2, CCNE1, TAB1, RB1	Prostaglandin biosynthesis, development, cell cycle, TGF-beta-interleukin 1- and WNT-1-signaling
Wald et al. (2011), Lajer et al. (2012)	hsa_miR_29a	Up and down	MCL1, DNMT3A, DNMT3B, BCL2, PIK3R1	Apoptosis, DNA methylation, PI3K-signaling
Wald et al. (2011), Lajer et al. (2012), Gao et al. (2013)	hsa_miR_155	Up and down	CEBPB, TAB2, TP53INP1, SMAD1, KRAS	Immune and inflammatory response, TGF-beta-TP53-signaling, cell growth, apoptosis, morphogenesis, development and immune responses, transformation
Miller et al. (2015), Wald et al. (2011)	hsa-miR-222	Up and down	CDKN1B, MMP1, KIT, PTEN, CDKN1C	Cell cycle, breakdown of extracellular matrix, proto-oncogene c-kit, tumor suppression
Lajer et al. (2011), (2012)	hsa-miR-125a	Down	ERBB3, CDKN1A, CD34, TP53, ERBB2	Cell cycle, EGF signaling, cell attachment, tumor suppression
Lajer et al. (2011), Miller et al. (2015)	hsa-miR-143	Down	KRAS, MAPK7, MYO6, DNMT3A, FNDC3B	Transformation, proliferation, differentiation, transcription regulation and development, intracellular vesicle and organelle transport, DNA methylation
Lajer et al. (2011), Miller et al. (2015)	hsa-miR-145	Down	BNIP3, STAT1, FSCN1, KLF5, SOX2	Apoptosis, cell viability, cell migration, motility, adhesion and cellular interactions, cell proliferation, embryonic development, cell fate, stem cell maintenance, epithelial-mesenchymal transition

(continued)

Table 2 (continued)

Reference	miRNA	Regulated in HPV+ compared to HPV-	Top-scoring targets (selected) based on number of validation methods (mirtarbase)	Target function
Lajer et al. (2011), Miller et al. (2015)	hsa-miR-199a	Down	MET, MTOR, GSK3B, WNT2, HIF1A	Proto-oncogene, responses to DNA damage and nutrient deprivation, cell cycle arrest and immunosuppressive effects, transformation, energy metabolism, neuronal cell development, and body pattern formation, oncogenesis and development, cell fate, embryogenesis, hypoxia pathway
Lajer et al. (2011), Miller et al. (2015)	hsa-miR-126	Down	VEGFA, SOX2, KRAS, PIK3R2, TERT	Proliferation and migration of vascular endothelial cells, embryonic development, cell fate, stem cell maintenance, epithelial-mesenchymal transition, transformation, PI3 K-signaling, telomere elongation
Wald et al. (2011), Lajer et al. (2012)	hsa_miR_181b	Down	TCL1A, TIMP3, PLAG1, BCL2, RNF2	Development of mature T cell leukemia, inhibition of the matrix metalloproteinases, apoptosis, development and cell proliferation
Lajer et al. (2012), Gao et al. (2013)	hsa_miR_31	Down	RHOA, SATB2, FOXP3, MMP16, HIF1AN	Tumor cell proliferation and metastasis, transcription regulation and chromatin remodeling, immunology, breakdown of extracellular matrix, oxygen sensing, HIF1A repression

Selected miRNA targets based on the most divers experimental methods used for validation according to mirtarbase.org (Chou et al. 2016) and their importance for HNSCC are given. Expression status of miRNA (up or down) refers to previous studies: Layer 2011 (Lajer et al. 2011), Wald 2011 (Wald et al. 2011), Layer 2012 (Lajer et al. 2011), Gao 2013 (Gao et al. 2013), Miller 2015 (Miller et al. 2015) number of key processes including genomic imprinting and X-chromosome inactivation, whereas methylation of adenine is restricted to prokaryotes. In normal development, gene expression is stably guided by DNA methylation during cell division and differentiation, which prevents differentiated cells to revert differentiation or to convert to another cell type. Gene expression can be affected by DNA methylation in two ways: Transcriptional proteins may be impeded in binding to a gene resulting in reduced gene expression. Second, methylated DNA may attract MBD (methyl-CpG-binding domain) proteins, thereby recruiting additional chromatin remodeling proteins like histone deacetylases. As a consequence, a compact, inactive chromatin structure is formed called heterochromatin, which links DNA methylation to histone modification, the third epigenetic processes affecting gene expression.

Histone proteins (2 copies each of the core histones H2A, H2B, H3, and H4) form a histone octamer, which is wrapped around by about 147 base pairs of DNA and forms a nucleosome core particle. Approximately 80 bases of DNA connect each nucleosome and linker histone proteins (e.g., H1) are involved in compaction of this chromatin structure. Histone proteins can be modified posttranslationally by acetylation, methylation, ubiquitination and phosphorylation of certain amino acids. These modifications affect molecular interactions between histones and between histones and DNA within the nucleosome core, which alters chromatin structure and thereby may affect gene expression in either an activating or inactivation manner.

DNA methylation and histone modifications in HNSCC and specific aspects for HPV-associated cancers are reviewed in other Chapters entitled "Risk factors for oral infection with Human Papilloma Virus" and "Predictive factors for outcome and quality of life in HPV-positive and HPV-negative HNSCC."

2 Conclusion

Viral proteins interacting with key cellular regulators are important and necessary to drive HPV-associated carcinogenesis, contrasting with HPV-ve tumors where (simplified) each step in carcinogenesis has to be facilitated by genetic or epigenetic alterations. Consequently, mutations are less frequently found in HPV-associated cancers, but it is still not completely resolved, whether these are only passenger mutations or important at certain steps in carcinogenic progression.

HPV-driven cancers and HPV+ve OPSCC were shown to have recurrent focal 3q26.3-qter amplifications (Klussmann et al. 2009), which includes important cancer-associated genes such as *TP63*, *SOX2*, as well as the oncogene *PIK3CA*. In contrast, *TP53* mutations, loss of chromosome arms 3p and 9p, and the amplification of 11q13 are prominently missing in HPV+ve tumors, while these changes are very common in HPV-ve tumors (Braakhuis et al. 2004). Importantly, the absence of chromosome 9p loss and the presence of HPV oncoproteins in HPV+ve tumors are requirements for overexpression of the $p16^{INK4a}$ gene, which serves as surrogate marker for HPV-associated cancers in the clinical setting. These molecular differences indicate different genetic progression models for both entities, but challenge the concept of field cancerization for HPV-related cancers.

Taken together, current molecular and clinical data clearly display HPV-related and HPV-unrelated HNSCC to be differential cancer subtypes. In addition, future research may provide evidence for additional subgroups, also within the HPV+ve HNSCC, which justify adapted therapy concepts for particular patient groups based on molecular ("omic-") diagnostics in addition to tests performed by classical pathology.

References

Balz V, Scheckenbach K, Gotte K, Bockmuhl U, Petersen I, Bier H (2003) Is the p53 inactivation frequency in squamous cell carcinomas of the head and neck underestimated? Analysis of p53 exons 2-11 and human papillomavirus 16/18 E6 transcripts in 123 unselected tumor specimens. Cancer Res 63(6):1188–1191

Bayo P, Jou A, Stenzinger A, Shao C, Gross M, Jensen A, Grabe N, Mende CH, Rados PV, Debus J, Weichert W, Plinkert PK, Lichter P, Freier K, Hess J (2015) Loss of SOX2 expression induces cell motility via vimentin up-regulation and is an unfavorable risk factor for survival of head and neck squamous cell carcinoma. Mol Oncol 9(8):1704–1719. doi:10.1016/j.molonc.2015.05.006

Berns K, Hijmans EM, Mullenders J, Brummelkamp TR, Velds A, Heimerikx M, Kerkhoven RM, Madiredjo M, Nijkamp W, Weigelt B, Agami R, Ge W, Cavet G, Linsley PS, Beijersbergen RL, Bernards R (2004) A large-scale RNAi screen in human cells identifies new components of the p53 pathway. Nature 428(6981):431–437. doi:10.1038/nature02371

Braakhuis BJ, Snijders PJ, Keune WJ, Meijer CJ, Ruijter-Schippers HJ, Leemans CR, Brakenhoff RH (2004) Genetic patterns in head and neck cancers that contain or lack transcriptionally active human papillomavirus. J Natl Cancer Inst 96(13):998–1006

Brcic L, Sherer CK, Shuai Y, Hornick JL, Chirieac LR, Dacic S (2012) Morphologic and clinicopathologic features of lung squamous cell carcinomas expressing Sox2. Am J Clin Pathol 138(5):712–718. doi:10.1309/AJCP05TTWQTWNLTN

Califano J, van der Riet P, Westra W, Nawroz H, Clayman G, Piantadosi S, Corio R, Lee D, Greenberg B, Koch W, Sidransky D (1996) Genetic progression model for head and neck cancer: implications for field cancerization. Cancer Res 56(11):2488–2492

Cancer Genome Atlas N (2015) Comprehensive genomic characterization of head and neck squamous cell carcinomas. Nature 517(7536):576–582. doi:10.1038/nature14129

Chou CH, Chang NW, Shrestha S, Hsu SD, Lin YL, Lee WH, Yang CD, Hong HC, Wei TY, Tu SJ, Tsai TR, Ho SY, Jian TY, Wu HY, Chen PR, Lin NC, Huang HT, Yang TL, Pai CY, Tai CS, Chen WL, Huang CY, Liu CC, Weng SL, Liao KW, Hsu WL, Huang HD (2016) miRTarBase 2016: updates to the experimentally validated miRNA-target interactions database. Nucleic Acids Res 44(D1):D239–D247. doi:10.1093/nar/gkv1258

Chung CH, Parker JS, Karaca G, Wu J, Funkhouser WK, Moore D, Butterfoss D, Xiang D, Zanation A, Yin X, Shockley WW, Weissler MC, Dressler LG, Shores CG, Yarbrough WG, Perou CM (2004) Molecular classification of head and neck squamous cell carcinomas using patterns of gene expression. Cancer Cell 5(5):489–500

Dickson MA, Hahn WC, Ino Y, Ronfard V, Wu JY, Weinberg RA, Louis DN, Li FP, Rheinwald JG (2000) Human keratinocytes that express hTERT and also bypass a p16 (INK4a)-enforced mechanism that limits life span become immortal yet retain normal growth and differentiation characteristics. Mol Cell Biol 20(4):1436–1447

Gao G, Gay HA, Chernock RD, Zhang TR, Luo J, Thorstad WL, Lewis JS Jr, Wang X (2013) A microRNA expression signature for the prognosis of oropharyngeal squamous cell carcinoma. Cancer 119(1):72–80. doi:10.1002/cncr.27696

Gerner EW, Meyskens FL Jr (2004) Polyamines and cancer: old molecules, new understanding. Nat Rev Cancer 4(10):781–792. doi:10.1038/nrc1454

Gu W, An J, Ye P, Zhao KN, Antonsson A (2011) Prediction of conserved microRNAs from skin and mucosal human papillomaviruses. Arch Virol 156(7):1161–1171. doi:10.1007/s00705-011-0974-3

Ha PK, Califano JA (2004) The role of human papillomavirus in oral carcinogenesis. Crit Rev Oral Biol Med 15(4):188–196

Hafkamp HC, Mooren JJ, Claessen SM, Klingenberg B, Voogd AC, Bot FJ, Klussmann JP, Hopman AH, Manni JJ, Kremer B, Ramaekers FC, Speel EJ (2009) P21 Cip1/WAF1 expression is strongly associated with HPV-positive tonsillar carcinoma and a favorable prognosis. Mod Pathol 22(5):686–698. doi:10.1038/modpathol.2009.23

Hanahan D, Weinberg RA (2000) The hallmarks of cancer. Cell 100(1):57–70

Hanahan D, Weinberg RA (2011) Hallmarks of cancer: the next generation. Cell 144(5):646–674. doi:10.1016/j.cell.2011.02.013

Hanna E, Shrieve DC, Ratanatharathorn V, Xia X, Breau R, Suen J, Li S (2001) A novel alternative approach for prediction of radiation response of squamous cell carcinoma of head and neck. Cancer Res 61(6):2376–2380

Huebbers CU, Preuss SF, Kolligs J, Vent J, Stenner M, Wieland U, Silling S, Drebber U, Speel EJ, Klussmann JP (2013) Integration of HPV6 and downregulation of AKR1C3 expression mark malignant transformation in a patient with juvenile-onset laryngeal papillomatosis. PLoS ONE 8(2):e57207. doi:10.1371/journal.pone.0057207

Jung AC, Briolat J, Millon R, de Reynies A, Rickman D, Thomas E, Abecassis J, Clavel C, Wasylyk B (2010) Biological and clinical relevance of transcriptionally active human papillomavirus (HPV) infection in oropharynx squamous cell carcinoma. Int J Cancer 126 (8):1882–1894. doi:10.1002/ijc.24911

Keck MK, Zuo Z, Khattri A, Stricker TP, Brown CD, Imanguli M, Rieke D, Endhardt K, Fang P, Bragelmann J, DeBoer R, El-Dinali M, Aktolga S, Lei Z, Tan P, Rozen SG, Salgia R, Weichselbaum RR, Lingen MW, Story MD, Ang KK, Cohen EE, White KP, Vokes EE, Seiwert TY (2015) Integrative analysis of head and neck cancer identifies two biologically distinct HPV and three non-HPV subtypes. Clin Cancer Res 21(4):870–881. doi:10.1158/1078-0432.CCR-14-2481

Klussmann JP, Gultekin E, Weissenborn SJ, Wieland U, Dries V, Dienes HP, Eckel HE, Pfister HJ, Fuchs PG (2003) Expression of p16 protein identifies a distinct entity of tonsillar carcinomas associated with human papillomavirus. Am J Pathol 162(3):747–753. doi:10.1016/S0002-9440(10)63871-0

Klussmann JP, Mooren JJ, Lehnen M, Claessen SM, Stenner M, Huebbers CU, Weissenborn SJ, Wedemeyer I, Preuss SF, Straetmans JM, Manni JJ, Hopman AH, Speel EJ (2009) Genetic signatures of HPV-related and unrelated oropharyngeal carcinoma and their prognostic implications. Clin Cancer Res 15(5):1779–1786. doi:10.1158/1078-0432.CCR-08-1463

Lajer CB, Nielsen FC, Friis-Hansen L, Norrild B, Borup R, Garnaes E, Rossing M, Specht L, Therkildsen MH, Nauntofte B, Dabelsteen S, von Buchwald C (2011) Different miRNA signatures of oral and pharyngeal squamous cell carcinomas: a prospective translational study. Br J Cancer 104(5):830–840. doi:10.1038/bjc.2011.29

Lajer CB, Garnaes E, Friis-Hansen L, Norrild B, Therkildsen MH, Glud M, Rossing M, Lajer H, Svane D, Skotte L, Specht L, Buchwald C, Nielsen FC (2012) The role of miRNAs in human papilloma virus (HPV)-associated cancers: bridging between HPV-related head and neck cancer and cervical cancer. Br J Cancer 106(9):1526–1534. doi:10.1038/bjc.2012.109

Lee RC, Feinbaum RL, Ambros V (1993) The C. elegans heterochronic gene lin-4 encodes small RNAs with antisense complementarity to lin-14. Cell 75(5):843–854

Leemans CR, Braakhuis BJ, Brakenhoff RH (2011) The molecular biology of head and neck cancer. Nat Rev Cancer 11(1):9–22. doi:10.1038/nrc2982

Lim X, Tan SH, Koh WL, Chau RM, Yan KS, Kuo CJ, van Amerongen R, Klein AM, Nusse R (2013) Interfollicular epidermal stem cells self-renew via autocrine Wnt signaling. Science 342 (6163):1226–1230. doi:10.1126/science.1239730

Lohavanichbutr P, Houck J, Fan W, Yueh B, Mendez E, Futran N, Doody DR, Upton MP, Farwell DG, Schwartz SM, Zhao LP, Chen C (2009) Genomewide gene expression profiles of HPV-positive and HPV-negative oropharyngeal cancer: potential implications for treatment choices. Arch Otolaryngol Head Neck Surg 135(2):180–188. doi:10.1001/archoto.2008.540

Martinez I, Wang J, Hobson KF, Ferris RL, Khan SA (2007) Identification of differentially expressed genes in HPV-positive and HPV-negative oropharyngeal squamous cell carcinomas. Eur J Cancer 43(2):415–432. doi:10.1016/j.ejca.2006.09.001

Miller DL, Davis JW, Taylor KH, Johnson J, Shi Z, Williams R, Atasoy U, Lewis JS Jr, Stack MS (2015) Identification of a human papillomavirus-associated oncogenic miRNA panel in human oropharyngeal squamous cell carcinoma validated by bioinformatics analysis of the Cancer Genome Atlas. Am J Pathol 185(3):679–692. doi:10.1016/j.ajpath.2014.11.018

Mirghani H, Ugolin N, Ory C, Lefevre M, Baulande S, Hofman P, St Guily JL, Chevillard S, Lacave R (2014) A predictive transcriptomic signature of oropharyngeal cancer according to HPV16 status exclusively. Oral Oncol 50(11):1025–1034. doi:10.1016/j.oraloncology.2014.07.019

Mooren JJ, Gultekin SE, Straetmans JM, Haesevoets A, Peutz-Kootstra CJ, Huebbers CU, Dienes HP, Wieland U, Ramaekers FC, Kremer B, Speel EJ, Klussmann JP (2014) P16 (INK4A) immunostaining is a strong indicator for high-risk-HPV-associated oropharyngeal carcinomas and dysplasias, but is unreliable to predict low-risk-HPV-infection in head and neck papillomas and laryngeal dysplasias. Int J Cancer 134(9):2108–2117. doi:10.1002/ijc.28534

Napier SS, Speight PM (2008) Natural history of potentially malignant oral lesions and conditions: an overview of the literature. J Oral Pathol Med 37(1):1–10. doi:10.1111/j.1600-0714.2007.00579.x

Opitz OG, Suliman Y, Hahn WC, Harada H, Blum HE, Rustgi AK (2001) Cyclin D1 overexpression and p53 inactivation immortalize primary oral keratinocytes by a telomerase-independent mechanism. J Clin Invest 108(5):725–732. doi:10.1172/JCI11909

Poeta ML, Manola J, Goldwasser MA, Forastiere A, Benoit N, Califano JA, Ridge JA, Goodwin J, Kenady D, Saunders J, Westra W, Sidransky D, Koch WM (2007) TP53 mutations and survival in squamous-cell carcinoma of the head and neck. N Engl J Med 357(25):2552–2561. doi:10.1056/NEJMoa073770

Preuss SF, Weinell A, Molitor M, Semrau R, Stenner M, Drebber U, Wedemeyer I, Hoffmann TK, Guntinas-Lichius O, Klussmann JP (2008a) Survivin and epidermal growth factor receptor expression in surgically treated oropharyngeal squamous cell carcinoma. Head Neck 30 (10):1318–1324. doi:10.1002/hed.20876

Preuss SF, Weinell A, Molitor M, Stenner M, Semrau R, Drebber U, Weissenborn SJ, Speel EJ, Wittekindt C, Guntinas-Lichius O, Hoffmann TK, Eslick GD, Klussmann JP (2008b) Nuclear survivin expression is associated with HPV-independent carcinogenesis and is an indicator of poor prognosis in oropharyngeal cancer. Br J Cancer 98(3):627–632. doi:10.1038/sj.bjc.6604192

Prigge ES, Toth C, Dyckhoff G, Wagner S, Muller F, Wittekindt C, Freier K, Plinkert P, Hoffmann J, Vinokurova S, Klussmann JP, von Knebel Doeberitz M, Reuschenbach M (2015) p16(INK4a)/Ki-67 co-expression specifically identifies transformed cells in the head and neck region. Int J Cancer 136(7):1589–1599. doi:10.1002/ijc.29130

Pyeon D, Newton MA, Lambert PF, den Boon JA, Sengupta S, Marsit CJ, Woodworth CD, Connor JP, Haugen TH, Smith EM, Kelsey KT, Turek LP, Ahlquist P (2007) Fundamental differences in cell cycle deregulation in human papillomavirus-positive and human papillomavirus-negative head/neck and cervical cancers. Cancer Res 67(10):4605–4619. doi:10.1158/0008-5472.CAN-06-3619

Qian K, Pietila T, Ronty M, Michon F, Frilander MJ, Ritari J, Tarkkanen J, Paulin L, Auvinen P, Auvinen E (2013a) Identification and validation of human papillomavirus encoded microRNAs. PLoS ONE 8(7):e70202. doi:10.1371/journal.pone.0070202

Qian X, Wagner S, Ma C, Klussmann JP, Hummel M, Kaufmann AM, Albers AE (2013b) ALDH1-positive cancer stem-like cells are enriched in nodal metastases of oropharyngeal squamous cell carcinoma independent of HPV status. Oncol Rep 29(5):1777–1784. doi:10.3892/or.2013.2340

Qian X, Wagner S, Ma C, Coordes A, Gekeler J, Klussmann JP, Hummel M, Kaufmann AM, Albers AE (2014) Prognostic significance of ALDH1A1-positive cancer stem cells in patients with locally advanced, metastasized head and neck squamous cell carcinoma. J Cancer Res Clin Oncol 140(7):1151–1158. doi:10.1007/s00432-014-1685-4

Reed AL, Califano J, Cairns P, Westra WH, Jones RM, Koch W, Ahrendt S, Eby Y, Sewell D, Nawroz H, Bartek J, Sidransky D (1996) High frequency of p16 (CDKN2/MTS-1/INK4A) inactivation in head and neck squamous cell carcinoma. Cancer Res 56(16):3630–3633

Reimers N, Kasper HU, Weissenborn SJ, Stutzer H, Preuss SF, Hoffmann TK, Speel EJ, Dienes HP, Pfister HJ, Guntinas-Lichius O, Klussmann JP (2007) Combined analysis of HPV-DNA, p16 and EGFR expression to predict prognosis in oropharyngeal cancer. Int J Cancer 120(8):1731–1738. doi:10.1002/ijc.22355

Rheinwald JG, Hahn WC, Ramsey MR, Wu JY, Guo Z, Tsao H, De Luca M, Catricala C, O'Toole KM (2002) A two-stage, p16(INK4A)- and p53-dependent keratinocyte senescence mechanism that limits replicative potential independent of telomere status. Mol Cell Biol 22(14): 5157–5172

Rietbergen MM, Braakhuis BJ, Moukhtari N, Bloemena E, Brink A, Sie D, Ylstra B, Baatenburg de Jong RJ, Snijders PJ, Brakenhoff RH, Leemans CR (2014) No evidence for active human papillomavirus (HPV) in fields surrounding HPV-positive oropharyngeal tumors. J Oral Pathol Med 43(2):137–142. doi:10.1111/jop.12123

Schlecht NF, Burk RD, Adrien L, Dunne A, Kawachi N, Sarta C, Chen Q, Brandwein-Gensler M, Prystowsky MB, Childs G, Smith RV, Belbin TJ (2007) Gene expression profiles in HPV-infected head and neck cancer. J Pathol 213(3):283–293. doi:10.1002/path.2227

Sewell A, Brown B, Biktasova A, Mills GB, Lu Y, Tyson DR, Issaeva N, Yarbrough WG (2014) Reverse-phase protein array profiling of oropharyngeal cancer and significance of PIK3CA mutations in HPV-associated head and neck cancer. Clin Cancer Res 20(9):2300–2311. doi:10.1158/1078-0432.CCR-13-2585

Slaughter DP, Southwick HW, Smejkal W (1953) Field cancerization in oral stratified squamous epithelium; clinical implications of multicentric origin. Cancer 6(5):963–968

Slebos RJ, Yi Y, Ely K, Carter J, Evjen A, Zhang X, Shyr Y, Murphy BM, Cmelak AJ, Burkey BB, Netterville JL, Levy S, Yarbrough WG, Chung CH (2006) Gene expression differences associated with human papillomavirus status in head and neck squamous cell carcinoma. Clin Cancer Res 12(3 Pt 1):701–709. doi:10.1158/1078-0432.CCR-05-2017

Smeets SJ, Braakhuis BJ, Abbas S, Snijders PJ, Ylstra B, van de Wiel MA, Meijer GA, Leemans CR, Brakenhoff RH (2006) Genome-wide DNA copy number alterations in head and neck squamous cell carcinomas with or without oncogene-expressing human papillomavirus. Oncogene 25(17):2558–2564. doi:10.1038/sj.onc.1209275

Smeets SJ, Brakenhoff RH, Ylstra B, van Wieringen WN, van de Wiel MA, Leemans CR, Braakhuis BJ (2009) Genetic classification of oral and oropharyngeal carcinomas identifies subgroups with a different prognosis. Cell Oncol 31(4):291–300. doi:10.3233/CLO-2009-0471

Smeets SJ, van der Plas M, Schaaij-Visser TB, van Veen EA, van Meerloo J, Braakhuis BJ, Steenbergen RD, Brakenhoff RH (2011) Immortalization of oral keratinocytes by functional inactivation of the p53 and pRb pathways. Int J Cancer 128(7):1596–1605. doi:10.1002/ijc.25474

Snijders PJ, van Duin M, Walboomers JM, Steenbergen RD, Risse EK, Helmerhorst TJ, Verheijen RH, Meijer CJ (1998) Telomerase activity exclusively in cervical carcinomas and a subset of cervical intraepithelial neoplasia grade III lesions: strong association with elevated messenger RNA levels of its catalytic subunit and high-risk human papillomavirus DNA. Cancer Res 58(17):3812–3818

Tabor MP, Brakenhoff RH, van Houten VM, Kummer JA, Snel MH, Snijders PJ, Snow GB, Leemans CR, Braakhuis BJ (2001) Persistence of genetically altered fields in head and neck cancer patients: biological and clinical implications. Clin Cancer Res 7(6):1523–1532

van der Waal I (2009) Potentially malignant disorders of the oral and oropharyngeal mucosa; terminology, classification and present concepts of management. Oral Oncol 45(4–5):317–323. doi:10.1016/j.oraloncology.2008.05.016

van Houten VM, Snijders PJ, van den Brekel MW, Kummer JA, Meijer CJ, van Leeuwen B, Denkers F, Smeele LE, Snow GB, Brakenhoff RH (2001) Biological evidence that human papillomaviruses are etiologically involved in a subgroup of head and neck squamous cell carcinomas. Int J Cancer 93(2):232–235. doi:10.1002/ijc.1313

van Houten VM, Tabor MP, van den Brekel MW, Kummer JA, Denkers F, Dijkstra J, Leemans R, van der Waal I, Snow GB, Brakenhoff RH (2002) Mutated p53 as a molecular marker for the diagnosis of head and neck cancer. J Pathol 198(4):476–486. doi:10.1002/path.1242

Wald AI, Hoskins EE, Wells SI, Ferris RL, Khan SA (2011) Alteration of microRNA profiles in squamous cell carcinoma of the head and neck cell lines by human papillomavirus. Head Neck 33(4):504–512. doi:10.1002/hed.21475

Walter V, Yin X, Wilkerson MD, Cabanski CR, Zhao N, Du Y, Ang MK, Hayward MC, Salazar AH, Hoadley KA, Fritchie K, Sailey CJ, Weissler MC, Shockley WW, Zanation AM, Hackman T, Thorne LB, Funkhouser WD, Muldrew KL, Olshan AF, Randell SH, Wright FA, Shores CG, Hayes DN (2013) Molecular subtypes in head and neck cancer exhibit distinct patterns of chromosomal gain and loss of canonical cancer genes. PLoS ONE 8(2):e56823. doi:10.1371/journal.pone.0056823

Whitfield ML, George LK, Grant GD, Perou CM (2006) Common markers of proliferation. Nat Rev Cancer 6(2):99–106. doi:10.1038/nrc1802

Wilkerson MD, Yin X, Hoadley KA, Liu Y, Hayward MC, Cabanski CR, Muldrew K, Miller CR, Randell SH, Socinski MA, Parsons AM, Funkhouser WK, Lee CB, Roberts PJ, Thorne L, Bernard PS, Perou CM, Hayes DN (2010) Lung squamous cell carcinoma mRNA expression subtypes are reproducible, clinically important, and correspond to normal cell types. Clin Cancer Res 16(19):4864–4875. doi:10.1158/1078-0432.CCR-10-0199

Winter SC, Buffa FM, Silva P, Miller C, Valentine HR, Turley H, Shah KA, Cox GJ, Corbridge RJ, Homer JJ, Musgrove B, Slevin N, Sloan P, Price P, West CM, Harris AL (2007) Relation of a hypoxia metagene derived from head and neck cancer to prognosis of multiple cancers. Cancer Res 67(7):3441–3449. doi:10.1158/0008-5472.CAN-06-3322

Zhang L, Poh CF, Williams M, Laronde DM, Berean K, Gardner PJ, Jiang H, Wu L, Lee JJ, Rosin MP (2012) Loss of heterozygosity (LOH) profiles–validated risk predictors for progression to oral cancer. Cancer Prev Res (Phila) 5(9):1081–1089. doi:10.1158/1940-6207.CAPR-12-0173

HPV Integration in Head and Neck Squamous Cell Carcinomas: Cause and Consequence

Ernst Jan M. Speel

Abstract

Human papillomaviruses (HPVs) are a necessary cause of anogenital squamous cell carcinomas (SCC) and a subgroup of head and neck SCC, i.e., those originating in the oropharynx. The key events in high-risk HPV (HRHPV)-associated neoplastic progression include persistent infection, deregulated expression of virus early genes in basal epithelial cells, local immune suppression and the accumulation of chromosomal alterations. Evidence for these events particularly comes from studies of uterine cervical carcinogenesis; primary premalignant HRHPV-positive lesions of the head and neck mucosa are seldomly detected. Integration of virus DNA into host chromosomes is considered an important driver of carcinogenesis and observed in 40 up to 90 % of uterine cervical SCC (UCSCC) and oropharyngeal SCC (OPSCC), dependent on the integration detection method used and HRHPV type. In OPSCC, > 90 % HPV-positive tumors are infected with HPV16. Ten up to 60 % of HPV-positive tumors thus contain extrachromosomal (episomal) virus. In this chapter, causes and consequences of HPV integration are summarized

E.J.M. Speel (✉)
Unit Molecular Oncopathology & Diagnostics, Department of Pathology, GROW-School for Oncology and Developmental Biology, Maastricht University Medical Center, P.O. Box 5800, 6202 AZ Maastricht, The Netherlands
e-mail: ernstjan.speel@mumc.nl

W. Golusiński et al. (eds.), *HPV Infection in Head and Neck Cancer*,
Recent Results in Cancer Research 206, DOI 10.1007/978-3-319-43580-0_4

from the literature, with special focus on the site of HPV integration in the cellular genome, and its effect on expression of viral oncogenes (particularly E6 and E7), on human (tumor) gene expression and on deregulation of cell proliferation, apoptosis and cell signaling pathways. Also data on DNA methylation, viral load and clinical outcome in relation to HPV integration are provided.

Keywords
Human papillomavirus · HPV · Head and neck squamous cell carcinoma (HNSCC) · Oropharyngeal carcinoma · Tonsillar carcinoma · Viral integration · E2 · E6 · E7 · FISH · PCR · NGS · Tumor genes

1 Human Papillomaviruses and Their Life Cycle

Human papillomaviruses (HPVs) are non-enveloped viruses, containing circular double-stranded DNA of approximately 8 kb. They are highly epitheliotropic and can infect both mucosal and cutaneous epithelia. The HPV family is classified into 5 genera and subdivided into 31 species and 120 types (zur Hausen 2002; Bernard et al. 2010). Each type is defined as a complete papillomavirus genome, whose L (ate) 1 gene nucleotide sequence is at least 10 % different from that of any other known type. I will focus here on the mucosal HPV types. Fifteen HPV types belonging to the α genus are linked to the development of malignant epithelial lesions, i.e., the so-called high-risk (HR) HPVs, including HPV16 and HPV18 which are found in ~50 % and ~20 % of uterine cervical malignancies, respectively (WHO IARC Monographs 2007). HPV16 is also the predominant type in oropharyngeal carcinomas (OPSCC) (Olthof et al. 2012). Differences in the capacity to deregulate cellular protein function by viral oncogenes E6 and E7 account for the carcinogenic properties of HRHPV in comparison with low-risk (LR) HPVs. LRHPV types, such as HPV6 and HPV11, are often found in benign mucosal lesions (e.g., anogenital and laryngeal papillomas) and are only sporadically associated with carcinomas (Olthof et al. 2012; Huebbers et al. 2013; Mooren et al. 2014).

To date, most information on the initiation of HPV-associated mucosal disease comes from studies on uterine cervical carcinogenesis, because patients with head and neck lesions containing HRHPV usually present with advanced disease and only seldomly with primary premalignant lesions (Mooren et al. 2014). The following events are more or less generally accepted to occur during the HPV life cycle (for reviews, see zur Hausen 2002; Woodman et al. 2007; Olthof et al. 2012, Groves and Coleman 2015 and references therein) (Fig. 1a):

(1) HPV tends to target the multilayered keratinocyte layers of the epidermis for infection and reproduction. In particular, the virus prefers to target functional epithelial appendages, such as hair follicles, several glands including salivary glands in the oral cavity and tonsillar crypts, as well as sites where stratified epithelium abuts columnar epithelium, such as in the uterine cervical transformation zone. These vulnerable sites lack the highly structured barrier function of the epithelium and have the heighted presence of epithelial reserve cells/stem cells (Egawa et al. 2015).
(2) HPV infects the basal cell layer of stratified epithelia via epithelial wounding/microlesions.
(3) Viral entry of cells requires active cell division and studies with HPV16 suggest that the L1 capsid protein binds to heparan sulfate proteoglycans (HSPGs) on segments of the basement membrane, which are exposed at sites of (micro)injury. Furthermore, the virion binds to α6 integrins, which initiate further intracellular signaling events. Binding to HSPGs induces conformational changes, L2 cleavage and binding of the exposed L2 N terminus to a newly identified L2-specific receptor, the annexin A2 heterotetramer. Subsequently, clathrin-, caveolin-, lipid raft-, flotillin-, cholesterol- and dynamin-independent endocytosis of HPV16 occurs (Schiller et al. 2010; Raff et al. 2013).
(4) Infection is associated with HPV early gene E1 and E2 expression and low-level amplification of the HPV episome (circular, extrachromosomal DNA). E2 furthermore binds to mitotic spindles enabling viral DNA partitioning during cell division (Van Tine et al. 2004a).
(5) Infected cells replicate and move into parabasal epithelial layers. E6 and E7 expression suppress differentiation and promote re-entering the cell cycle.
(6) Infected cells move to the upper epithelial layers, replicate their viral genome to high copy number and express E4 and the late genes L1 and L2 allowing encapsulation of episomes into infectious virus particles and shedding from the cornified surface. Recognizable lesions that are going through these usually non-neoplastic productive HPV infections are classified as low-grade intraepithelial lesion (LSIL) or cervical intraepithelial neoplasia 1 (CIN1). These lesions often regress due to the action of the immune system.
(7) In ~5 % of cases, infections may become persistent (lesions classified as high-grade SIL, or CIN 2/3) leading to local immune suppression, accumulation of chromosome alterations in the infected host cells (Southern et al. 2001; Hopman et al. 2004, 2006), deregulated expression of HPV early genes and consequently reduced virus production. 0.3–1.2 % of initial infections will eventually progress to invasive cancer (WHO 2014).

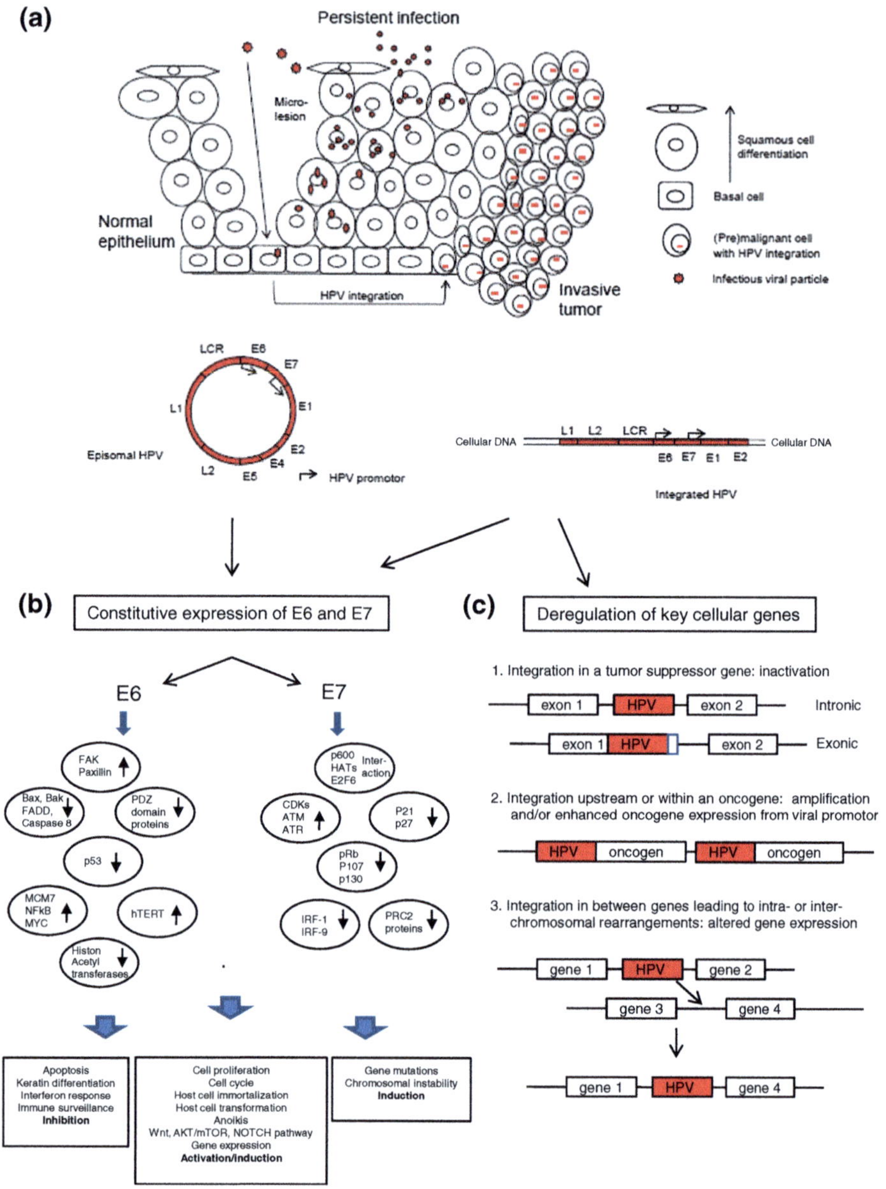
(a)
Persistent infection
Micro-
lesion
Normal
epithelium
HPV integration
Invasive
tumor
Squamous cell
differentiation
Basal cell
(Pre)malignant cell
with HPV integration
Infectious viral particle
LCR
E6
E7
E1
E2
E4
E5
L2
L1
Episomal HPV
HPV promotor
Cellular DNA
L1 L2 LCR
E6 E7 E1 E2
Cellular DNA
Integrated HPV
(b)
Constitutive expression of E6 and E7
E6
E7
FAK
Paxillin
Bax, Bak
FADD,
Caspase 8
PDZ
domain
proteins
p53
MCM7
NFkB
MYC
hTERT
Histon
Acetyl
transferases
p600
HATs
E2F6
Inter-
action
CDKs
ATM
ATR
P21
p27
pRb
P107
p130
IRF-1
IRF-9
PRC2
proteins
Apoptosis
Keratin differentiation
Interferon response
Immune surveillance
Inhibition
Cell proliferation
Cell cycle
Host cell immortalization
Host cell transformation
Anoikis
Wnt, AKT/mTOR, NOTCH pathway
Gene expression
Activation/induction
Gene mutations
Chromosomal instability
Induction
(c)
Deregulation of key cellular genes
1. Integration in a tumor suppressor gene: inactivation
exon 1
HPV
exon 2
Intronic
exon 1
HPV
exon 2
Exonic
2. Integration upstream or within an oncogene: amplification
and/or enhanced oncogene expression from viral promotor
HPV
oncogen
HPV
oncogen
3. Integration in between genes leading to intra- or inter-
chromosomal rearrangements: altered gene expression
gene 1
HPV
gene 2
gene 3
gene 4
gene 1
HPV
gene 4

◀ **Fig. 1** **a** Schematic overview of HPV infection and integration during the development of HPV-positive tumors (modified from Woodman et al. 2007; Cornet et al. 2015). HPV is thought to access the basal cells through micro lesions in the squamous cell epithelium. Following infection, the early HPV genes E1, E2, E4, E5, E6 and E7 are expressed and the viral DNA replicates from episomal DNA. In the *upper layers* of the epithelium, the viral genome is replicated further, and the late genes L1 and L2, and E4 are expressed. L1 and L2 allow encapsulation of the viral genomes to form progeny virions in the nucleus. The shed virus can then initiate a new infection. In the transition to (micro)invasive cancer, viral DNA often integrates in 1 or more copies into the host genomic DNA, with often associated loss or disruption of E2, and subsequent upregulation of E6 and E7 oncogene expression. LCR, long control region. **b** The subsequent upregulation of E6 and E7 oncoproteins results in deregulation of cell signaling pathways, which, among others, leads to increased cellular proliferation and inhibition of apoptosis (modified from Olthof et al. 2012; Groves and Coleman 2015). **c** Multiple mechanisms by which HPV integration into the host genome may directly lead to deregulation of the key cellular tumor suppressor genes and proto-oncogenes (modified from Rusan et al. 2015)

2 Mechanisms Involved in and Approaches to Detect HPV Integration

Persistent infection may also result in integration of the HRHPV genome or parts thereof into the host genome. Although in premalignant CIN lesions the time and frequency of integration has been heavily debated, it is now believed that it occurs relatively late in the progression of high-grade dysplasia to (micro)invasive anogenital carcinomas (Klaes et al. 1999; Hopman et al. 2004; Vinokurova et al. 2008; Rusan et al. 2015). HPV16 integration could also be detected in OPSCC and in tumor adjacent dysplasia in some of these cases (Hafkamp et al. 2003; Mooren et al. 2014). So far, in situ localization of a persistent HRHPV infection in the oropharynx/palatine tonsils has been extremely difficult to find and detect in the normal population (Klingenberg et al. 2010), and analysis of tissue biopsies of a population with a high chance of HPV infection (e.g., people having many sex partners, oral sex or who are immunosuppressed) is probably required to successfully identify such infections. In contrast, LRHPV infections are easy to detect, for example in laryngeal papillomas, but in these cases viral integration is a seldom finding (Huebbers et al. 2013; Mooren et al. 2014).

Because viral integration requires the breakage of both the viral and the host DNA, the integration rate is believed to be linked to the levels of DNA damage (Chen et al. 2014). DNA damage can be caused by both endogenous and exogenous factors, including inflammation induced either by the virus itself (E6 and E7 expression) or by co-infections with other agents (both resulting in production of excessive amounts of reactive oxygen and nitrate species), environmental agents and other factors (Wei et al. 2009; Lace et al. 2015; Visalli et al. 2016). In this respect, the activation of DNA damage repair mechanisms as well as the accumulation of chromosomal alterations may also contribute to the viral integration process (Southern et al. 2001; Hopman et al. 2004, 2006).

In uterine cervical squamous cell carcinomas (UCSCC), which are HPV positive in 95–100 % of cases, different HRHPV types tend to integrate at different frequencies, such as HPV16 at 50–80 %, HPV18 at >90 %, HPV31 and −33 at

15–40 % and HPV45 at > 80 % (Wentsenzen et al. 2004; Vinokurova et al. 2008; Olthof et al. 2012; Groves and Coleman 2015). In OPSCC HPV, positivity range from 20 to 90 % in different studies and depend among others on the geographical location, sample preparation and detection methods used (Olthof et al. 2012). 90–95 % of virus-positive OPSCC are infected with HPV16, and integration percentages range between 40 and 80 % dependent on the methods used to identify integrated HPV.

Along with the many HPV detection methods available to date (Snijders et al. 2010), a number of approaches have been developed to specifically detect integrated HPV. On the one hand, approaches have been designed to only identify integration events that are transcriptionally active detecting virus–host fusion transcripts, such as RNA in situ hybridization (ISH) (Van Tine et al. 2004b), 3′ RACE–PCR [also known as "Amplification of Papillomavirus Oncogene Transcripts" (APOT) PCR] (Klaes et al. 1999; Lace et al. 2011; Olthof et al. 2014, 2015; Vojtechova et al. 2016) and RNASeq (Akagi et al. 2014; Ojesina et al. 2014; Parfenov et al. 2014; Hu et al. 2015). On the other hand, procedures have been used to detect integrated HPV genomes (regardless of their transcriptional activity), including DNA (F)ISH (Cooper et al. 1991; Hopman et al. 2004; Hafkamp et al. 2008), Southern blotting (Cullen et al. 1991; Cooper et al. 1991; Vojtechova et al. 2016), detection of integrated papillomavirus sequences (DIPS) PCR (Luft et al. 2001; Peter et al. 2010; Huebbers et al. 2013; Li et al. 2013; Olthof et al. 2014, 2015), restriction-site PCR (Thorland et al. 2000), quantitative PCR (Peitsaro et al. 2002; Nagao et al. 2002; Ziegert et al. 2003) and DNASeq (Xu et al. 2013; Akagi et al. 2014; Parfenov et al. 2014, Chandrani et al. 2015; Hu et al. 2015). These analyses have contributed significantly to our current knowledge on the frequency of HPV integration in UCSCC and OPSCC and its impact on cancer development and progression as well as on viral (onco)gene and human gene expression. However, all these assays also have their (dis)advantages and differ in their detection sensitivities, which have to be taken into account when comparing reported data and generating general conclusions on these issues (below).

3 Identification of HPV Integration Sites in the Human Genome

Identification of sites in the human cellular genome where HPV integration events occur is a longstanding field of interest in HPV research. Molecular studies have provided evidence that often 1 and sometimes >1 integration site(s) can be detected in UCSCC and OPSCC (Hopman et al. 2004; Hafkamp et al. 2008; Peter et al. 2010; Mooren et al. 2013; Akagi et al. 2014; Ojesina et al. 2014; Parfenov et al. 2014; Hu et al. 2015). HPV integration sites appear to be distributed all over the human genome in both UCSCC and OPSCC, and lie often within, or close to, fragile sites (Wentsenzen et al. 2004; Akagi et al. 2014; Ojesina et al. 2014; Olthof et al. 2014, 2015; Parfenov et al. 2014; Hu et al. 2015). Furthermore, a number of cytogenetic bands have been identified as integration hotspots, including 3q28, 4q13.3, 8q24.21, 13q22.1 and 17q21.2 accounting for integration sites of >20 % of UCSCC analyzed (Schmitz et al. 2012; Olthof et al. 2014; Chandrani et al. 2015). In addition, Parfenov et al. (2014) and Hu et al. (2015) reported that integration in both UCSCC and OPSCC is often in regions of microhomology (1–10 bp) among the viral and host genome, indicating that fusion between viral and human DNA may have occurred by microhomology-mediated DNA repair pathways. Most frequently integration is detected into genic regions and to a lesser extent in miRNA regions. Parfenov et al. (2014) reported that in 54 % of OPSCC HPV integrated into a known gene (e.g., RAD51B), and in 17 % within 20 kb of a gene. Similarly, Olthof et al. identified in 29 OPSCC 37 HPV16 integration sites, 27 of which were in known or predicted genes, including 17 with a known role in tumorigenesis, such as BCL2, FANCC, HDAC2 and TP63. Hu et al. (2015) reported integration hot spots (range 4.9–9.7 %) in POU5F1B, FHIT, KLF12, KLF5, LRP1B, LEPREL1, HMGA2, DLG2 and SEMA3D, whereas Ojesina et al. (2014) found virus breakpoints in MYC, ERBB2, TP63, FANCC, RAD51B and CEACAM5, both in UCSCC. Also in 7 often used HPV16-positive HNSCC cell lines 2–7 integration sites per nucleus were identified, with integration in genes (DIAPH2, TP63, C9orf156) and intergenic regions (Olthof et al. 2014). Akagi et al. (2014) were able to confirm these observations in cell lines as well as primary tumor specimens and, moreover, found that sites of integration cluster near sites of structural alterations (amplifications, deletions) in the genome. These findings have also been described previously for UCSCC (Lockwood et al. 2007; Peter et al. 2010; Ojesina et al. 2014). As a result, Akagi et al. (2014) proposed a viral genome looping model to explain HPV-driven amplifications and rearrangements that occur at sites of integration, which may be further propagated throughout the genome. It consists of the following steps: (1) host genome and viral episome are nicked, (2) linear HPV genome integrates in cellular genome, (3) circular DNA containing both host and viral sequences is formed, (4) this template is amplified by rolling circle amplification and (5) integrated concatemers of viral–host sequences are generated that might spread further in the genome. Indeed, in the HPV16-positive HNSCC cell lines described by Olthof et al. (2015), FISH experiments provided evidence for multiplication and translocation events of chromosomes harboring integrated viral DNA sequences as well as genomic instability. It should be noted, however, that the looping model is particularly based on analysis of tumor cell lines, which might also have accumulate additional chromosomal alterations induced by long-term cultivation. It would be interesting to compare the used cell lines with early passages and the primary tumor tissue to examine this in more detail.

Taken together, these data suggest that HPV integration is not simply a random event, but rather has a preference for less protected and more accessible chromosomal regions such as transcribed tumor genes and fragile sites. It will be interesting to further explore (1) whether integration takes place in genes, which are highly expressed during carcinogenesis or (2) whether integration itself is rather random but may affect the expression of interrupted genes or (3) whether both may occur simultaneously. In this respect, Kraus Christiansen et al. (2015) recently reported that integration sites seem to coincide with DNA that is transcriptionally active in mucosal epithelium, as judged after relating data of integration sites to DNase hypersensitivity and H3K4me3 methylation. These results might point to integration being rather an early event in carcinogenesis than a late product of chromosomal instability, which is in agreement with data of Hopman et al. (2006) showing that integration already can occur in diploid CIN lesions.

4 Consequences of Viral Integration: Viral Gene Expression

In vitro studies have suggested that HPV integration events occur in cells that also contain non-integrated episomes resulting in repression of integrant-derived transcription of E6 and E7 by expression of the E2 transcriptional regulator from the episome (Bechtold et al. 2003; Pett et al. 2006; Groves and Coleman 2015). Only after episome clearance, for example by a host anti-virus response (Herdman et al. 2006), an upregulated expression of E6 and E7 oncoproteins from the integrated viral DNA might be detected, which leads to a selective growth advantage over cells harboring episomal DNA (Jeon and Lambert 1995). There is, however, discussion on the height of the E6 and E7 expression levels and how they are exactly regulated in HPV-positive lesions. The general view is that viral DNA often integrates in 1 or more copies into the host genomic DNA (see above). During this process, the viral episome is most often opened within the E2 open reading frame (preferential site of integration), frequently leading to deletion of E4 and E5 and part of E2 and L2 (zur Hausen 2002; Wentsenzen et al. 2004; Olthof et al. 2012, 2013). Olthof et al. and Parfenov et al. (2014) also detected disruption of the viral episome in the E1 gene, which also leads to E2 loss. The subsequent upregulation of E6 and E7 oncoproteins results in deregulation of cell signaling pathways, which, among others, leads to increased cellular proliferation and inhibition of apoptosis and finally· to a transformed cell state (zur Hausen 2002; Ganguly and Parihar 2009; Moody and Laimins 2010; Pim and Banks 2010; Olthof et al. 2012) (Fig. 1b). Transformation is continuously dependent upon E6/E7 expression and can be reversed by the reintroduction of E2 (Adams et al. 2014) or by downregulation of E6/E7 using short-hairpin RNAs (Rampias et al. 2009). HPV breakpoints have also been mapped outside the E2 and E1 open reading frame (Akagi et al. 2014; Hu et al. 2015), most frequently in the L1 and L2 genes. In these cases, however, methylation of the E2-binding sites in the LCR promotor, preventing E2 to bind to the LCR promotor, might be responsible for de-repression of E6 and E7 expression (Reuschenbach et al. 2015). This might also be the case in tumors that harbor multiple copies of the HPV genome in stretches or concatenates in the human genome (Olthof et al. 2014; Groves and Coleman 2015). Another possibility might be that viral gene expression is influenced by nearby cellular regulatory sequences (Rusan et al. 2015).

In contrast to this view, a study in primary keratinocytes immortalized with HPV16 genomes has shown that disruption of the E2 gene sequence upon viral integration does not result in increased expression of the viral E6 and E7 oncogenes (Lace et al. 2011). In addition, a publication by Häfner et al. (2008) using APOT-PCR has shown no correlation between the integration state of the viral genome and the expression of the viral gene E6 in a collection of 55 HPV16-positive UCSCC samples. Recently, Olthof et al. (2014, 2015) have provided evidence that also in 7 HPV-positive HNSCC cell lines as well as in 75 primary OPSCC HPV physical status (extrachromosomal episomes or host DNA integrated) does not affect the levels of viral E2, E6 and E7 gene transcripts. Therefore, constitutive rather than a high-level expression of viral oncogene transcripts appears to be required in HPV-related OPSCC, enough to ensure the viral oncogenes to consistently deregulate cellular proteins and cell signaling pathways, including cell proliferation (pRb pathway), apoptosis and DNA damage response (p53 pathway) (Wiest et al. 2002; zur Hausen 2002; Hafkamp et al. 2009; Leemans et al. 2011; Pim and Banks 2010; Rieckmann et al. 2013; Arenz et al. 2014) (Fig. 1b).

5 Consequences of Viral Integration: Human Gene Expression

Besides its promotion of stable viral gene expression and subsequent deregulation of cell signaling pathways, HPV integration may also confer a selective growth advantage to the host cells through a direct effect on the host genome (i.e., by affecting the key cellular genes). Olthof et al. (2014) had mRNA expression profiling data of 6 OPSCC with proven HPV16 integration in gene sequences, including the known tumor-related genes FANCC, HDAC2, SYNPO2 and TRAF3. Viral integration, however, did not lead to significantly different expression of the interrupted gene in comparison with OPSCC having integration in another DNA sequence or showing solely viral episomes. This is in contrast to a study of Huebbers et al. (2013) showing that integration of low-risk HPV6 in the AKR1C3 gene resulted in loss of gene expression in a laryngeal carcinoma. In this case, however, the other gene copy was lost in the tumor as shown by array CGH analyses. In the 6 OPSCC studied by Olthof et al. (2014), no loss or amplification of the chromosomal regions containing the virally interrupted genes has been detected by array CGH, indicating that one or more expressed gene copies are still present in these tumors, which can mask a possible effect of the integration on gene expression. On the other hand, this might also point to the fact that viral integration is not per se meant to deregulate the interrupted gene in the cell, as also can be concluded by the finding of HPV16 integrated in intergenic sequences of 10 OPSCC in this study.

In UCSCC, however, Ojesina et al. (2014) found significantly elevated host gene expression levels at sites of integration compared with expression levels of the same genes in tumors without integration. This was associated in a number of cases with copy number gains, but not at all sites, indicating that expression may also be driven by alternative mechanisms, such as the viral promotor of the integrant, other regulatory sequences and proteins, or decreased E6/E7 expression (Rusan et al. 2015).

Figure 1c shows several mechanisms by which HPV integration may directly affect gene expression, previously presented by Rusan et al. (2015), i.e., (1) integration in a tumor suppressor gene resulting in loss of gene function, (2) integration adjacent to an oncogene leading to gene amplification and expression or enhanced expression from the viral promotor and (3) intra- or interchromosomal rearrangements followed by altered expression of genes in involved regions. Examples of (1) are described above and may involve additional loss of the chromosome without the HPV integrant (Huebbers et al. 2013) or amplification or loss of gene components leading to truncated proteins, as has been found for the double-strand break DNA repair pathway gene RAD51B (Khoury et al. 2013; Ojesina et al. 2014; Parfenov et al. 2014). HPV integration upstream near or within the NR4A2 or MYC oncogenes in UCSCC and OPSCC are examples of (2) (Ferber et al. 2003; Wentsenzen et al. 2004; Ojesina et al. 2014; Parfenov et al. 2014), and examples of HPV insertion associated with chromosomal rearrangements, gene amplification and increased expression have been described by Akagi et al. (2014), Parfenov et al. (2014) and Olthof et al. (2015) involving the TP63 gene, a transcription factor with a role in epithelial development and highly expressed in squamous cell carcinomas (SCC).

In summary, recent as well as older literature has provided evidence that at least in a part of UCSCC and OPSCC HPV integration has a direct effect on the host genome and human gene expression, further underscored by recurrent integration events in specific genes. However, more studies are needed to fully explore the molecular mechanisms underlying human as well as viral gene expression as a result of HPV integration in anogenital and head and neck cancers.

6 HPV Integration in Relation to Viral Load, Methylated Genes and Outcome

A number of studies have examined other parameters in relation to HPV integration, although different methods have been used to determine the viral physical status. Olthof et al. (2014) examined whether tumors with episomal virus have a higher viral load than those with integration as determined by APOT and/or DIPS-PCR. For this purpose qPCR was performed on 73 OPSCC samples. Viral load ranged from 3.4×10^{-6} up to 97 HPV DNA copies per cell. When comparing the average viral load in cases with or without integration, no significant differences were seen (7 vs. 8.5 HPV DNA copies/cell). Furthermore, no correlation was found between the mean log2 expression levels of the viral genes E2, E6 or E7 and the viral load. This was also the case in 7 HPV16-positive HNSCC cell lines containing 2–7 integration sites, in which the viral load ranged from 1-739 HPV DNA copies/referencee gene (Beta-globin) copy (Olthof et al. 2015).

In two studies, methylation of human genes as well as E2-binding sites in the HPV LCR DNA, respectively, were examined and compared with the HPV integration status of head and neck cancers. In the first study, Parfenov et al. (2014) showed that DNA methylation profiles are distinct for HPV-positive tumors with integration than for those without integration. Differentially methylated genes included the tumor suppressors BARX2 and IRX4, and the oncogenes SIM2 and CTSE. The mechanism by which integration alters the methylation profile, however, remains to be elucidated (Rusan et al. 2015). In the second study, Reuschenbach et al. (2015) detected differential methylation levels in the HPV16 (LCR) E2-binding sites E2BS3 and E2BS4 depending on the viral DNA physical status, i.e., (1) complete methylation (>80 %) associated with the presence of integrated HPV genomes with an intact E2 gene; (2) intermediate methylation levels (20–80 %) with predominantly episomal HPV genomes with intact E2; and (3) no methylation (<20 %) with a disrupted E2 gene. Patients with high methylation levels tended to have a worse 5-year overall survival compared with patients with intermediate methylation (hazard ratio: 3.23). The authors therefore concluded that further studies are warranted to determine whether the E2BS methylation status may represent a prognostic marker.

A number of studies analyzed if tumors with HPV integration show a worse outcome as compared to tumors with episomal virus present. Parfenov et al. (2014) explored in primary head and neck cancers whether HPV integration was associated with clinical outcome or other clinical features (anatomic site, tumor stage, age, smoking status), but did not find significant associations. An explanation could be the relatively small sample size of the study. Vojtechova et al. (2016) recently analyzed a series of 186 tonsillar carcinomas showing integration in 43 % of cases as assessed by E2 mRNA mapping, which in a subset of tumors corresponded to APOT and Southern blotting data. These authors also did not find a statistically significant difference in disease-specific survival between patients with HPV-positive integrated vs. extrachromosomal/mixed forms of the virus. Finally, in cervical cancer patients treated with radiotherapy, Shin et al. (2014) found a trend toward decreased disease-free survival in patients with only HPV integrated forms versus patients with both integrated and episomal HPV. In conclusion, further studies are required to elucidate the relationship between HPV physical status (integrated vs. episomal vs. mixed integrated/episomal) and survival in both OPSCC and UCSCC.

Taken together, HPV integration affects both the viral and host genome, which may lead to deregulation of viral oncoproteins, critical cellular (cancer) genes as well as changes in DNA methylation, transcription and accumulation of chromosomal alterations (see also chapter "Molecular patterns and biology of HPV associated HNSCC" by Brakenhoff RH, Wagner S, Klussmann JP). More genome-wide studies with larger tumor series are necessary to further explore viral integration events, their impact on genomic alterations and the clinical implications of these findings.

References

Adams AK, Wise-Draper TM, Wells SI (2014) Human papillomavirus induced transformation in cervical and head and neck cancers. Cancers 6:1793–1820 doi:10.3390/cancers6031793

Akagi K, Li J, Broutian TR, Padilla-Nash H, Xiao W, Jiang B, Rocco JW, Teknos TN, Kumar B, Wangsa D, He D, Ried T, Symer DE, Gillison ML (2014) Genomewide analysis of HPV integration in human cancers reveals recurrent, focal genomic instability. Genome Res 24: 185–199

Arenz A, Ziemann F, Mayer C, Wittig A, Dreffke K, Preising S, Wagner S, Klussmann JP, Engenhart-Cabillic R, Wittekindt C (2014) Increased radiosensitivity of HPV-positive head and neck cancer cell lines due to cell cycle dysregulation and induction of apoptosis. Strahlenther Onkol 190:839–846

Bechtold V, Beard P, Raj K (2003) Human papillomavirus type 16 E2 protein has no effect on transcription from episomal viral DNA. J Virol 77:2021–2028

Bernard HU, Burk RD, Chen Z et al (2010) Classification of papillomaviruses (PVs) based on 189 PV types and proposal of taxonomic amendments. Virology 401:70–79

Chandrani P, Kulkarni V, Iyer P, Upadhyay P, Chaubal R, Das P, Mulherkar R, Singh R, Dutt A (2015) NGS-based approach to determine the presence of HPV and their sites of integration in human cancer genome. Br J Cancer 112:1958–1965

Chen Y, Williams V, Filippova M, Filippov V, Duerksen-Hughes P (2014) Viral carcinogenesis: factors inducing DNA damage and viral integration. Cancers 6:2155–2186. doi:10.3390/cancers6042155

Cooper K, Herrington CS, Stickland JE, Evans MF, McGee JO (1991) Episomal and integrated human papillomavirus in cervical neoplasia shown by non-isotopic in situ hybridisation. J Clin Pathol 44:990–996

Cornet I, Kaanders JHAM, Kremer B, Speel EJM (2015) Hoofdhalskanker en HPV: hoe op maat te behandelen? Kanker Breed 7:26–29

Cullen AP, Reid R, Campion M, Lörincz AT (1991) Analysis of the physical state of different human papillomavirus DNAs in intraepithelial and invasive cervical neoplasm. J Virol 65: 606–612

Egawa N, Egawa K, Griffin H, Doorbar J (2015) Human papillomaviruses; epithelial tropisms and the development of neoplasia. Viruses 7:3863–3890

Ferber MJ, Thorland EC, Brink AA, Rapp AK, Phillips LA, McGovern R, Gostout BS, Cheung TH, Chung TK, Fu WY, Smith DI (2003) Preferential integration of human papillomavirus type 18 near the c-myc locus in cervical carcinoma. Oncogene 22:7233–7242

Ganguly N, Parihar SP (2009) Human papillomavirus E6 and E7 oncoproteins as risk factors for tumorigenesis. J Biosci 34:113–123

Groves IJ, Coleman N (2015) Pathogenesis of human papillomavirus-associated mucosal disease. J Pathol 235:527–538

Hafkamp HC, Speel EJM, Haesevoets A, Bot FJ, Dinjens WNM, Ramaekers FCS, Hopman AHN, Manni JJ (2003) A subset of head and neck squamous cell carcinomas exhibits integration of HPV 16/18 DNA and overexpression of $p16^{INK4A}$ and p53 in the absence of mutations in exons 5–8. Int J Cancer 107:394–400

Hafkamp HC, Manni JJ, Haesevoets A, Voogd AC, Schepers M, Bot FJ, Hopman AHN, Ramaekers FCS, Speel EJM (2008) Marked differences in survival rate between smokers and non-smokers with HPV 16-associated tonsillar carcinomas. Int J Cancer 122:2656–2664

Hafkamp HC, Mooren JJ, Claessen SHM, Klingenberg B, Voogd AC, Bot FJ, Klussmann JP, Hopman AHN, Manni JJ, Kremer B, Ramaekers FCS, Speel EJM (2009) P21Cip1/WAF1 expression is strongly associated with HPV-positive tonsillar carcinoma and a favorable prognosis. Modern Pathol 22:686–698

Häfner N, Driesch C, Gajda M, Jansen L, Kirchmayr R, Runnebaum IB, Dürst M (2008) Integration of the HPV16 genome does not invariably result in high levels of viral oncogene transcripts. Oncogene 27:1610–1617

Herdman MT, Pett MR, Roberts I, Alazawi WO, Teschendorff AE, Zhang XY, Stanley MA, Coleman N (2006) Interferon-β treatment of cervical keratinocytes naturally infected with human papillomavirus 16 episomes promotes rapid reduction in episome numbers and emergence of latent integrants. Carcinogenesis 27:2341–2353

Hopman AHN, Smedts F, Dignef W, Ummelen M, Sonke G, Mravunac M, Vooijs GP, Speel EJM, Ramaekers FCS (2004) Transition of high grade cervical intraepithelial neoplasia to micro-invasive carcinoma is characterized by integration of HPV 16/18 and numerical chromosome abnormalities. J Pathol 202:23–33

Hopman AHN, Theelen W, Hommelberg P, Kamps MA, Herrington CS, Morrison LE, Speel EJM, Smedts F, Ramaekers FCS (2006) Genomic integration of oncogenic HPV and gain of the Human Telomerase Gene *TERC* at 3q26 are strongly associated events in the progression of uterine cervical dysplasia to invasive cancer. J Pathol 210:412–419

Hu Z, Zhu D, Wang W, Li W, Jia W, Zeng X, Ding W, Yu L, Wang X, Wang L, Shen H, Zhang C, Liu H, Liu X, Zhao Y, Fang X, Li S, Chen W, Tang T, Fu A, Wang Z, Chen G, Gao Q, Li S, Xi L, Wang C, Liao S, Ma X, Wu P, Li K, Wang S, Zhou J, Wang J, Xu X, Wang H, Ma D (2015) Genome-wide profiling of HPV integration in cervical cancer identifies clustered genomic hot spots and a potential microhomology-mediated integration mechanism. Nat Genet 47:158–163

Huebbers CU, Preuss SF, Kolligs J, Vent J, Stenner M, Wieland U, Silling S, Drebber U, Speel EJM, Klussmann JP (2013) Integration of HPV6 and downregulation of AKR1C3 expression mark malignant transformation in a patient with juvenile-onset laryngeal papillomatosis. PLoS ONE 8(2):e57207. doi:10.1371/journal.pone.0057207

Jeon S, Lambert PF (1995) Integration of human papillomavirus type 16 DNA into the human genome leads to increased stability of E6 and E7 mRNAs: implications for cervical carcinogenesis. Proc Natl Acad Sci USA 92:1654–1658

Khoury JD, Tannir NM, Williams MD, Chen Y, Yao H, Zhang J, Thompson EJ, Network TCGA, Meric-Bernstam F, Medeiros LJ, Weinstein JN, Su X (2013) Landscape of DNA virus associations across human malignant cancers: analysis of 3,775 cases using RNA-Seq. J Virol 87:8916–8926

Klaes R, Woerner SM, Ridder R, Wentzensen N, DuerstM Schneider A, Lotz B, Melsheimer P, von Knebel Doeberitz M (1999) Detection of high-risk cervical intraepithelial neoplasia and cervical cancer by amplification of transcripts derived from integrated papillomavirus oncogenes. Cancer Res 59:6132–6136

Klingenberg B, Hafkamp HC, Haesevoets A, Manni JJ, Slootweg PJ, Weissenborn SJ, Klussmann JP, Speel EJM (2010) $p16^{INK4A}$ overexpression is frequently detected in tumor-free tonsil tissue without association with HPV. Histopathology 56:957–967

Kraus Christiansen I, Kjetil Sandve G, Schmitz M, Dürst M, Hovig E (2015) Transcriptionally active regions Are the Preferred Targets for Chromosomal HPV Integration in Cervical Carcinogenesis. PLoS ONE 10(3):e0119566. doi:10.1371/journal.pone.0119566

Lace MJ, Anson JR, Klussmann JP, Wang DH, Smith EM, Haugen TH, Turek LP (2011) Human papillomavirus type 16 (HPV-16) genomes integrated in head and neck cancers and in HPV-16-immortalized human keratinocyte clones express chimeric virus cell mRNAs similar to those found in cervical cancers. J Virol 85:1645–1654

Lace MJ, Anson JR, Haugen TH, Dierdorff JM, Turek LP (2015) Interferon treatment of human keratinocytes harboring extrachromosomal, persistent HPV-16 plasmid genomes induces de novo viral integration. Carcinogenesis 36:151–159

Leemans CR, Braakhuis BJ, Brakenhoff RH (2011) The molecular biology of head and neck cancer. Nat Rev Cancer 11:9–22

Li H, Yang Y, Zhang R, Cai Y, Yang X, Wang Z, Li Y, Cheng X, Ye X, Xiang Y, Zhu B (2013) Preferential sites for the integration and disruption of human papillomavirus 16 in cervical lesions. J Clin Virol 56:342–347

Lockwood WW, Coe BP, Williams AC, MacAuley C, Lam WL (2007) Whole genome tiling path aray CGH analysis of segmental copy number alterations in cervical cancer cell lines. Int J Cancer 120:436–443

Luft F, Klaes R, Nees M, Dürst M, Heilmann V, Melsheimer P, von Knebel Doeberitz M (2001) Detection of integrated papillomavirus sequences by ligation-mediated PCR (DIPS-PCR) and molecular characterization in cervical cancer cells. Int J Cancer 92:9–17

Moody CA, Laimins LA (2010) Human papillomavirus oncoproteins: pathways to transformation. Nat Rev Cancer 10:550–560

Mooren JJ, Kremer B, Claessen SMH, Voogd AC, Bot FJ, Klussmann JP, Huebbers CU, Hopman AHN, Ramaekers FCS, Speel EJM (2013) Chromosome stability in tonsillar squamous cell carcinomas is associated with HPV 16 integration and indicates a favourable prognosis. Int J Cancer 132:1781–1789

Mooren JJ, Gultekin SE, Straetmans JM, Haesevoets A, Peutz-Kootstra CJ, Huebbers CU, Dienes HP, Wieland U, Ramaekers FC, Kremer B, Speel EJ, Klussmann JP (2014) P16 (INK4A) immunostaining is a strong indicator for high-risk-HPV-associated oropharyngeal carcinomas and dysplasias, but is unreliable to predict low-risk-HPV-infection in head and neck papillomas and laryngeal dysplasias. Int J Cancer 134:2108–2117

Nagao S, Yoshinouchi M, Miyagi Y, Hongo A, Kodama J, Itoh S, Kudo T (2002) Rapid and sensitive detection of physical status of human papillomavirus type 16 DNA by quantitative real-time PCR. J Clin Microbiol 40:863–867

Ojesina AI, Lichtenstein L, Freeman SS, Pedamallu CS, Imaz-Rosshandler I, Pugh TJ, Cherniack AD, Ambrogio L, Cibulskis K, Bertelsen B, Romero-Cordoba S, Treviño V, Vazquez-Santillan K, Guadarrama AS, Wright AA, Rosenberg MW, Duke F, Kaplan B, Wang R, Nickerson E, Walline HM, Lawrence MS, Stewart C, Carter SL, McKenna A, Rodriguez-Sanchez IP, Espinosa-Castilla M, Woie K, Bjorge L, Wik E, Halle MK, Hoivik EA, Krakstad C, Gabiño NB, Gómez-Macías GS, Valdez-Chapa LD, Garza-Rodríguez ML, Maytorena G, Vazquez J, Rodea C, Cravioto A, Cortes ML, Greulich H, Crum CP, Neuberg DS, Hidalgo-Miranda A, Escareno CR, Akslen LA, Carey TE, Vintermyr OK, Gabriel SB, Barrera-Saldaña HA, Melendez-Zajgla J, Getz G, Salvesen HB, Meyerson M (2014) Landscape of genomic alterations in cervical carcinomas. Nature 506:371–375

Olthof NC, Straetmans JMJAA, Snoeck R, Ramaekers FCS, Kremer B, Speel EJM (2012) Next generation treatment strategies for HPV-related head and neck squamous cell carcinomas: where do we go? Rev Med Virol 22:88–105

Olthof NC, Speel EJM, Kolligs J, Haesevoets A, Henfling M, Ramaekers FCS, Preuss SF, Drebber U, Wieland U, Silling S, Lam WL, Vucic EA, Kremer B, Klussmann JP, Huebbers CU (2014) Comprehensive analysis of HPV 16 integration in OSCC reveals no significant impact of physical status on viral oncogene and virally disrupted human gene expression. PLoS ONE 9(2):e88718. doi:10.1371/journal.pone.0088718

Olthof NC, Huebbers CU, Kolligs J, Henfling M, Ramaekers FC, Cornet I, van Lent-Albrechts JA, Stegmann AP, Silling S, Wieland U, Carey TE, Walline HM, Gollin SM, Hoffmann TK, de Winter J, Kremer B, Klussmann JP, Speel EJM (2015) Viral load, gene expression and mapping of viral integration sites in HPV16-associated HNSCC cell lines. Int J Cancer 136: E207–E218

Parfenov M, Pedamallu CS, Gehlenborg N, Freeman SS, Danilova L, Bristow CA, Lee S, Hadjipanayis AG, Ivanova EV, Wilkerson MD, Protopopov A, Yang L, Seth S, Song X, Tang J, Ren X, Zhang J, Pantazi A, Santoso N, Xu AW, Mahadeshwar H, Wheeler DA, Haddad RI, Jung J, Ojesina AI, Issaeva N, Yarbrough WG, Hayes DN, Grandis JR, El-Naggar AK, Meyerson M, Park PJ, Chin L, Seidman JG, Hammerman PS, Kucherlapati R, Network Cancer Genome Atlas (2014) Characterization of HPV and host genome interactions in primary head and neck cancers. Proc Natl Acad Sci U S A 111:15544–15549

Peitsaro P, Johansson B, Syrjanen S (2002) Integrated human papillomavirus type 16 is frequently found in cervical cancer precursors as demonstrated by a novel quantitative real-time PCR technique. J Clin Microbiol 40:886–891

Peter M, Stransky N, Couturier J, Hupe P, Barillot E, de Cremoux P, Cottu P, Radvanyi F, Sastre-Garau X (2010) Frequent genomic structural alterations at HPV insertion sites in cervical carcinoma. J Pathol 221:320–330

Pett MR, Herdman MT, Palmer RD, Yeo GS, Shivji MK, Stanley MA, Coleman N (2006) Selection of cervical keratinocytes containing integrated HPV16 associates with episome loss and an endogenous antiviral response. Proc Natl Acad Sci USA 103:3822–3827

Pim D, Banks L (2010) Interaction of viral oncoproteins with cellular target molecules: infection with high-risk vs low-risk human papillomaviruses. APMIS 118:471–493

Raff AB, Woodham AW, Raff LM, Skeate JG, Yan L, Da Silva DM, Schelhaas M, Kast WM (2013) The evolving field of human papilloma virus receptor research: a review of binding and entry. J Virol 87:6062–6072

Rampias T, Sasaki C, Weinberger P, Psyrri A (2009) E6 and E7 gene silencing and transformed phenotype of human papillomavirus 16-positive oropharyngeal cancer cells. J Natl Cancer Inst 101:412–423

Reuschenbach M, Huebbers CU, Prigge ES, Bermejo JL, Kalteis MS, Preuss SF, Seuthe IM, Kolligs J, Speel EJM, Olthof N, Kremer B, Wagner S, Klussmann JP, Vinokurova S, von Knebel Doeberitz M (2015) Methylation status of HPV16 E2-binding sites classifies subtypes of HPV-associated oropharyngeal cancers. Cancer 121:1966–1976

Rieckmann T, Tribius S, Grob TJ, Meyer F, Busch CJ, Petersen C, Dikomey E, Kriegs M (2013) HNSCC cell lines positive for HPV and p16 possess higher cellular radiosensitivity due to an impaired DSB repair capacity. Radiother Oncol 107:242–246

Rusan M, Li YY, Hammerman PS (2015) Genomic landscape of human papillomavirus-associated cancers. Clin Cancer Res 21:2009–2019

Schiller JT, Day PM, Kines RC (2010) Current understanding of the mechanism of HPV infection. Gynecol Oncol 118:S12–17

Schmitz M, Driesch C, Jansen L, Runnebaum IB, Durst M (2012) Non-random integration of the HPV genome in cervical cancer. PLoS ONE 7(6):e39632. doi:10.1371/journal.pone.0039632

Shin HJ, Joo J, Yoon JH, Yoo CW, Kim JY (2014) Physical status of human papillomavirus integration in cervical cancer is associated with treatment outcome of the patients treated with radiotherapy. PLoS ONE 9(1):e78995. doi:10.1371/journal.pone.0078995

Snijders PJF, Heideman DAM, Meijer CJLM (2010) Methods for HPV detection in exfoliated cell and tissue specimens. APMIS 118:520–528

Southern SA, Noya F, Meyers C, Broker TR, Chow LT, Herrington CS (2001) Tetrasomy is induced by human papillomavirus type 18 E7 gene expression in keratinocyte raft cultures. Cancer Res 61:4858–4863

Thorland EC, Myers SL, Persing DH, Sarkar G, McGovern RM, Gostout BS, Smith DI (2000) Human papillomavirus type 16 integrations in cervical tumors frequently occur in common fragile sites. Cancer Res 60:5916–5921

Van Tine BA, Dao LD, Wu SY, Sonbuchner TM, Lin BY, Zou N, Chiang CM, Broker TR, Chow LT (2004a) Human papillomavirus (HPV) origin-binding protein associates with mitotic spindles to enable viral DNA partitioning. Proc Natl Acad Sci U S A 101:4030–4035

Van Tine BA, Kappes JC, Banerjee NS, Knops J, Lai L, Steenbergen RD, Meijer CL, Snijders PJ, Chatis P, Broker TR, Moen PT Jr, Chow LT (2004b) Clonal selection for transcriptionally active viral oncogenes during progression to cancer. J Virol 78:11172–11186

Vinokurova S, Wentzensen N, Kraus I, Klaes R, Driesch C, Melsheimer P, Kisseljov F, Dürst M, Schneider A, von Knebel Doeberitz M (2008) Type-dependent integration frequency of human papillomavirus genomes in cervical lesions. Cancer Res 68:307–313

Visalli G, Riso R, Facciolà A, Mondello P, Caruso C, Picerno I, Di Pietro A, Spataro P, Bertuccio MP (2016) Higher levels of oxidative DNA damage in cervical cells are correlated with the grade of dysplasia and HPV infection. J Med Virol 88:336–344

Vojtechova Z, Sabol I, Salakova M, Turek L, Grega M, Smahelova J, Vencalek O, Lukesova E, Klozar J, Tachezy R (2016) Analysis of the integration of human papillomaviruses in head and neck tumours in relation to patients' prognosis. Int J Cancer 138:386–395

Wei L, Gravitt PE, Song H, Maldonado AM, Ozbun MA (2009) Nitric oxide induces early viral transcription coincident with increased DNA damage and mutation rates in human papillomavirus-infected cells. Cancer Res 69:4878–4884
Wentzensen N, Vinokurova S, von Knebel Doeberitz M (2004) Systematic review of genomic integration sites of human papillomavirus genomes in epithelial dysplasia and invasive cancer of the female lower genital tract. Cancer Res 64:3878–3884
Wiest T, Schwarz E, Enders C, Flechtenmacher C, Bosch FX (2002) Involvement of intact HPV16 E6/E7 gene expression in head and neck cancers with unaltered p53 status and perturbed pRb cell cycle control. Oncogene 21:1510–1517
World Health Organization (2007) Human papillomaviruses: IARC Monographs on the evaluation of carcinogenic risks to humans. International Agency for Research on Cancer, Lyon
World Health Organization (2014) Cancers of the female reproductive organs. In: Stewart BW, Wild CP (eds) World cancer report 2014. Lyon, IARC, pp 465–481
Woodman CBJ, Collins SI, Young LS (2007) The natural history of cervical HPV infection. Nat Rev Cancer 7:11–22
Xu B, Chotewutmontri S, Wolf S, Klos U, Schmitz M, Dürst M, Schwarz E (2013) Multiplex identification of human papillomavirus 16 DNA integration sites in cervical carcinomas. PLoS ONE 8(6):e66693. doi:10.1371/journal.pone.0066693
Ziegert C, Wentzensen N, Vinokurova S, Kisseljov F, Einenkel J, Hoeckel M, Knebel Doeberitz M (2003) A comprehensive analysis of HPV integration loci in anogenital lesions combining transcript and genome-based amplification techniques. Oncogene 22:3977–3984
zur Hausen H (2002) Papillomaviruses and cancer: from basic studies to clinical application. Nat Rev Cancer 2:342–350

Risk Factors for Oral Infection with Human Papillomavirus

Pawel Golusinski

Abstract

Human papillomavirus has been identified as a causative factor for a subset of head and neck carcinomas (HNSCC). The majority of the HPV-positive tumors arises in the oropharyngeal region, and at present, the infection of the human papilloma type 16 is the major cause of the oropharyngeal cancer development. Patients with HPV DNA-positive tumors have been shown to be younger in age and are less likely to have a history of tobacco smoking or alcohol use. The tumors referred to the HPV positivity have been proven to more likely confer better prognosis. Seven percent of the population between ages of 14 and 69 are infected by HPV at any given time within the oral mucosa. However, only about 1 % of those infections is associated with the high-risk cancerogenous types of the virus. Up to date few risk factors of HPV infection have been identified including age, gender and the sexual behavior. Tobacco smoking and immunosuppression have also been reported to play a role in HPV infection.

Keywords

Oral HPV infection · Risk factors · Sexual behavior

P. Golusinski (✉)
Department of Biology and Environmental Studies,
Poznan University of Medical Sciences, Poznan, Poland
e-mail: pawel.golusinski@wco.pl

P. Golusinski
Department of Head and Neck Surgery, Greater Poland Cancer Centre,
Poznan University of Medical Sciences, Poznan, Poland

W. Golusiński et al. (eds.), *HPV Infection in Head and Neck Cancer*,
Recent Results in Cancer Research 206, DOI 10.1007/978-3-319-43580-0_5

1 Introduction

Human papillomavirus has been identified as a causative factor for a subset of head and neck carcinomas (HNSCC). The majority of the HPV-positive tumors arises in the oropharyngeal region, most commonly in the palatine tonsil. HPV has also been detected within the oral cavity, hypopharynx, larynx, paranasal sinuses and nasopharynx, however, to a far lesser extent (Gillison et al. 2015). Whereas the incidence of oral cavity cancers has slightly decreased in a previous decade, oropharyngeal cancer (OPC) incidence is constantly increasing in particular in some subpopulations (Gillison et al. 2015; Chaturvedi et al. 2011; Schantz and Yu 2002). The declining incidence of oral cavity cancers may be attributed to reductions in tobacco use in the western world. Reasons underlying the increasing incidence of oropharyngeal cancers suggest a dominant role for HPV infection. In Sweden, the proportion of HPV DNA-positive tonsil tumors increased from 28 % in the 1970s to 68 % in the 2000s (Hammarstedt et al. 2006), and in the same time in the USA the similar trend has been reported (Schantz and Yu 2002). In fact, at present, the infection of the human papilloma type 16 is considered to be the major cause of the oropharyngeal cancer development (Chaturvedi et al. 2011; Lewis et al. 2015). Patients with HPV DNA-positive tumors have been shown to be younger in age by 3–5 years and are less likely to have a history of tobacco smoking or alcohol use than patients who developed the tumor with no HPV DNA involvement (Gillison 2007). Furthermore, the tumors referred to the HPV positivity have been proven to more likely confer better prognosis (Gillison et al. 2000; D'Souza et al. 2007; Schwartz et al. 2001).

Other factors apart from the age describing the HPV-positive OPC patients are better socioeconomical status, the risky sexual behavior (Gillison et al. 2008).

Mucosal HPVs are known to be transmitted by sexual contacts, and in fact, HPV infection is the most common sexually transmitted disease in the world (Jay and Moscicki 2000). To picture the scale of that phenomenon one can imagine that more than a half of all the sexually active individuals in the world will have a genital HPV infection at least once in their lifetime. Seven percent of the population between ages of 14 and 69 are infected by HPV at any given time within the oral mucosa. However, only about 1 % of those infections is associated with the high-risk cancerogenous types of the virus (Gillison et al. 2008).

2 Age and Gender

Age at diagnosis for HPV-related OPC significantly declined over time. This fact is coherent with the younger age of HPV-related OPC contrasted to individuals with the HPV-negative OPC. The incidence trends by birth cohort and results from age-period-cohort models for both HPV-related and HPV-unrelated OPCs, clearly support a dominant role for birth cohort effects on the observed incidence patterns. It is crucial to mention that in fact in last years the diagnosis and screening for

OPCs has not significantly changed, so observation that HPV-related OPCs were diagnosed at younger ages may have also be a result of the increasing incidence among recent birth cohorts (Fig. 1).

Gillisson et al. (2012) conducted a cross-sectional study, on the statistically representative sample of the civilian non-institutionalized US population (National Health and Nutrition Examination Survey (NHANES) 2009–2010). Men and women aged 14–69 years ($N = 5579$) examined at mobile examination centers were involved in the study. Participants provided a 30 second oral rinse and gargle with mouthwash. The prevalence of oral HPV infection followed a bimodal pattern with age (Fig. 2), with a first peak in prevalence observed among those aged 30–34 years and a second, higher peak among those aged 60–64 years. Whether these peaks are caused by increased duration of infection over an individual's lifespan or whether they are caused by an increase in acquisition at older ages is an important epidemiological question. One of the hypotheses is the trend of changing sexual practices with oral sex being performed more by men and women that are currently aged 30–49 years compared to older generations. The second peak, however, cannot be entirely explained by sexual behaviors and could have also

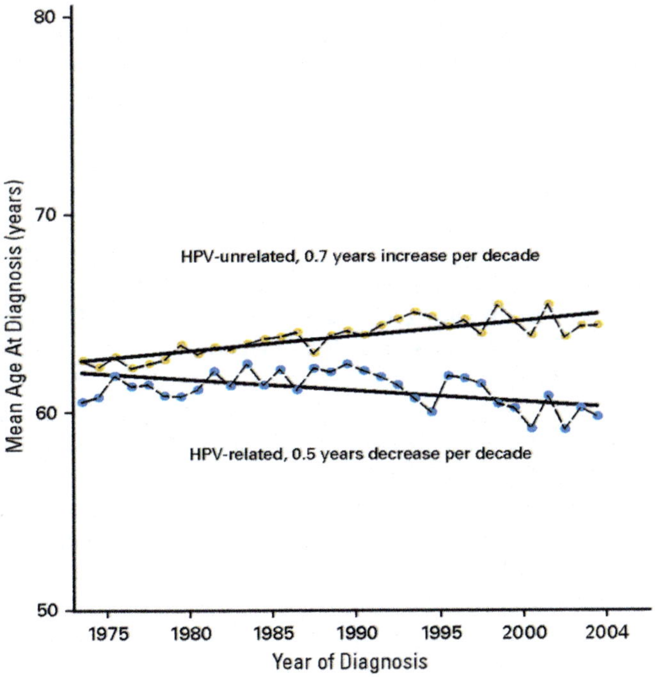

Fig. 1 Age-adjusted incidence by calendar year of diagnosis for human papillomavirus (HPV)-related sites (including base of tongue, lingual tonsil, tonsil, oropharynx, and Waldeyer ring) and HPV-unrelated sites (including other and unspecified parts of tongue). Chaturvedi et al. J Clin Oncol 2008

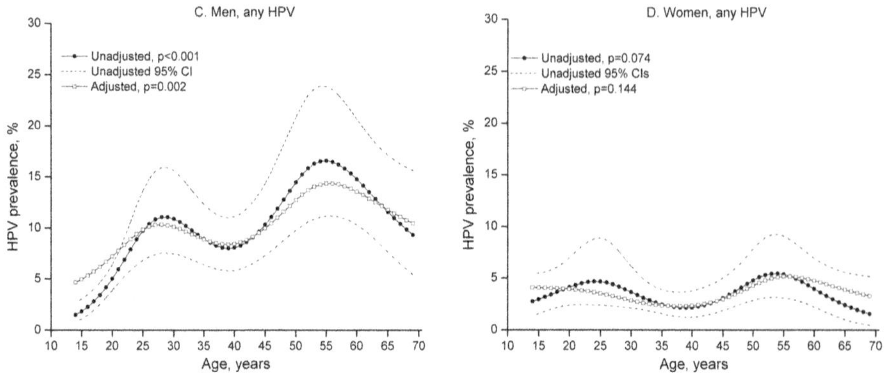

Fig. 2 Modeled HPV prevalence across age in the US population aged 14–69. Gillisson et al. JAMA 2012

arisen from a combination of increased incidence, reactivation of latent infections due to age-related loss of immunity, differences in sexual behaviors across birth cohorts, or increased persistence among older individuals.

Men had a significantly higher prevalence than women for overall oral HPV infection. The age and gender have also been confirmed as independent risk factors for HPV infection in a multivariable analysis, when the other significant risk factors including the number of the life time sexual partners and current smoking intensity have been considered.

The prevalence of oral HPV infection was significantly higher among men than among women, even after accounting for higher-risk behaviors reported by men. Significant interactions were observed between sex and age. Therefore, multivariable analyses were performed stratified by sex. A significant bimodal distribution across age was observed for men, but not for women (Fig. 2).

Chaturvedi et al. (2015) analyzed data for NHANES 2010–2012 represented by 219,608,892 individuals. Overall oral HPV infection was 6.8 %, but significantly higher among men than among women. (10.5 vs. 3.1 %, $P < 0.001$). The groups of oncogenic HPV and HPV 16 only were also more numerous among men than among women (Fig. 3). The prevalence of the oral HPV infection was similar in groups of NHANES 2010–2012 and 2009–2010.

In unadjusted analyses, demographic factors significantly associated with oral oncogenic HPV prevalence among men included older age (with a bimodal pattern), race/ethnicity, high school or equivalent education, marital status, current smoking (including serum cotinine levels) and marijuana use. Among women, age, race/ethnicity and serum cotinine levels were associated with oral oncogenic HPV prevalence. However, despite these factors, the gender remains the independent risk factor for oncogenic HPV infection. The analysis of US population of men and women separately across the subgroups defined by other key risk factors including age, tobacco smoking and number of the lifetime sexual partners has revealed

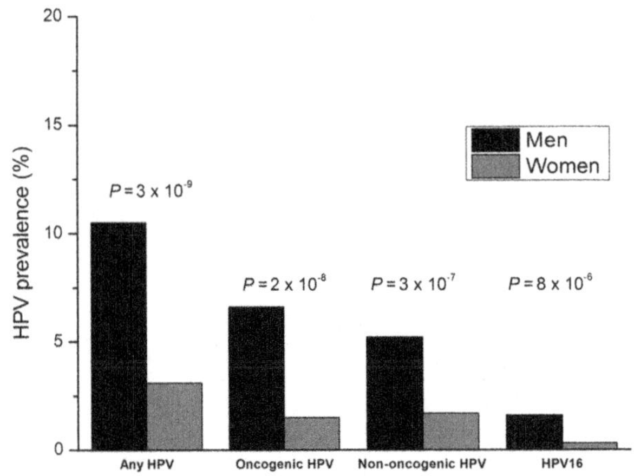

Fig. 3 Prevalence of any HPV infection, oncogenic HPV infection, non-oncogenic HPV infection and HPV type 16 infection among men (*black bars*) and women (*gray bars*). Chaturvedi Clin Cancer Res 2015

further contrasts. The prevalence of oncogenic infection was significantly higher among men than among women across all subgroups (Figs. 4 and 5).

The difference in a prevalence of the burden of oncogenic infections among men and women correlating with the incidence on the HPV-related OPC in these groups is evident. The explanation of that fact seems to be attributable to both behavioral

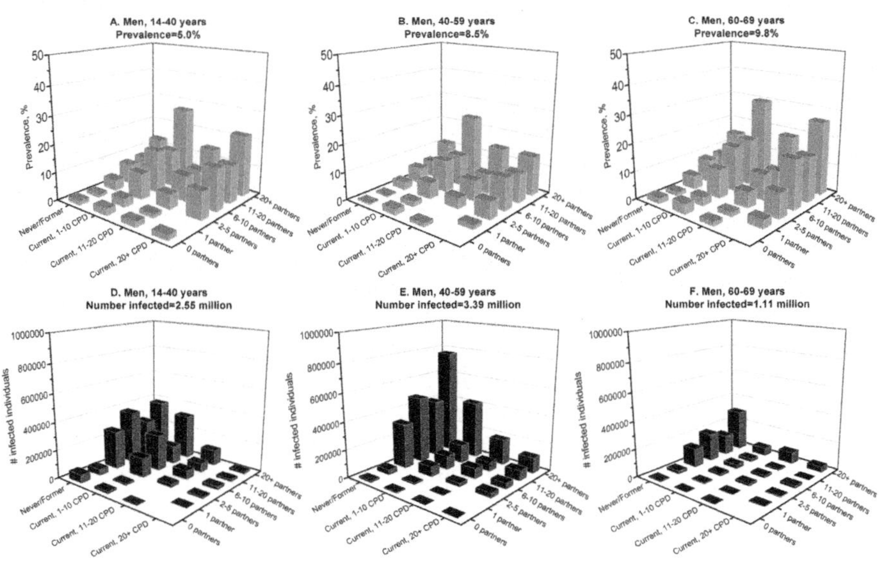

Fig. 4 Burden of oral oncogenic HPV infection among men in the USA

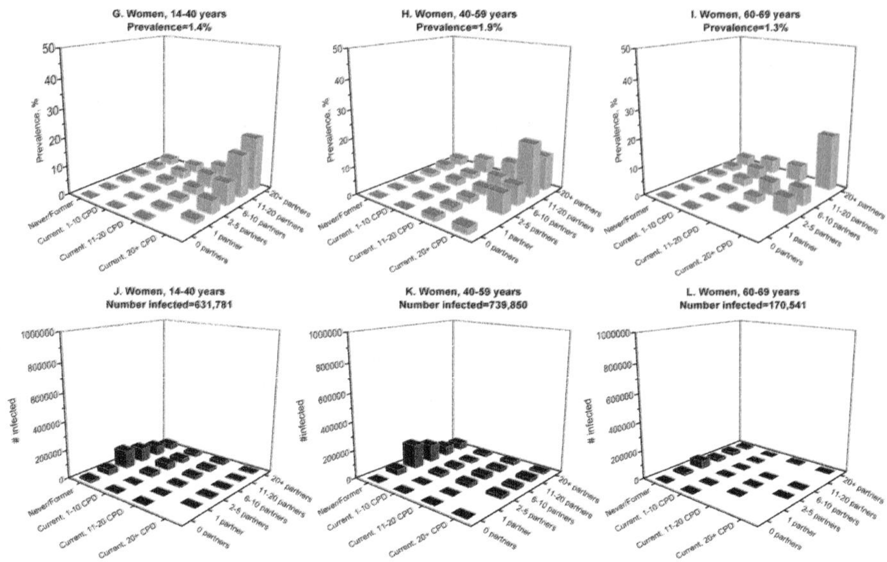

Fig. 5 Burden of oral oncogenic HPV infection among women in the USA. Chaturvedi Clin Cancer Res 2015

and biological differences between men and women. The majority of oral oncogenic HPV infections among are attributable to sexual behavior. Yet, men had substantially higher prevalence than women. This higher prevalence among men is partly explained by the significantly higher number of lifetime sexual partners reported by men. However, only 18 % of the male–female difference in prevalence can be clearly explained by differences in risk behaviors (i.e., smoking and number of sexual partners) between men and women.

The biological differences between genders may also contribute to the increased susceptibility of men to oral HPV infection. The immune responses to parasitic, bacterial and viral infections, but also vaccination, have been determined to vary between men and women. Men are characterized by generally weaker immune response (Klein 2000). Most of the available data come from the studies of anogenital HPV infections equally prevalent among men and women in younger ages. The data support the hypothesis that the seroconversion rates following genital HPV infection among men are lower and there are lower antibody titers upon seroconversion (Markowitz et al. 2009). Moreover, some studies clearly confirmed the absence of acquired immunity against reinfection among men (Lu et al. 2012) and the absence of age-related declines in genital HPV prevalence among men (Giuliano et al. 2011). Genital and oral HPV viral loads among men are also significantly higher than among women (Chaturvedi et al. 2014).

3 Sexual Behavior

Oral HPV infection, associated with the development of OPC, is predominantly sexually transmittable. The analysis of the multiple heterogenous populations in different parts of the world clearly indicated that more than 90 % of all oncogenic HPV infections are transmitted by the given form of the sexual contact and revealed that infection is an uncommon phenomenon in sexually inexperienced individuals. The infection prevalence is eightfold higher among sexually experienced individuals and increased significantly with number of sexual partners. Lifetime number of oral sexual partners has been previously considered to be the behavioral measure most strongly, consistently and specifically associated with oropharyngeal cancer (Marur et al. 2010). The risk of infection by sexual contact is, however, multifactorial. It depends on both the number of sexual partners during lifetime and the form of sexual contacts. Gillison et al. (2012) has performed a comprehensive analysis of the NHANES 2009–2010 study group in terms of sexual behavior. She analyzed the type of the sexual contact (any form of sexual contact, vaginal, oral or anal), the lifetime number of sexual partners, number of sexual partners within last 12 months but also the frequency of particular contacts and sexual orientation.

The analysis revealed that oral HPV prevalence was more than eightfold higher among individuals who reported ever having had sex versus not. Prevalence of HPV increased with lifetime or recent number of partners for any kind of sex, vaginal sex or oral sex. One in five individuals with more than 20 lifetime sexual partners was infected. Prevalence was higher among individuals who first performed oral sex at 18 years or younger.

A recent analysis of the NHANES data (2009–2012) (Chaturvedi et al. 2015) demonstrated the per sexual partner increase in high-risk oral HPV prevalence to be threefold greater for men than for women, consistent with reported higher transmission rates for HPV from female to male than vice versa. Also noted was a plateau in prevalence among men at approximately 15 oral sexual partners in contrast to approximately five partners among women (Fig. 7).

Thus, the prevalence of oral HPV infection continues to increase among men with more than five partners, but not among women. This sex difference may reflect reduced seroconversion rates among men versus women after genital HPV

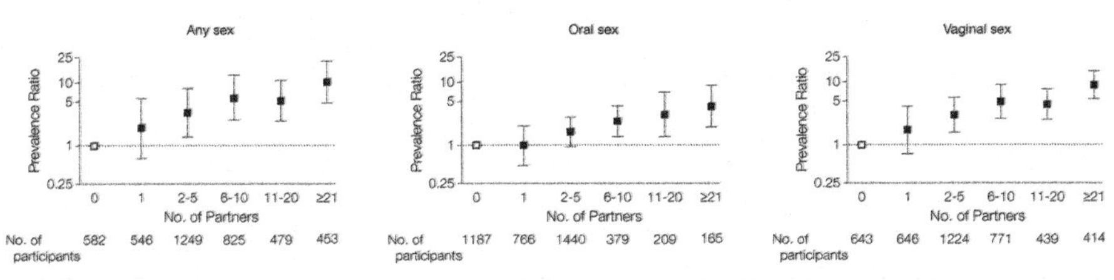

Fig. 6 Association of number of lifetime sexual partners with prevalent oral HPV infection. Gillisson et al. JAMA 2012

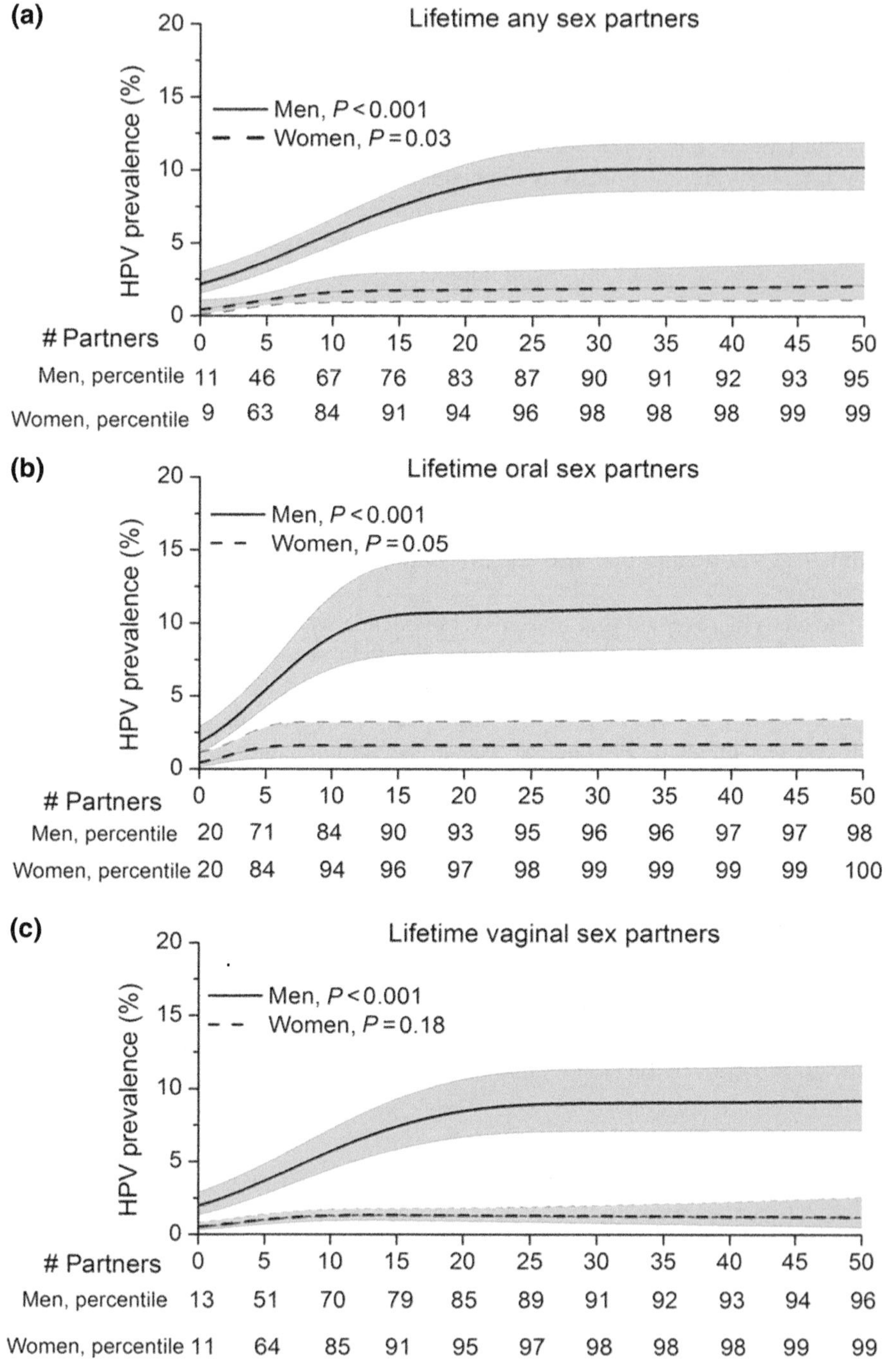

Fig. 7 Gender, sexual behavior and oral HPV. Chaturvedi Clin Cancer Res 2015

infection Giuliano et al. 2015, resulting in greater protection against subsequent oral infections among women. Natural seroconversion to genital HPV16 infection reduces risk of subsequent infection among women by approximately 50 % Ho et al. 2002. Thus, increased oral sexual behaviors among recent birth cohorts of men and women would result in greater prevalence increases for oral HPV infection and consequent accelerated rates for HPV-positive OPC in men versus women over the last several decades in the USA.

Kreimer et al. (2013) analyzed the 1626 men aged 18–73 years coming from Brazil, Mexico and the USA who were HIV-negative and reported no history of anogenital cancer and were recruited into the *HPV Infection in Men* (*HIM*) cohort study. According to their analysis, marital status was strongly associated with risk of acquiring any and oncogenic oral HPV infections, with married or cohabiting men at a significantly reduced risk in both categories. Marital status seems to be more predictive of oral HPV acquisition than lifetime number of sexual partners does. Also in multivariable models, the effect estimates for marital status remained unchanged after adjustment for lifetime number of sexual partners. The sexual orientation was also associated with risk of oral HPV infection in our study, with bisexual men at the highest risk. These findings suggest that marital status and sexual orientation could reflect a participant's likelihood of engaging in risky sexual behaviors and partnerships, or differences in a participant's sexual network, and that these characteristics might be more predictive of risk than lifetime number of sexual partners.

4 Smoking

Smoking and use of other forms of tobacco are the strongest causative risk factors for the development of the squamous cell carcinoma of the head and neck. Because of significant decrease in smoking in the western world in the past decade, the incidence of the tobacco-related HNSCC is slightly lower. However, use of tobacco products may also have an impact on the development of HPV-related head and neck tumors by facilitating the oral HPV infection. For the cervical cancer where the HPV infection is the necessary cause, the tobacco smoking is an established co-existing risk factor (Bosch and de Sanjose 2007).

There is an evidence that current tobacco smoking may be an important risk factor for the HPV infection. Fakhry et al. (2014), in large cross-sectional populations-based study, showed the significant dose-dependent relationship between tobacco smoking and HPV infection.

Current tobacco users were more likely than nonusers to be male, younger less educated and have higher number of lifetime oral partners. Oral HPV16 prevalence was greater in current tobacco users compared with newer/former tobacco users. In HIM cohort study (Kreimer et al. 2013), cigarette smoking was significantly associated with acquisition of oral HPV in healthy men; the risk of acquiring an oncogenic oral HPV infection was nearly three times higher in current smokers

(HR = 2·80) and more than two times higher in former smokers (HR = 2·31) than in those who had never smoked. However, the effect of the tobacco smoke as a factor facilitating oral HPV infection remains unclear, and it has been proven to have the local and systemic immunosuppressive and proinflammatory effect. The direct contact of the carcinogens in the tobacco smoke with the oral mucosa is likely to increase the likelihood of HPV infection.

5 HIV and Immunosuppression

The life expectancy of HIV-infected individuals has significantly increased in last years, mainly due to effective antiretroviral therapy (ART) significantly reducing viral-related malignancies such as Kaposi Sarcoma and Non-Hodgkin's lymphoma. The longer lifespan is, however, associated with higher probability of development of HPV-associated malignancies. Several cross-sectional studies have observed that HIV-infected individuals have a 2–3 fold higher odds of prevalent oral HPV infection compared to HIV-uninfected individuals, even after adjustment for sexual behavior and other relevant factors (Beachler et al. 2012; Kreimer et al. 2004). Beachler in his study (Beachler and D'Souza 2013) analyzed HIV-infected individuals from previous studies and found an overall oral HPV DNA prevalence to be between 20 and 45 %. Oncogenic oral HPV DNA with the predominance of HPV 16 was reported in between 12 and 26 %.

The mechanism of the increased HPV prevalence in HIV-positive individuals is most likely to be associated with HIV-related immunosuppression. Advanced stage of HIV disease, characterized by low CD4 T cell count and high HIV viral load, has also been associated with increased oral HPV prevalence which may reflect a loss of viral control in those with compromised immune systems. The direct effect of immunosuppression on oral HPV persistence is currently less understood, but research on other HPV-associated cancers suggests immunosuppression may act more on the earlier stages of the HPV carcinogenesis process (Palefsky 2006). The hypothesis of the immunosuppression as a factor facilitating the infection and persistence of the virus has been also supported by the increased prevalence among solid organ transplant recipients, another immunosuppressed population (Grulich et al. 2007). Reduced CD4 T cell count was nonsignificantly related to the higher risk of development of oropharyngeal cancer in several independent studies (Clifford et al. 2005; Silverberg et al. 2011; Engels et al. 2008). Engels et al. found a higher risk of oral cavity/pharynx cancer in individuals with AIDS relative to HIV-infected individuals who have not developed AIDS (Engels et al. 2008).

However, effective antiretroviral therapy has greatly improved the life expectancy of HIV-infected individuals while reducing viral-related malignancies such as Kaposi Sarcoma and Non-Hodgkin's lymphoma, and the incidence rates of HPV-associated malignancies have remained stable. A preliminary study suggested ART use was associated with increased six-month oral HPV persistence (D'Souza et al. 2007), and other studies have suggested ART use is associated with an increase in oral lesions/warts (Anaya-Saavedra et al. 2013; Greenspan et al. 2001). However, these studies may be prone to confounding by indication, as ART is more likely to be indicated for sicker individuals.

The data from cervical HPV analysis have indicated that ART reduces the incidence of cervical HPV, decreases the incidence of squamous epithelial lesions and increases the regression of these lesions (Adler et al. 2012). However, if ART use does not fully recover oral HPV-specific immunity, it may not be able to substantially modify the elevated oral HPV incidence or persistence seen in HIV-infected individuals. Therefore, HPV-associated OPC could pose a further increasing threat for immune-competent HIV-infected individuals, if ART improves survival but did not improve control of oral HPV infections.

6 Conclusions

- Oral HPV infection has dramatically altered the landscape of HNC in numerous populations worldwide. The prevalence, despite significant variation in numerous geographical locations, is constantly increasing.
- The sexual behavior is the most important risk factor for oral oncogenic HPV infection
- The higher risk for HPV-positive cancer among men is attributable to both behavioral and biological differences between men and women.
- Oral HPV16 prevalence is greater in current tobacco users compared with newer/former tobacco users.
- The prevalence among HIV-positive individuals is significantly higher most likely due to HIV-related immunosuppression.

References

Adler DH, Kakinami L, Modisenyane T et al (2012) Increased regression and decreased incidence of human papillomavirus-related cervical lesions among HIV-infected women on HAART. AIDS 26:1645–1652

Anaya-Saavedra G, Flores-Moreno B, Garcia-Carranca A, Irigoyen-Camacho E, Guido-Jimenez M, Ramirez-Amador V (2013) HPV oral lesions in HIV-infected patients: the impact of long-term HAART. J Oral Pathol Med 42:443–449

Beachler DC, D'Souza G (2013) Oral human papillomavirus infection and head and neck cancers in HIV-infected individuals. Curr Opin Oncol 25:503–510

Beachler DC, Weber KM, Margolick JB et al (2012) Risk factors for oral HPV infection among a high prevalence population of HIV-positive and at-risk HIV-negative adults. Cancer Epidemiol Biomarkers Prev 21:122–133

Bosch FX, de Sanjose S (2007) The epidemiology of human papillomavirus infection and cervical cancer. Dis Markers 23:213–227

Chaturvedi AK, Engels EA, Pfeiffer RM et al (2011) Human papillomavirus and rising oropharyngeal cancer incidence in the United States. J Clin Oncol 29:4294–4301

Chaturvedi AK, Graubard BI, Pickard RK, Xiao W, Gillison ML (2014) High-risk oral human papillomavirus load in the US population, National health and nutrition examination survey 2009–2010. J Infect Dis 210:441–447
Chaturvedi AK, Graubard BI, Broutian T et al (2015) NHANES 2009–2012 findings: association of sexual behaviors with higher prevalence of oral oncogenic human papillomavirus infections in U.S. men. Cancer Res 75:2468–2477
Clifford GM, Polesel J, Rickenbach M et al (2005) Cancer risk in the Swiss HIV cohort study: associations with immunodeficiency, smoking, and highly active antiretroviral therapy. J Natl Cancer Inst 97:425–432
D'Souza G, Kreimer AR, Viscidi R et al (2007) Case-control study of human papillomavirus and oropharyngeal cancer. N Engl J Med 356:1944–1956
Engels EA, Biggar RJ, Hall HI et al (2008) Cancer risk in people infected with human immunodeficiency virus in the United States. Int J Cancer 123:187–194
Fakhry C, Gillison ML, D'Souza G (2014) Tobacco use and oral HPV-16 infection. JAMA 312:1465–1467
Gillison ML (2007) Current topics in the epidemiology of oral cavity and oropharyngeal cancers. Head Neck 29:779–792
Gillison ML, Koch WM, Capone RB et al (2000) Evidence for a causal association between human papillomavirus and a subset of head and neck cancers. J Natl Cancer Inst 92:709–720
Gillison ML, D'Souza G, Westra W et al (2008) Distinct risk factor profiles for human papillomavirus type 16-positive and human papillomavirus type 16-negative head and neck cancers. J Natl Cancer Inst 100:407–420
Gillison ML, Broutian T, Pickard RK et al (2012) Prevalence of oral HPV infection in the United States, 2009–2010. JAMA 307:693–703
Gillison ML, Chaturvedi AK, Anderson WF, Fakhry C (2015) Epidemiology of human papillomavirus-positive head and neck squamous cell carcinoma. J Clin Oncol 33:3235–3242
Giuliano AR, Lee JH, Fulp W et al (2011) Incidence and clearance of genital human papillomavirus infection in men (HIM): a cohort study. Lancet 377:932–940
Giuliano AR, Nyitray AG, Kreimer AR et al (2015) EUROGIN 2014 roadmap: Differences in human papillomavirus infection natural history, transmission and human papillomavirus-related cancer incidence by gender and anatomic site of infection. Int J Cancer 136:2752–2760
Greenspan D, Canchola AJ, MacPhail LA, Cheikh B, Greenspan JS (2001) Effect of highly active antiretroviral therapy on frequency of oral warts. Lancet 357:1411–1412
Grulich AE, van Leeuwen MT, Falster MO, Vajdic CM (2007) Incidence of cancers in people with HIV/AIDS compared with immunosuppressed transplant recipients: a meta-analysis. Lancet 370:59–67
Hammarstedt L, Lindquist D, Dahlstrand H et al (2006) Human papillomavirus as a risk factor for the increase in incidence of tonsillar cancer. Int J Cancer 119:2620–2623
Ho GY, Studentsov Y, Hall CB et al (2002) Risk factors for subsequent cervicovaginal human papillomavirus (HPV) infection and the protective role of antibodies to HPV-16 virus-like particles. J Infect Dis 186:737–742
Jay N, Moscicki AB (2000) Human papillomavirus infections in women with HIV disease: prevalence, risk, and management. AIDS Read 10:659–668
Klein SL (2000) The effects of hormones on sex differences in infection: from genes to behavior. Neurosci Biobehav Rev 24:627–638
Kreimer AR, Alberg AJ, Daniel R et al (2004) Oral human papillomavirus infection in adults is associated with sexual behavior and HIV serostatus. J Infect Dis 189:686–698
Kreimer AR, Pierce Campbell CM, Lin HY et al (2013) Incidence and clearance of oral human papillomavirus infection in men: the HIM cohort study. Lancet 382:877–887
Lewis A, Kang R, Levine A, Maghami E (2015) The new face of head and neck cancer: the HPV epidemic. Oncology (Williston Park) 29:616–626
Lu B, Viscidi RP, Wu Y et al (2012) Prevalent serum antibody is not a marker of immune protection against acquisition of oncogenic HPV16 in men. Cancer Res 72:676–685

Markowitz LE, Sternberg M, Dunne EF, McQuillan G, Unger ER (2009) Seroprevalence of human papillomavirus types 6, 11, 16, and 18 in the United States: National health and nutrition examination survey 2003–2004. J Infect Dis 200:1059–1067

Marur S, D'Souza G, Westra WH, Forastiere AA (2010) HPV-associated head and neck cancer: a virus-related cancer epidemic. Lancet Oncol 11:781–789

Palefsky J (2006) Biology of HPV in HIV infection. Adv Dent Res 19:99–105

Schantz SP, Yu GP (2002) Head and neck cancer incidence trends in young Americans, 1973–1997, with a special analysis for tongue cancer. Arch Otolaryngol Head Neck Surg 128:268–274

Schwartz SR, Yueh B, McDougall JK, Daling JR, Schwartz SM (2001) Human papillomavirus infection and survival in oral squamous cell cancer: a population-based study. Otolaryngol Head Neck Surg 125:1–9

Silverberg MJ, Chao C, Leyden WA et al (2011) HIV infection, immunodeficiency, viral replication, and the risk of cancer. Cancer Epidemiol Biomarkers Prev 20:2551–2559

Part II
HPV Testing

HPV-Related Head and Neck Squamous Cell Carcinomas

Andrzej Marszałek and Łukasz Szylberg

Abstract

Since more than 5 years, it becomes evident that there is a new group of patients with squamous cell carcinomas of the head and neck area, namely human papillomavirus (HPV)-related (caused) tumors. As clinical statistics indicate, those patients have better prognosis, even despite more advanced stage compared to those with HPV-negative tumors. In fact, as a surrogate of HPV infection for clinical studies, an immunohistochemical expression of p16 protein is used. In the following chapter, the spectrum of squamous cell carcinomas variants with indication of the percentage cases with proved HPV infection will be presented.

Keywords

HPV-carcinomas · Histopathology · Classification

1 Introduction

As presented in the key paper by Marur et al. (2010), it becomes evident a new entity of head and neck squamous cell carcinomas. This new group related to infection by human papillomavirus (HPV) has a growing epidemiologic tendency. Those tumors were attributed to the oropharynx (including base of tongue and

A. Marszałek (✉)
Department of Oncologic Pathology and Prophylactics, Greater Poland Cancer Center, Poznan University of Medical Sciences, Poznan, Poland
e-mail: andrzej.marszalek@wco.pl

Ł. Szylberg
Department of Clinical Pathomorphology, Collegium Medicum in Bydgoszcz, Nicolaus Copernicus University in Torun, Torun, Poland

W. Golusiński et al. (eds.), *HPV Infection in Head and Neck Cancer*,
Recent Results in Cancer Research 206, DOI 10.1007/978-3-319-43580-0_6

tonsils). According to their histology, they tend to be non-keratinized squamous cell carcinomas. The clinical data indicate that gender predilection, e.g., male-to-female ratio, remains the same as in classical type as 3:1. Those tumors tend to be diagnosed in younger generation, even by 20–30 years. Additionally, HPV-related cancers although with more dynamic biology were diagnosed at earlier stage and treated with better outcome, regardless of the way of treatment (e.g., surgery, chemotherapy, radiotherapy, and multimodal therapeutic approach) (Pai et al. 2009; Gray et al. 2015; Betiol et al. 2013; Fakhry et al. 2014). The incidence of this aforementioned tumor type is growing. The most common type of primary head and neck region cancer is squamous cell carcinoma (Pannone et al. 2011). But according to its morphology changing between cases, there were introduced some subtypes (Table 1). In the following part, there were presented most important morphological and clinical data to subtypes of squamous cell carcinomas (El-Mofty 2012). A special attention will be paid to the occurrence of cases (Fig. 1) with proved HPV correlation (Figs. 2 and 3).

Table 1 Squamous cell carcinoma in head and neck region

"Classical-type" variants
Verrucous carcinoma
Basaloid squamous cell carcinoma
Spindle cell (sarcomatoid) squamous cell carcinoma
Papillary squamous cell carcinoma
Adenosquamous carcinoma
Lymphoepitheliomatous carcinoma
Sinonasal non-keratinizing carcinoma
Adenoid squamous (acantholytic) carcinoma
HPV-associated oropharyngeal squamous cell carcinoma

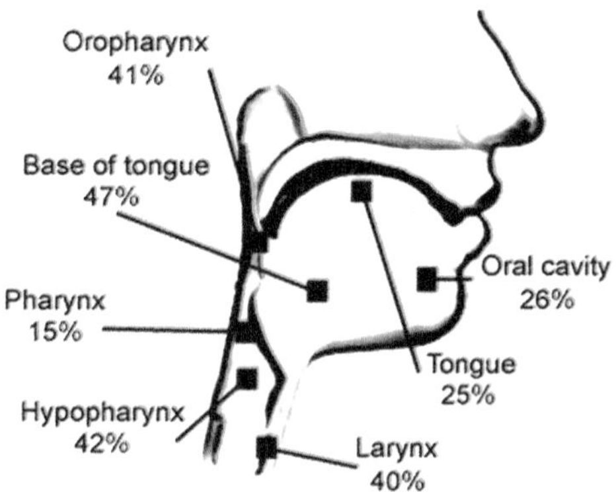

Fig. 1 Epidemiological distribution of HPV-positive cancers in head and neck region in Europe (according to Abogunrin et al. BMC Cancer, 2014; **14**, 1)

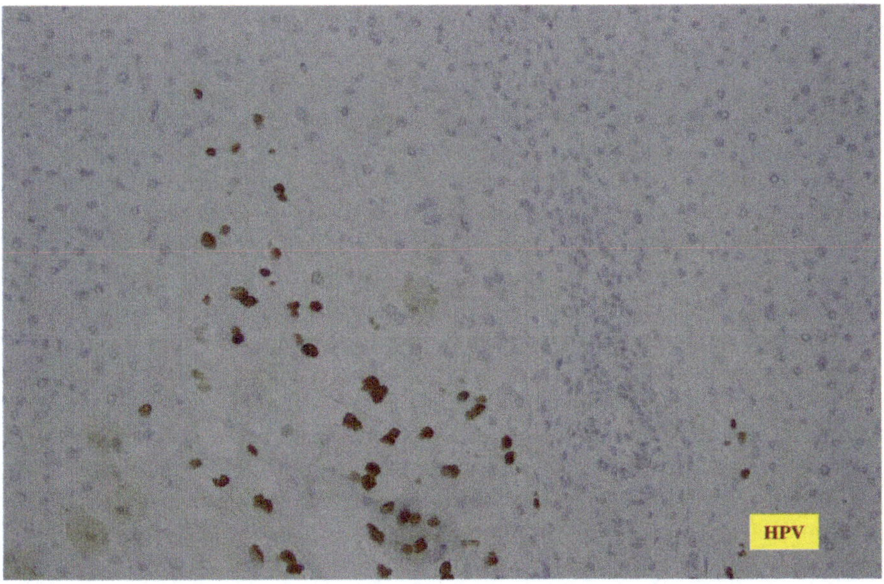

Fig. 2 Immunohistochemical visualization of HPV antigen expressed in squamous cell carcinoma

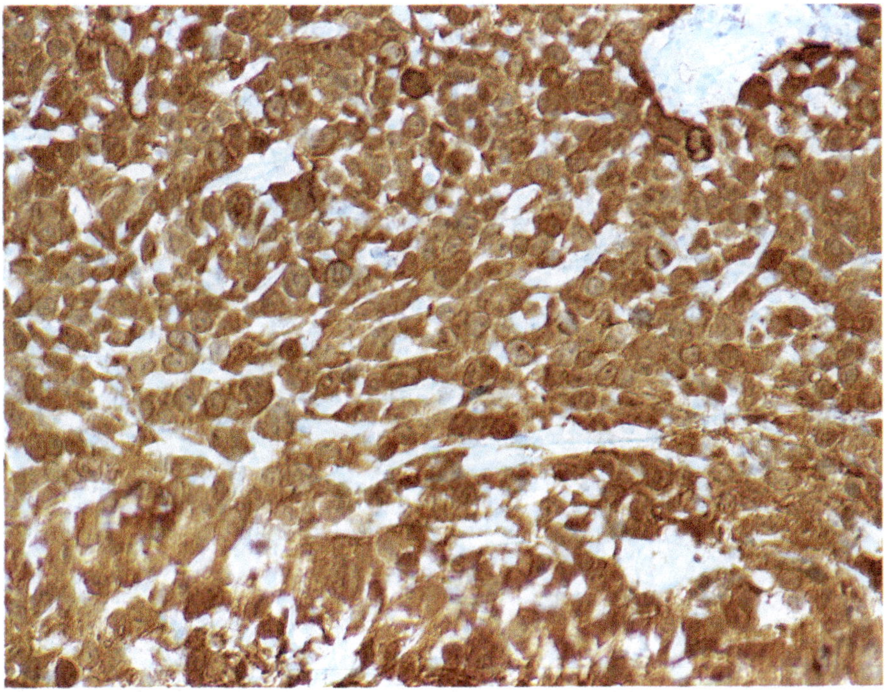

Fig. 3 Immunohistochemical visualization of overexpression of p16 in squamous cell carcinoma

2 Squamous Cell Carcinoma: "Classic" Type ("Classic" SCC)

The so-called classical type of SCC (with some histologically visible evidence of keratinization) of head and neck region consists of about 1 % of all malignancies in humans. However, it comprises more then 90 % of all malignancies in larynx. This type of tumor occurs usually in adults with peak from 6th to 7th decade. It is much more common in males, reaching incidence of 1/10,000 population, while among females, it is diagnosed as common as 1/100,000. But the most common male-to-female ratio is presented as 6:1. This classical type of tumor is attributed to the typical (in common sense) risk factors such as tobacco smoking (or exposure to tobacco smoke in environment) and alcohol abuse (Pai et al. 2009). In this "classical" variant, a very common alteration of p53 is found—especially in those associated with exposure to alcohol and tobacco. There are also correlations with long-standing gastroesophageal reflux, as well as radiation exposure. In some reports, there were indicated genetic risk factors, including Lynch syndrome, Bloom syndrome, and Li–Fraumeni syndrome. In classic SCC, an epidermal growth factor receptor (EGFR) overexpression is commonly found. It is related to more aggressive outcome. However, immunohistochemically estimated p16-positive cases along with low EGFR have better prognosis (Alexandrov et al. 2013). Morphologic examination reveals its occurrence in almost all anatomical areas. It could be

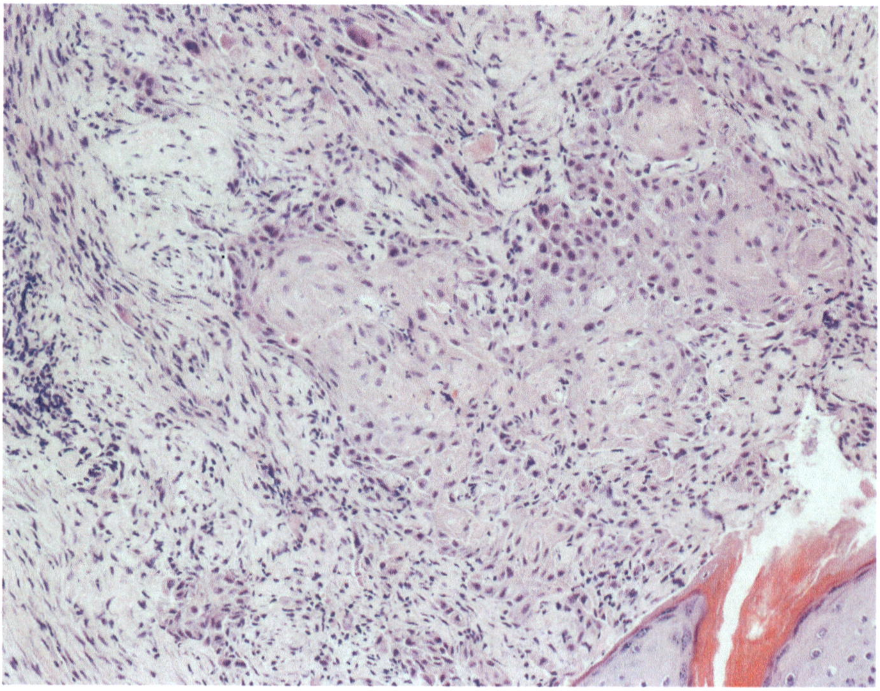

Fig. 4 Histological picture of classical squamous cell carcinoma

supraglottic (this localization predominates in Europe), glottic (predominate in US patients), subglottic, and transglottic. Macroscopically, those tumors either could be ulcerative or might grow endophytically or as flat or even polypoid masses; verrucous and exophytic lesions are also described (Cardesa et al. 2011).

On microscopic examination, it could be keratinizing or non-keratinized SCC (Fig. 4).

3 Squamous Cell Carcinoma: "Verrucous" Type ("Verrucous" SCC)

Verrucous type of SCC consists of about 3% of all SCC in head and neck region. This type of SCC is clearly correlated with HPV infection (Orvidas et al. 1998). It is most commonly found in oral cavity and then in larynx. In oral localization, it is found more common in females than in males, while in all other places male patients predominate (Orvidas et al. 1999). This tumor type has a distinct morphology. Macroscopically, it is described as broad-based warty mass that could be very large (even up to 10 cm of diameter). Microscopically, it also has distinct features such as clearly visible large club-shaped rete pegs (Fig. 5). In all tumors, there is abundant keratin. But usually, there is no pleomorphism of tumor cells.

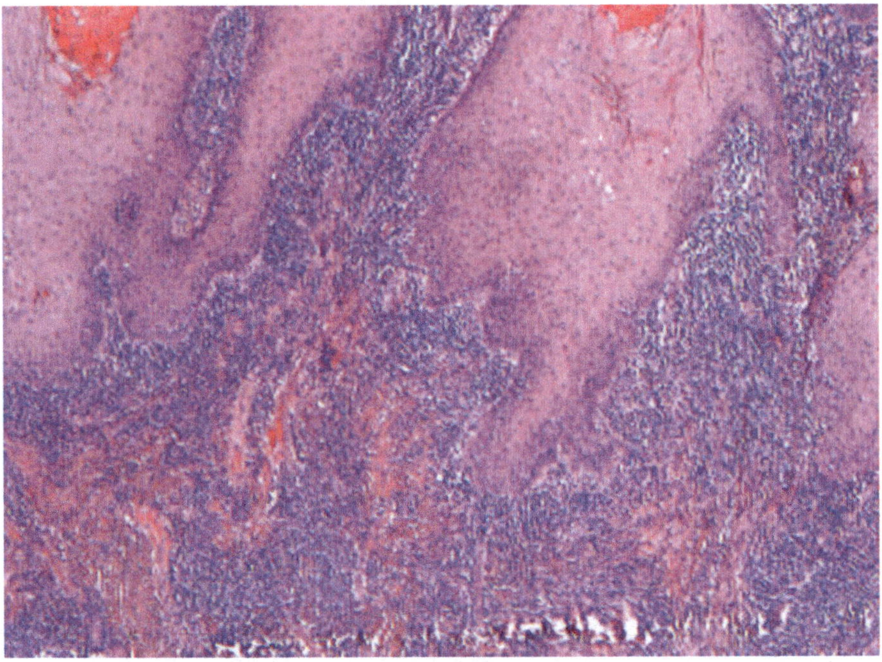

Fig. 5 Verrucous variant of squamous cell carcinoma

Additionally, usually there is no mitotic activity found. Those lately mentioned features are related to very good prognosis with a 5-year survival rate of about 75 % cases (Santoro et al. 2011; Teymoortash et al. 2014).

4 Squamous Cell Carcinoma: "Spindle Cell" ("Sarcomatoid") Type ("Spindle Cell" SCC)

Sarcomatoid SCC according to its microscopic morphology resembling spindle cells of mesenchymal origin should be first differentially diagnosed with pleomorphic high-grade sarcoma. But primary sarcomas of this morphology in such localization are extremely rare. On the other hand, as in those tumors a coincidence of immunohistochemical markers for mesenchymal origin (positivity for vimentin) and ectodermal/epithelial origin (positive reactions with different types of cytokeratins) is found, and they could be called "collision" squamous cell carcinoma—highlighting their peculiar histology (Bishop et al. 2014). Sarcomatoid SCC consists of about 3 % of SCC in head and neck area. Some reports indicate radiation as their possible risk factor. Such tumors could be found in larynx. Next, in order of incidence is oral cavity, then nasal cavity (Stransky et al. 2011). According to gender differences, male cases are far more common than female. Macroscopically, they usually form polypoid mass of about 2 cm diameter. Microscopic pictures

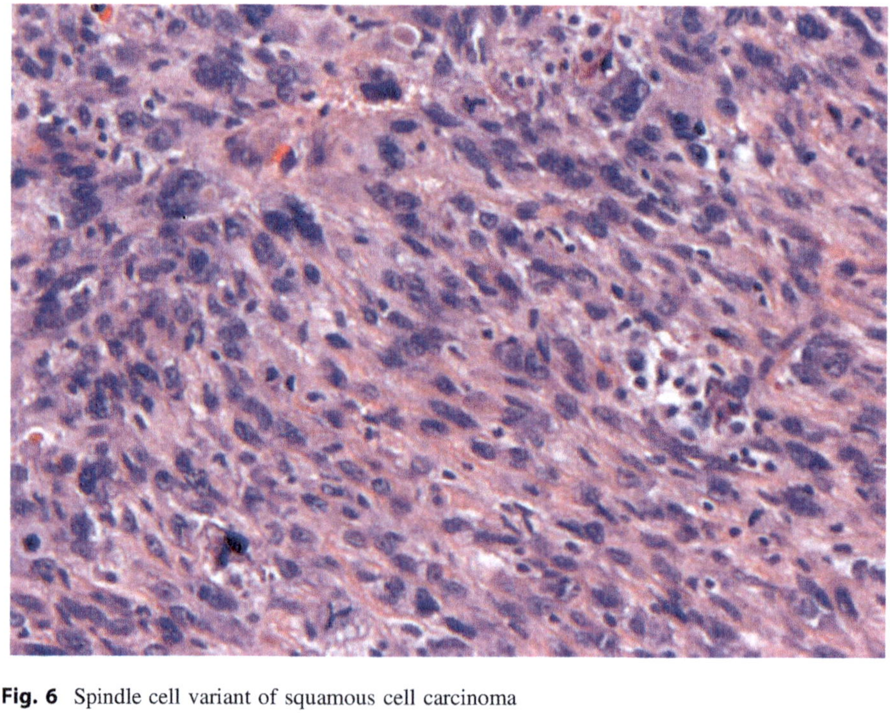

Fig. 6 Spindle cell variant of squamous cell carcinoma

have some tips enabling its diagnosis include a biphasic morphology. There are areas of squamous cell carcinoma differentiation along with area of atypical spindle cells (resembling mesenchymal tumors, for instance fibrosarcoma or any other sarcoma). These tumors are usually hypercellular with prominent pleomorphism and high mitotic activity (Fig. 6). According to clinical data, the 5-year survival could reach 80 %.

5 Basaloid Squamous Cell Carcinoma (BSCC)

BSCC is uncommon variant of "classic" SCC. It occurs in less than 1 % of squamous cell carcinoma in the head and neck region. BSCC is associated with conventional risk factors such as smoking and alcohol abuse (Marur et al. 2010). These lesions are typically aggressive variant of squamous cancer with early lymph node metastasis (68 % of patients have regional metastases at presentation) and poor prognosis with 2-*year survival* rates of less than 40 %. It has predilection for hypopharynx and larynx and less frequently oropharynx, but also occurs in other sites such as lung. Microscopically, BSCC has biphasic pattern which includes basaloid component and often areas with typical squamous differentiation (Fakhry et al. 2014). The basaloid cells are pleomorphic with minimal cytoplasm and hyperchromatic nuclei. They form demarcated nests of small basaloid cells with

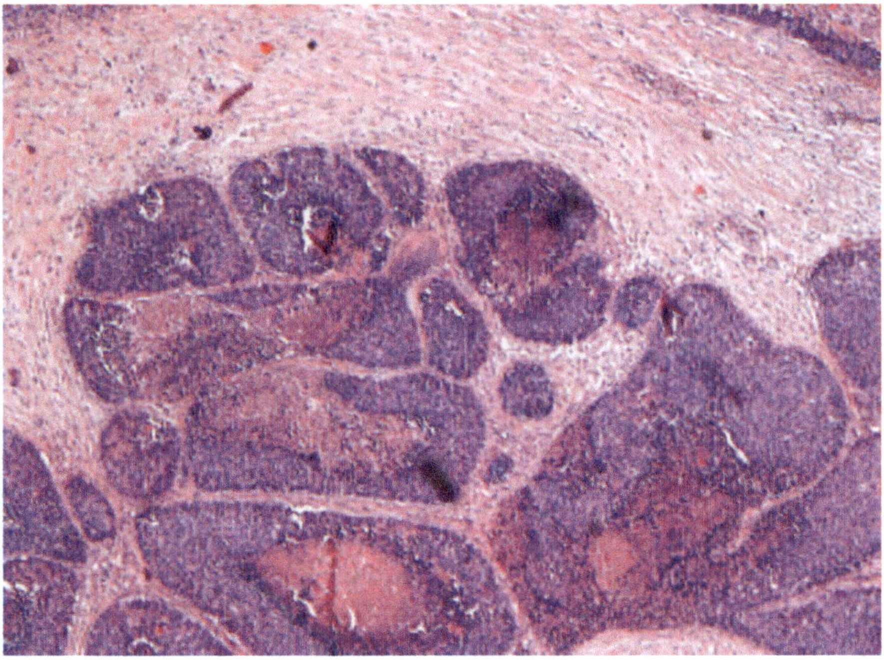

Fig. 7 Basaloid variant of squamous cell carcinoma with clearly visible comedonecrosis

peripheral palisading and show numerous mitotic figures. Comedonecrosis is common (Fig. 7). Stromal hyalinization may be present. Pseudoglandular spaces resembling adenoid cystic carcinoma may occur. HPV-16 is detectable in majority (more than 75 % of cases) of oropharyngeal BSCC (El-Mofty 2012). The absence of HPV-16 in these tumors is associated with a decreased overall survival. HPV-positive tumors affected younger patients.

6 Papillary Squamous Cell Carcinoma (PSCC)

True papillary carcinomas are rare. PSCC is usually confused with other exophytic mucosal malignancies, such as verrucous carcinoma and squamous cell carcinoma with verrucous features. PSCC occurs in less than 1 % of squamous cell carcinoma in the head and neck region and has a favorable prognosis with 5-*year survival* rates more than 70 % (Marur et al. 2010). These lesions have predilection for larynx and less frequently oral and nasal mucosa. Microscopically, PSCC is composed of exophytic papillary squamous proliferation overlying a thin fibrovascular core. Neoplastic cells may resemble immature basaloid cells or dysplastic cells with variable keratosis. There is significant cytologic atypia, but stromal invasion may not be prominent (Mehrad et al. 2013). A very limited number of studies have investigated the significance of HPV in PSCC of the head and neck. Studies revealed transcriptionally active HPV in more than 50 % of tumors (El-Mofty 2012). The majority of HPV-positive tumors arise in the oropharynx and demonstrate non-keratinizing morphology. HPV-related tumors showed a trend toward better survival.

7 Adenosquamous Carcinoma (AdSC)

Adenosquamous carcinoma (AdSC) is a rare variant of SCC, characterized by mixed differentiation; with both SCC and adenocarcinoma. It occurs in less than 1 % of squamous cell carcinoma in the head and neck region. It has predilection for larynx and, in descending frequency, the oral cavity, sinonasal tract, oropharynx, and hypopharynx (Masand et al. 2011). These lesions are typically aggressive with early lymph node metastasis and poor prognosis with 2-*year survival* rates of less than 55%. AdSC is more common among men (male-to-female ratio of 6:1). Microscopically, AdSC has two distinct histological components. In the majority of cases, SCC predominates and can be in situ or invasive. The adenocarcinomatous component can form tubules, ducts, or glandular structures and typically produce mucin. The adenocarcinoma usually occurs in the deeper parts of the tumor. Mixture of adenocarcinoma and squamous cell carcinoma may resemble mucoepidermoid carcinoma (El-Mofty 2012). The relationship with HPV has not been well studied (Chen et al. 2012). Based on the very limited number of HPV-positive AdSC tumors, particularly in the oropharynx, they may have a more favorable prognosis.

8 Nasopharyngeal Carcinoma/Lymphoepithelioma (NPC)

NPC is a rare entity in the so-called Western world. But it is diagnosed more commonly in China. Such an incidence is attributed to the main risk factors such as infection with Epstein–Barr Virus (EBV). Additional risk factors consist of nitrosamines and smoking (Gray et al. 2015). NPC could develop in rather young patients, with peak between 4th and 6th decade. Almost all SCC is more common in males than in females. NPC might have a variable macroscopic presentation. Histologically, it could be keratinized or non-keratinized SCC. However, they could be described as undifferentiated carcinomas as well (Molinolo et al. 2009; Galbiatti et al. 2014). The microscopic tips useful in diagnosis include the following: diffuse cells areas with local syncytial arrangement. In classical cases, there is no keratinization and no necrosis. Lack of necrosis is used as one of the key diagnostic features. However, under microscopic examination the presence of brisk mitoses and apoptosis is easily found (Fig. 8). The prognosis in those patients is accompanied with 65 % 5-year survival.

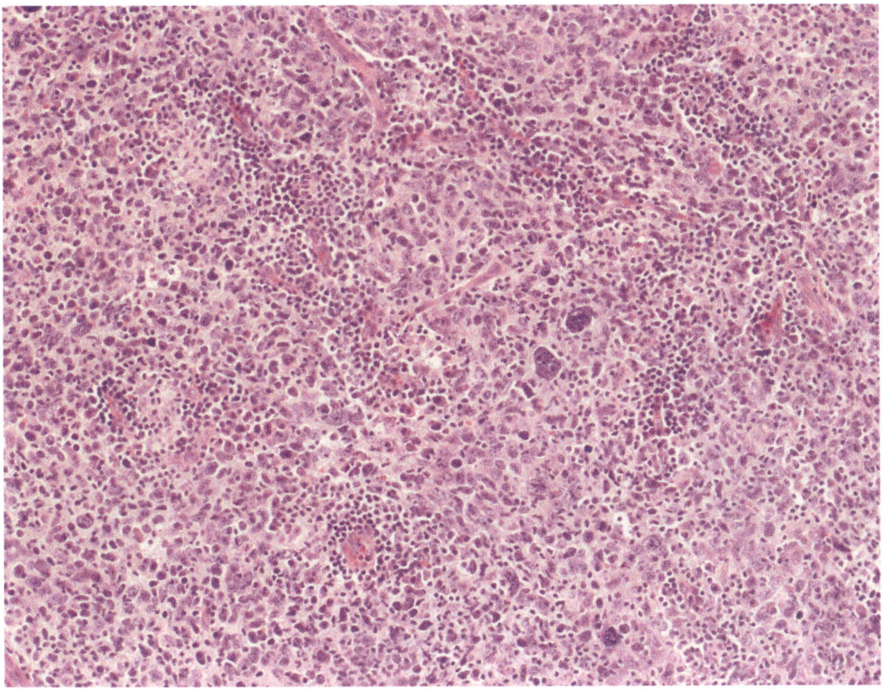

Fig. 8 Nasopharyngeal carcinoma (lymphoepithelioma)

9 Sinonasal Undifferentiated Carcinoma (Anaplastic) (SNUC)

SNUC is a rare entity accompanied with highly aggressive biology. Risk factors are probably smoking (as 85 % of patients are smokers) and possibly radiation. SNUC is mainly diagnosed in nasal cavity (Masand et al. 2011; Galbiatti et al. 2014). But it could occur in sinuses as well. Peak incidence occurs in 6th decade with far more common predilection for male patients. The tumor has macroscopically fungating and infiltrative pattern of growth. At diagnosis, tumor mass is usual over 4 cm in diameter. On microscopic examination, it is a hypercellular tumor with very high mitotic activity. Cells present high pleomorphisms (Fig. 9). There is prominent necrosis (Machado et al. 2010; Mandapathil et al. 2014). As a common finding, one can see lymphatic and perineural invasion. No squamous nor glandular differentiation is found. The prognosis is very poor. Some authors indicate the presence of p16 overexpression, but probably not related to HPV infection.

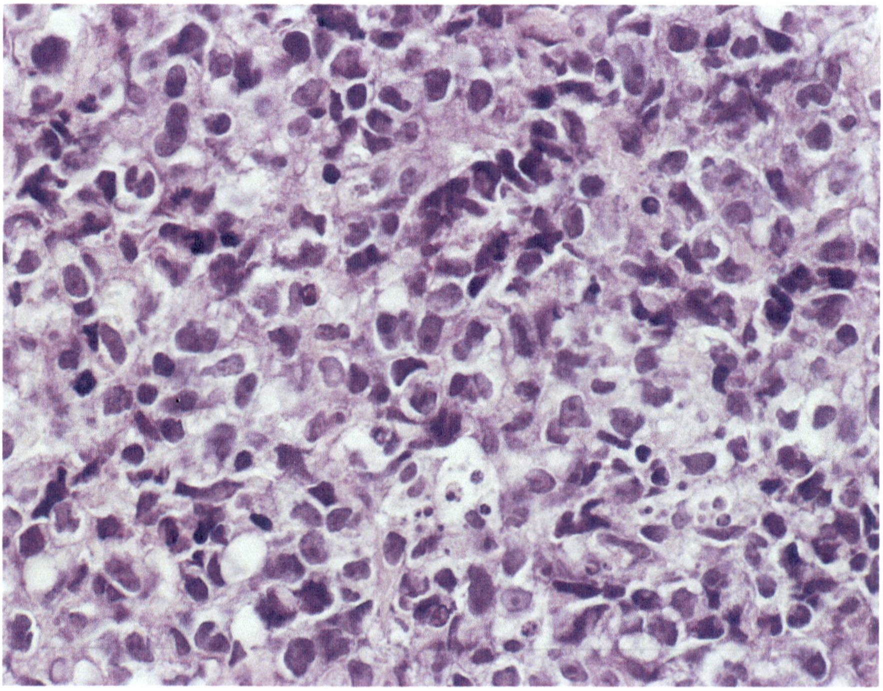

Fig. 9 Sinonasal undifferentiated carcinoma (SNUC)

10 Conclusions

Primary squamous cell carcinoma is the most common diagnosis in head and neck region. According to clinical observation and morphology along with tumor biology, recently there were described new entities. The classical risk factors include tobacco and alcohol exposure; however, there are evidences that some tumors have also other inducing factors such as viral infections. The spectrum of SCC based on morphology presented above could help understand different outcomes of SCC variants.

References

Abogunrin S et al (2014) Prevalence of human papillomavirus in head and neck cancers in European populations: a meta-analysis. BMC Cancer 14:968. doi: 10.1186/1471-2407-14-968

Alexandrov LB et al (2013) Signatures of mutational processes in human cancer. Nature 500: 415–421

Betiol J et al (2013) Impact of HPV infection on the development of head and neck cancer. Brazilian J Med Biol Res 46:217–226

Bishop JA et al (2014) Use of p40 and p63 immunohistochemistry and human papillomavirus testing as ancillary tools for the recognition of head and neck sarcomatoid carcinoma and its distinction from benign and malignant mesenchymal processes. Am J Surg Pathol 38:257–264

Cardesa A et al (2011) The Kaiser's cancer revisited: was Virchow totally wrong? Virchows Arch 458:649–57

Chen ZW et al (2012) Equivocal p16 immunostaining in squamous cell carcinoma of the head and neck: staining patterns are suggestive of HPV status. Head Neck Pathol 6:422–429

El-Mofty SK (2012) HPV-related squamous cell carcinoma variants in the head and neck. Head Neck Pathol 6(Suppl 1):S55–S62

Fakhry C et al (2014) Human papillomavirus and overall survival after progression of oropharyngeal squamous cell carcinoma. J Clin Oncol 32:3365–3373

Galbiatti ALS et al (2014) Gene expression profile of 5-fluorouracil metabolic enzymes in laryngeal cancer cell line: predictive parameters for response to 5-fluorouracil-based chemotherapy. Biomed Pharmacother 68:515–519

Gray ST et al (2015) Treatment outcomes and prognostic factors, including human papillomavirus, for sinonasal undifferentiated carcinoma: a retrospective review. Head Neck 37:366–374

Machado J et al (2010) Low prevalence of human papillomavirus in oral cavity carcinomas. Head Neck Oncol 2:6

Mandapathil M et al (2014) Salvage surgery for head and neck squamous cell carcinoma. Eur Arch Otorhinolaryngol 271:1845–1850

Marur S et al (2010) HPV-associated head and neck cancer: a virus-related cancer epidemic. Lancet Oncol 11:781–789

Masand RP et al (2011) Adenosquamous carcinoma of the head and neck: relationship to human papillomavirus and review of the literature. Head Neck Pathol 5:108–116

Mehrad M et al (2013) Papillary squamous cell carcinoma of the head and neck: clinicopathologic and molecular features with special reference to human papillomavirus. Am J Surg Pathol 37:1349–1356

Molinolo AA et al (2009) Dysregulated molecular networks in head and neck carcinogenesis. Oral Oncol 45:324–34

Orvidas LJ et al (1998) Verrucous carcinoma of the larynx: a review of 53 patients. Head Neck 20:197–203

Orvidas LJ et al (1999) Intranasal verrucous carcinoma: relationship to inverting papilloma and human papillomavirus. Laryngoscope 109:371–375

Pai S et al (2009) Molecular pathology of head and neck cancer: implications for diagnosis, prognosis, and treatment. Annu Rev Pathol 4:49–70

Pannone G et al (2011) The role of human papillomavirus in the pathogenesis of head & neck squamous cell carcinoma: an overview. Infect Agent Cancer 6:4

Santoro A et al (2011) A troubling diagnosis of verrucous squamous cell carcinoma ("the bad kind" of keratosis) and the need of clinical and pathological correlations: a review of the literature with a case report. J Skin Cancer

Stransky N et al (2011) The mutational landscape of head and neck squamous cell carcinoma. Science 333:1157–1160

Teymoortash A et al (2014) Verrucous carcinoma: a retrospective diagnosis in three historic patients. Eur Arch Otorhinolaryngol 271:631–633

HPV Testing of Head and Neck Cancer in Clinical Practice

Max Robinson

Abstract

The pathology laboratory has a central role in providing human papillomavirus (HPV) tests for patients with head and neck cancer. There is an extensive literature around HPV testing and a large number of proprietary HPV tests, which makes the field difficult to navigate. This review provides a concise contemporary overview of the evidence around HPV testing in head and neck cancer and signposts key publications, guideline documents and the most commonly used methods in clinical practice.

Keywords

HPV · Molecular diagnostics · Head and neck · p16 · Immunohistochemistry · In situ hybridisation

1 Introduction

The diagnosis of human papillomavirus (HPV)-related squamous cell carcinoma (SCC) mandates the use of laboratory tests. Ideally, the laboratory tests should provide evidence that HPV is driving the malignant process. Specifically, the malignant cells should contain an oncogenic HPV genotype and show evidence of viral transcription, with production of E6/E7 oncoproteins causing detrimental effects on cell behaviour, namely uncontrolled cell proliferation, loss of DeoxyriboNucleic

M. Robinson (✉)
Oral Pathology, Centre for Oral Health Research, Newcastle University, Framlington Place, Newcastle upon Tyne NE2 4BW, UK
e-mail: max.robinson@newcastle.ac.uk

W. Golusiński et al. (eds.), *HPV Infection in Head and Neck Cancer*,
Recent Results in Cancer Research 206, DOI 10.1007/978-3-319-43580-0_7

Acid (DNA) damage checkpoints and the acquisition of cell immortality (Leemans et al. 2011). Consequently there are numerous biomarkers that can be used to indicate HPV infection, from detection of HPV DNA, RiboNucleic Acid (RNA) and protein to demonstrating changes in endogenous gene and protein expression that can be used as indirect, surrogate markers of HPV infection. The adoption of HPV tests in clinical practice has mainly been driven by the availability of tests that can easily be incorporated into the diagnostic laboratory work flow, that is, formulated for the detection of the target molecule in formalin-fixed paraffin-embedded (FFPE) tissue or alcohol-preserved cytology samples (Schache et al. 2014). Nevertheless, the clinical acceptability of a particular test also depends on how accurately it classifies patient samples. The accuracy of the HPV test could be assessed against an accepted 'reference' or 'gold-standard' analytical test, or perhaps more clinically relevant, the ability of the test to identify patients with clinically significant HPV-related disease, such that the result informs patient prognosis or allows them access to clinical trials recruiting patients with HPV-related SCC (Bhatia and Burtness 2015). The literature around HPV testing is extensive and there are numerous proprietary tests that are licensed in vitro diagnostic devices (IVDs) that have regulatory approval (CE marking and/or US Food and Drug Administration (FDA) approval). The market for HPV testing has grown around applications in cervical cancer (screening, diagnosis, test of cure) and has latterly been evaluated in head and neck cancers.

2 Indications for HPV Testing in the Head and Neck Cancer

HPV testing is recommended for oropharyngeal SCC (palatine tonsils, tongue base, soft palate, posterior pharyngeal wall) where the information is used in prognostication and for enrolment into clinical trials (The Royal College of Pathologists, UK; College of American Pathologists; National Comprehensive Cancer Network, USA). In the clinical scenario of a lump in the neck that turns out to be SCC, viral tests directed at HPV and Epstein Barr virus (EBV) are useful for locating the putative primary site. A similar strategy can be used to link distant metastases to an index primary tumour (Weichert et al. 2009; Huang et al. 2012). HPV-positive SCCs are usually located in the oropharynx, whereas EBV-positive SCCs are typically discovered in the nasopharynx. There are exceptions to the rule, there have been several reports of HPV-positive nasopharyngeal carcinoma (Maxwell et al. 2010; Robinson et al. 2013; Stenmark et al. 2014), however, the prognostic implications are unclear as most studies have included too few cases to demonstrate any significant difference when compared to EBV-positive nasopharygeal carcinoma (Robinson et al. 2013; Stenmark et al. 2014). Whilst cancers at other site in the head and neck region rarely harbour HPV (Mehanna et al. 2016), there is evidence emerging that these HPV-positive carcinomas have similar outcomes to HPV-related oropharyngeal SCC (Salazar et al. 2014; Chung et al. 2014). Larger, appropriately powered studies are required to confirm these findings; however, in the future it is possible that HPV testing may be recommended for other sites in the head and neck region, perhaps all sites. Furthermore, there have been reports of HPV-associated oral intraepithelial neoplasia (Woo et al. 2013; McCord et al. 2013). The biological significance of the HPV infection in this setting is uncertain due to the small number of cases and lack of extended follow-up data. Consequently, HPV testing in the pathology laboratory is likely to increase in the future as new data emerge and new clinical applications are proposed.

3 The Detection of HPV in Formalin-Fixed Paraffin-Embedded Biopsies Using Test Algorithms

Laboratory tests have characteristic features which determine their accuracy in the clinical setting. To date there is no single test that is considered the 'gold standard' for classifying HPV status in FFPE tissue. Combinations of tests, in algorithms, have been proposed to mitigate for the known limitations of individual tests and produce optimal sample classification.

3.1 VU University Medical Centre HPV Test Algorithm

This algorithm (Fig. 1) was first proposed in the seminal article by Smeets et al. (2007) and was built around the ability of a battery of tests to approximate to an analytical reference test, defined as reverse transcriptase polymerase chain reaction (RT-PCR) for HPV-16 E6/E7 on fresh-frozen tissue. Whilst an RT-PCR specifically developed for FFPE material showed perfect correlation with the reference test, it was considered to be too technically demanding to be used in the diagnostic laboratory. Nevertheless, the combination of p16 immunohistochemistry (IHC) followed by consensus PCR, using the GP5+/GP6+ primer pairs, for the p16 positive cases, showed almost perfect correlation with the reference test and was subsequently validated in a larger cohort (n = 86) with an accuracy of 98 % (Rietbergen et al. 2013a). The testing strategy also correlated with patient outcome, patients with p16-positive/HPV DNA-positive tumours had the best chance of survival following treatment (73.5 % vs. 40.7 % 5-year survival; Rietbergen et al. 2013b), and this has been validated in an independent cohort (Rietbergen et al. 2015). The testing strategy has been incorporated into a multi-parameter classifier that is publically available at www.predictcancer.org. The validated test algorithm uses p16 IHC (CINtec Histology, Roche mtm laboratories) and a 'non-proprietary' GP5+/GP6+ PCR enzyme immunoassay with genotyping using Luminex bead array.

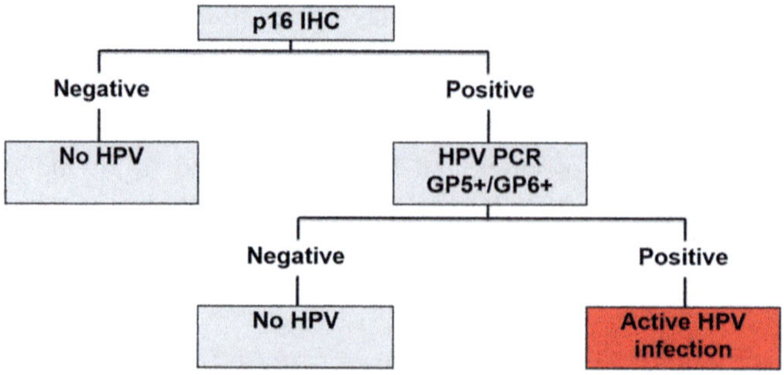

Fig. 1 VU University Medical Centre HPV test algorithm

3.2 The Johns Hopkins Medical Institutions HPV Test Algorithm

This algorithm (Fig. 2) was developed by The Johns Hopkins Medical Institutions, USA (Singhi and Westra 2010; Westra 2014) and was used in the landmark paper by Ang et al. (2010) demonstrating that patients with HPV-related oropharyngeal SCC had better prognosis than patients with HPV-negative disease (82.4 % vs. 57.1 % 3 years survival). The testing strategy incorporates upfront screening with p16 immunohistochemistry (CINtec Histology, Roche mtm laboratories) followed by two tiers of HPV DNA in situ hybridisation. The first tier employs an HPV-16-specific probe, which theoretically would identify the majority of HPV-positive cases (around 95 % of HPV-related oropharyngeal SCCs are HPV-16 positive) and a second tier containing a 'cocktail' of HPV probes to detect uncommon oncogenic HPV genotypes (HPV-16, -18, -31, -33, -35, -39, -45, -51, -52, -56, -58, -59, -68 DAKO Genpoint). Similar reagents are available from other suppliers: INFORM HPVIII Family 16 probes (Roche Ventana Medical Systems Ltd) are supplied as a cocktail and detect HPV-16, -18, -31, -33, -35, -39, -45, -51, -52, -56, -58, -66. Leica Biosystems supply a high-risk HPV probe set (cocktail) that detects HPV-16, -18, -31, -33, -51. Due to licensing restrictions, single genotype-specific probes available in the USA are not for sale in Europe. There is evidence that the testing strategy closely matches the analytical reference test (Schache et al. 2011); furthermore, the clinical importance as a prognostic classifier has been demonstrated in numerous independent cohort studies (Bhatia and Burtness 2015). As a result, the College of American Pathologists and the US National Comprehensive Cancer Network (NCCN) recommend 'either immunohistochemistry for analysis of p16 expression or HPV in situ hybridisation for detection of HPV DNA in tumour cell nuclei' for cancer of the oropharynx and the 'occult primary' in the head and neck region (College of American Pathologists; National Comprehensive Cancer Network, USA). In the UK the Royal College of Pathologists includes p16 IHC and HPV DNA in situ hybridisation in the datasets for reporting mucosal malignancies of the pharynx (The Royal College of Pathologists,

UK). The tests are also being used in clinical trials to identify patients with HPV-positive and HPV-negative SCC (Bhatia and Burtness 2015).

One of the inherent problems of using algorithms is that a few cases are inevitably classified in the two indeterminate categories: p16 positive/HPV DNA negative and p16 negative/HPV DNA positive (Table 1). Very few cases are classified in the latter group, which are likely to represent transient HPV infection, without activation of oncogenic effects, or simple interpretative errors. By contrast, the p16-positive/HPV DNA-negative cases represent a dilemma because there is evidence that patients with tumours in this category have similar favourable survival to patients with p16-positive/HPV DNA-positive tumours (Lewis et al. 2010), whereas in other studies this group of patients had unfavourable survival profiles that tracked with the p16-negative/HPV DNA-negative cases (Perrone et al. 2011; Rietbergen et al. 2013b). Interpretation of these data is limited by the small number of patients in the subgroup analysis and further studies are required.

4 p16 Immunohistochemistry

CINtec Histology and CINtec Cytology (p16 clone E6H4, Roche mtm laboratories) are the only p16 products that are register as in IVDs, effectively making them the only reagents that can be used for clinical diagnosis. Other antibody clones are available, but are 'research-use-only' (RUO) products. CINtec kits are supplied as 'ready-to-use' (RTU) products for the Ventana Benchmark autostainer (Roche Ventana Medical Systems Ltd) or as dispensable kits for use on other proprietary automated staining platforms or in manual assays. The assay should be optimised and validated in an appropriately accredited pathology laboratory. Ideally analyte controls should be included on the slides to be tested, and proprietary cell lines controls are available for this purpose (HistoCyte Laboratories Ltd, www.histocyte.com). Alternatively, known positive (e.g. oropharyngeal SCC or cervical

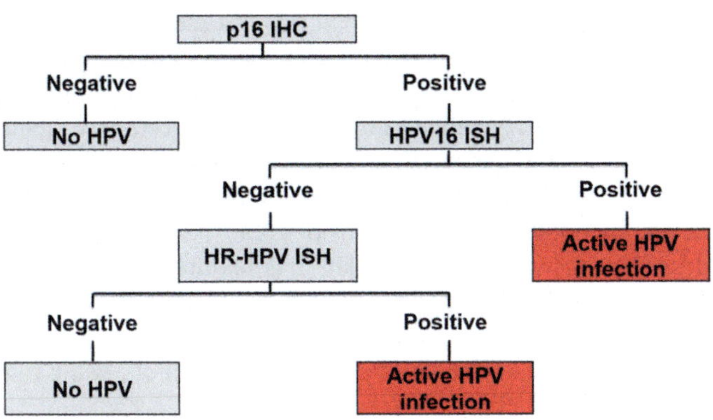

Fig. 2 The Johns Hopkins Medical Institutions HPV test algorithm

Table 1 Classification of oropharyngeal squamous cell carcinomas using p16 IHC and HPV DNA-specific tests

	No. of cases	p16+ HPV DNA+ (%)	p16− HPV DNA− (%)	p16+ HPV DNA− (%)	p16− HPV DNA+ (%)
Singhi and Westra (2010)	256	71	24	5	ND
Ang et al. (2010)	315	61	30	7	2
Lewis et al. (2010)	239	58	20	20	2
Thavaraj et al. (2011)	142	53	35	11	1
Jordan et al. (2012)	232	60	27	12	2
Rietbergen et al. (2013b)	841	19	77	4	ND

intraepithelial neoplasia grade 3) and negative tissue samples can be identified from tissue surplus to diagnostic requirements. Internal positive controls (tissue elements in the sample of interest that show expression of the target molecule) include reticulated tonsil epithelium, which shows patchy moderate staining, and follicular dendritic cells in secondary lymphoid follicles are weakly positive and occasionally fibroblasts showing weak-to-moderate staining. Multinucleated giant cells, if present, are also p16 positive (Schache et al. 2014). Carcinomas that contain oncogenic HPV typically show intense nuclear and cytoplasmic staining in the majority of the malignant cells (Fig. 3a). Westra's description in the Ang et al. (2010) paper is 'strong and diffuse nuclear and cytoplasmic staining in 70 % or more of the tumor cells'. Jordan et al. (2012) refined the 'cut-off' by comparison with an analytical reference test (RT-PCR for HPV-16, -18, -33 E6/E7 on FFPE tissue) and indicated that the optimum intensity was ≥2 (Scale 0-3), the optimum percentage of tumour cells staining was ≥35 % and the optimum H score (product of intensity and percentage; 0–300) was >60. Accepting a minimum intensity score of 2, at least 30 % of the tumour needed to be positive to show the best correlation with the reference test, and an intensity score of 3 suggests only 20 % of the tumour needs to be p16 positive. In clinical practice, the majority of cases are easily classified in a binary fashion (positive vs. negative), which accounts for the excellent inter-observer agreement for the assay (Thavaraj et al. 2011; Jordan et al. 2012). Clinical trials registering HPV-related oropharyngeal cancers have tended to adopt the >70 % cut-off described above (Bhatia and Burtness 2015). Infrequently, cases with weak staining confined to the cytoplasm of the majority of cells or nuclear staining alone are encountered and are considered to be p16 negative according to the criteria described above. While p16 IHC has features that make interpretation easy, it is recognised to be only an approximation of the HPV status. p16 IHC is considered to be highly sensitive, but lacks specificity, meaning there are occasions when p16 is overexpressed in the absence of HPV infection, using even the most sensitive HPV-specific tests. p16 is an endogenous gene, and increased expression is documented in other tumour types that have no association with HPV infection. With this in mind, there is a case to be made that p16 IHC testing should always be supported by HPV-specific tests (Perrone et al. 2011; Robinson et al. 2012; Rietbergen et al. 2013b), and there is a counter-argument that p16 IHC alone is satisfactory for prognostication and clinical trial recruitment (Ang et al. 2010; Lewis et al. 2010; Bhatia and Burtness 2015).

5 Detection of HPV DNA

Detection of HPV DNA can be achieved by either target amplification (polymerase chain reaction) or signal amplification (in situ hybridisation), but each method has inherent flaws. Non-quantitative PCR techniques tend to be too sensitive (producing false positive results), which can be ameliorated by employing quantitative PCR techniques (Schache et al. 2011). Assessment of PCR products on gels can be

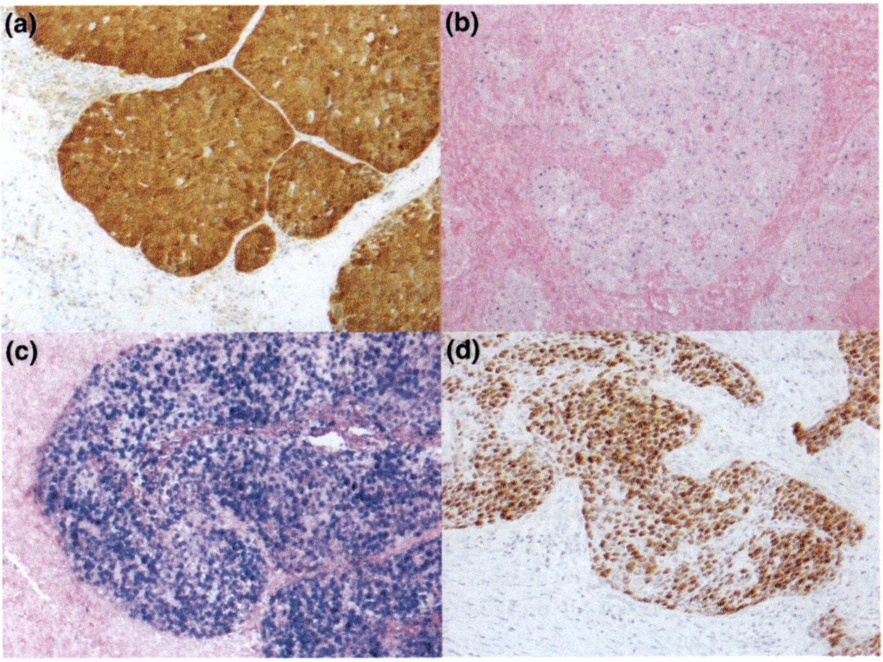

Fig. 3 Photomicrographs showing a typical p16 IHC-positive result (**a** CINtec histology, Roche mtm laboratories). High-risk HPV DNA ISH (INFORM HPV III Family 16, Roche Ventana Medical Systems Ltd) showing a punctate (**b**) and a diffuse (**c**) pattern of staining. High-risk HPV RNA ISH (RNAscope, Advanced Cell Diagnostics) showing brown reaction product in the malignant cells (**d**)

subjective, and adjusting detection thresholds in quantitative PCR determines the sensitivity and specificity of the assay. DNA in situ hybridisation is characterised by high specificity, but limited sensitivity, the limiting factor being the abundance of HPV copies and the availability of the target for hybridisation (Robinson et al. 2010). Interpretation of DNA in situ hybridisation shows good inter-observer agreement (Thavaraj et al. 2011; Jordan et al. 2012), and discordance is characterised by weak signals that are often patchy across the tissue section. For negative cases, it is essential that slide-based analyte controls are employed as there are no internal controls to quality assure the adequacy of the staining. Proprietary cell line controls (HistoCyte Laboratories Ltd www.histocyte.com) and tumour xenografts are available (HPV 3 in 1 control, Roche Ventana Medical Systems Ltd). Alternatively, known positive and negative tissue samples can be used as described above. Positive results vary from single punctate signals in the nucleus (Fig 3b), thought to represent single copies of the HPV integrated into the host genome, to cases that have a diffuse pattern of staining located in the nucleus and cytoplasm (Fig. 3c).

6 Detection of HPV RNA

There is evidence that HPV RNA in situ hybridisation (RNAscope, Advanced Cell Diagnostics) shows excellent agreement with the analytical reference test (RT-PCR for HPV-16, -18, -33 E6/E7 on fresh-frozen tissue; Schache et al. 2013; Mirghani et al. 2015) and encodes similar prognostic information for patients with oropharyngeal SCC as demonstrated by the other tests described above (Ukpo et al. 2011; Schache et al. 2013). The technique has several features that make it particularly useful for the detection of oncogenic HPV: Firstly, the patented hybridisation and amplification events produce highly sensitive and specific colorimetric signals (Fig. 3d). Second, the small size of the oligonucleotide probes facilitates the detection of partially degraded RNA in FFPE tissue. Third, HPV E6/E7 RNA is an abundant target in infected malignant cells. Fourth, the technique is based on the detection of HPV RNA, which is the target molecule for the analytical reference test (RT-PCR for HPV E6/E7 on fresh-frozen material). Nevertheless, the product is currently a 'research-use-only' (RUO) product; however, the manufacturers are seeking accreditation for clinical use.

In summary, providing the oncology team with the apposite molecular information to render a specific diagnosis is a contemporary theme in modern pathology and underpins the concept of stratified or personalised medicine. For HPV-related head and neck cancer, there are commercially available reagents with appropriate accreditation (IVD status, CE marking/FDA approved). Many pathology laboratories are able to deliver the tests to internationally recognised standards (ISO15189:2012). The tests produce consistent results on automated staining platforms with appropriate analyte controls. External quality assurance is available through College of American Pathologists Proficiency Testing/External Quality Assurance (CAP PT/EQA), UK National External Quality Assurance Scheme (UKNEQAS) and Nordic Immunohistochemical Quality Control (NordiQC). Tests are interpreted by informed pathologists cognisant of the features of the tests and the 'cut-offs'. The tests can be easily incorporated into the laboratory work flow with relatively short turnaround times. In the context of the patient pathway, these ancillary tests represent a minimal additional cost. Notwithstanding the above, it is important that the international community work together to define a compendium of recommended tests, provide guidance on the selection and interpretation of the tests and the clinical implications of the diagnosis. In the future, as clinical trials recruiting patients with known HPV status report their findings, it is feasible that the HPV testing landscape will make the transition from simple diagnostic tools for use in prognostication to predictive biomarkers, perhaps mandating less toxic treatment for patients with HPV-related head and neck cancer and directing targeted intensified therapy for patients with HPV-negative tumours. The ultimate hope is that this method of molecular classification will drive better outcomes for patients with head and neck cancer.

References

Ang KK, Harris J, Wheeler R, Weber R, Rosenthal DI, Nguyen-Tan PF et al (2010) Human papillomavirus and survival of patients with oropharyngeal cancer. N Engl J Med 363 (1):24–35

Bhatia A, Burtness B (2015) Human papillomavirus-associated oropharyngeal cancer: defining risk groups and clinical trials. J Clin Oncol 33(29):3243–3250

Chung CH, Zhang Q, Kong CS, Harris J, Fertig EJ, Harari PM et al (2014) p16 protein expression and human papillomavirus status as prognostic biomarkers of nonoropharyngeal head and neck squamous cell carcinoma. J Clin Oncol 32(35):3930–3938

College of American Pathologists (2012) Protocol for the examination of specimens from patients with carcinomas of the pharynx. College of American Pathologists, USA

Huang SH, Perez-Ordonez B, Liu FF, Waldron J, Ringash J, Irish J et al (2012) Atypical clinical behavior of p16-confirmed HPV-related oropharyngeal squamous cell carcinoma treated with radical radiotherapy. Int J Radiat Oncol Biol Phys 82(1):276–283

ISO15189:2012. http://www.iso.org/iso/catalogue_detail?csnumber=56115 (Accessed 06.03.2016)

Jordan RC, Lingen MW, Perez-Ordonez B, He X, Pickard R, Koluder M et al (2012) Validation of methods for oropharyngeal cancer HPV status determination in US cooperative group trials. Am J Surg Pathol 36(7):945–954

Leemans CR, Braakhuis BJ, Brakenhoff RH (2011) The molecular biology of head and neck cancer. Nat Rev Cancer 11(1):9–22

Lewis JS Jr (2012) p16 Immunohistochemistry as a standalone test for risk stratification in oropharyngeal squamous cell carcinoma. Head Neck Pathol 6(Suppl 1):S75–S82

Lewis JS Jr, Thorstad WL, Chernock RD, Haughey BH, Yip JH, Zhang Q et al (2010) p16 positive oropharyngeal squamous cell carcinoma: an entity with a favorable prognosis regardless of tumor HPV status. Am J Surg Pathol 34(8):1088–1096

Maxwell JH, Kumar B, Feng FY, McHugh JB, Cordell KG, Eisbruch A et al (2010) HPV-positive/p16-positive/EBV-negative nasopharyngeal carcinoma in white North Americans. Head Neck 32(5):562–567

McCord C, Xu J, Xu W, Qiu X, McComb RJ, Perez-Ordonez B et al (2013) Association of high-risk human papillomavirus infection with oral epithelial dysplasia. Oral Surg Oral Med Oral Pathol Oral Radiol 115(4):541–549

Mehanna H, Franklin N, Compton N, Robinson M, Powell N, Biswas-Baldwin N et al (2016) Regional and geographic variability in human papillomavirus-associated oropharyngeal cancer: individual patient data and samples from four multi-national randomised trials. Head Neck. doi:10.1002/hed.24336

Mirghani H, Casiraghi O, Amen F, He M, Ma XJ, Saulnier P et al (2015) Diagnosis of HPV-driven head and neck cancer with a single test in routine clinical practice. Mod Pathol 28 (12):1518–1527

National Cancer Comprehensive Network (2014) Clinical practice guidelines in oncology: head and neck cancers. National Cancer Comprehensive Network, USA

Perrone F, Gloghini A, Cortelazzi B, Bossi P, Licitra L, Pilotti S (2011) Isolating p16-positive/HPV-negative oropharyngeal cancer: an effort worth making. Am J Surg Pathol 35(5):774–777

Rietbergen MM, Leemans CR, Bloemena E, Heideman DA, Braakhuis BJ, Hesselink AT, Witte BI, Baatenburg de Jong RJ, Meijer CJ, Snijders PJ, Brakenhoff RH (2013a) Increasing prevalence rates of HPV attributable oropharyngeal squamous cell carcinomas in the Netherlands as assessed by a validated test algorithm. Int J Cancer 132(7):1565–1571

Rietbergen MM, Brakenhoff RH, Bloemena E, Witte BI, Snijders PJ, Heideman DA, et al (2013b) Human papillomavirus detection and comorbidity: critical issues in selection of patients with oropharyngeal cancer for treatment De-escalation trials. Ann Oncol 24(11):2740–2745

Rietbergen MM, Witte BI, Velazquez ER, Snijders PJ, Bloemena E, Speel EJ, Brakenhoff RH, Kremer B, Lambin P, Leemans CR (2015) Different prognostic models for different patient populations: validation of a new prognostic model for patients with oropharyngeal cancer in Western Europe. Br J Cancer 112(11):1733–1736

Robinson M, Sloan P, Shaw R (2010) Refining the diagnosis of oropharyngeal cancer using human papillomavirus testing. Oral Oncol 46(7):492–496

Robinson M, Schache A, Sloan P, Thavaraj S (2012) HPV specific testing: a requirement for oropharyngeal squamous cell carcinoma patients. Head Neck Pathol. 6(Suppl 1):S83–S90

Robinson M, Suh YE, Paleri V, Devlin D, Ayaz B, Pertl L et al (2013) Oncogenic human papillomavirus-associated nasopharyngeal carcinoma: an observational study of correlation with ethnicity, histological subtype and outcome in a UK population. Infect Agent Cancer. 8(1):30

Royal College of Pathologists (2013) Dataset for the reporting of mucosal malignancies of the pharynx. Royal College of Pathologists, UK

Salazar CR, Anayannis N, Smith RV, Wang Y, Haigentz M Jr, Garg M et al (2014) Combined P16 and human papillomavirus testing predicts head and neck cancer survival. Int J Cancer 135 (10):2404–2412

Schache AG, Liloglou T, Risk JM, Filia A, Jones TM, Sheard J et al (2011) Evaluation of human papilloma virus diagnostic testing in oropharyngeal squamous cell carcinoma: sensitivity, specificity, and prognostic discrimination. Clin Cancer Res 17(19):6262–6271

Schache AG, Liloglou T, Risk JM, Jones TM, Ma XJ, Wang H et al (2013) Validation of a novel diagnostic standard in HPV-positive oropharyngeal squamous cell carcinoma. Br J Cancer 108(6):1332–1339

Schache A, Croud J, Robinson M, Thavaraj S (2014) Human papillomavirus testing in head and neck squamous cell carcinoma: best practice for diagnosis. Methods Mol Biol 1180:237–255

Singhi AD, Westra WH (2010) Comparison of human papillomavirus in situ hybridization and p16 immunohistochemistry in the detection of human papillomavirus-associated head and neck cancer based on a prospective clinical experience. Cancer 116(9):2166–2173

Smeets SJ, Hesselink AT, Speel EJ, Haesevoets A, Snijders PJ, Pawlita M et al (2007) A novel algorithm for reliable detection of human papillomavirus in paraffin embedded head and neck cancer specimen. Int J Cancer 121(11):2465–2472

Stenmark MH, McHugh JB, Schipper M, Walline HM, Komarck C, Feng FY et al (2014) Nonendemic HPV-positive nasopharyngeal carcinoma: association with poor prognosis. Int J Radiat Oncol Biol Phys 88(3):580–588

Thavaraj S, Stokes A, Guerra E, Bible J, Halligan E, Long A et al (2011) Evaluation of human papillomavirus testing for squamous cell carcinoma of the tonsil in clinical practice. J Clin Pathol 64(4):308–312

Ukpo OC, Flanagan JJ, Ma XJ, Luo Y, Thorstad WL, Lewis JS Jr (2011) High-risk human papillomavirus E6/E7 mRNA detection by a novel in situ hybridization assay strongly correlates with p16 expression and patient outcomes in oropharyngeal squamous cell carcinoma. Am J Surg Pathol 35(9):1343–1350

Weichert W, Schewe C, Denkert C, Morawietz L, Dietel M, Petersen I (2009) Molecular HPV typing as a diagnostic tool to discriminate primary from metastatic squamous cell carcinoma of the lung. Am J Surg Pathol 33(4):513–520

Westra WH (2014) Detection of human papillomavirus (HPV) in clinical samples: evolving methods and strategies for the accurate determination of HPV status of head and neck carcinomas. Oral Oncol 50(9):771–779

Woo SB, Cashman EC, Lerman MA (2013) Human papillomavirus-associated oral intraepithelial neoplasia. Mod Pathol 26(10):1288–1297

Variation of HPV Subtypes with Focus on HPV-Infection and Cancer in the Head and Neck Region

Gunnar Wichmann

Abstract

The human papillomavirus (HPV) comprises a heterogeneous group of double-strand DNA viruses with variable potential to infect human epithelial cells and trigger neoplastic transformation. Its 8 kb genome encodes proteins required for virus replication and self-organized formation of infectious particles but also for early proteins E6 and E7 able to trigger neoplastic transformation. E6 and E7 of high-risk (HR) HPV subtypes can bind to p53 or release E2F and abrogate replication control. Due to variable amino acid sequence (AAS) in the binding sites of E6 and E7 particular HR-HPV variants within subtypes are essentially heterogeneous in efficacy triggering neoplastic transformation and cancer development. This could explain differences in the clinical course of HPV-driven head and neck cancer.

Keywords

Human papilloma virus (HPV) · HPV subtypes · HPV variants · HPV16 E6 variants · HPV16 AA · Head and neck squamous cell carcinoma (HNSCC)

1 Introduction

Molecular evidence provides support for a role for the human papillomavirus (HPV), particularly HPV16, to be deeply involved in the pathogenesis not only of squamous cell carcinomas (SCC) and adenocarcinoma (ADC) of the uterine cervix

G. Wichmann (✉)
ENT-Research Laboratory, Clinic of Otolaryngology, Head and Neck Surgery and Department of Head Medicine and Oral Health, University of Leipzig, Liebigstr. 21, 04103 Leipzig, Germany
e-mail: gunnar.wichmann@medizin.uni-leipzig.de

W. Golusiński et al. (eds.), *HPV Infection in Head and Neck Cancer*, Recent Results in Cancer Research 206, DOI 10.1007/978-3-319-43580-0_8

and other anogenital carcinoma but also of a subgroup of head and neck squamous cell carcinoma (HNSCC), especially those arising in oropharynx (Gillison et al. 2000) and, to be more precisely, in epithelia adjacent to lymphoid tissue of Waldeyer's throat ring, in particular the palatine and lingual tonsils. HPV comprises a heterogeneous group of double-strand DNA viruses with a variable potential to infect the epithelia of various parts of the body and cause a variety of diseases and clinical pictures. The HPV genome consists of a non-coding region Long Control Region (LCR) and 8 protein-coding genes (L1, L2, E1, E2, E4, E5, E6 and E7) summing up to a total length of about 7900 base pairs (Smith et al. 2011). HPV is classified into five groups (A to E), and A (the group of mucosal and genital HPV) includes the subtypes found to be present in benign and malignant tumors of the mucosa. The phylogenetic tree of group A includes three sub-entities of HPV detected in cancer of the uterine cervix, vulva, penis, but also HNSCC. According to the Papillomavirus Nomenclature Committee, a new HPV type is defined by a nucleotide sequence (NS) variation of more than 10 % compared to an already known HPV type in the L1 open reading frame. Those types differing in 2–10 % are considered subtypes, whereas intratype variants vary by 2 % in the L1 region (Bernard et al. 1994; Pande et al. 2008). The subgroups of significance for head and neck cancer are A7 (e.g, HPV18, HPV39, HPV45), A10 (e.g, HPV6, HPV11) and, of most relevance for HNSCC, A9 with the subtypes HPV16, HPV31, HPV33, HPV35, HPV52 and HPV58. The HPV subtypes of the three groups essentially differ in their potential to infect epithelial cells of the stratified epithelium of the mucosa of the head and neck region and to trigger their neoplastic transformation. HPV16 is the most relevant for HNSCC and comprises about 90 % of HPV in HNSCC (Kreimer et al. 2005).

2 Function of Oncogenic HPV Proteins

The HPV genome of about 7.9 kb codes not only for those genes required for the replication of the virus and self-organized formation of infectious particles but also encodes for proteins either causing diminished immune responses (E5) or able to trigger neoplastic transformation of the infected cell. Neoplastic transformation of epithelial cells is specifically caused by the two HPV proteins E6 and E7 of high-risk (HR-) HPV subtypes (Muñoz et al. 2003; Klussmann et al. 2009). The E6 and E7 proteins of HR-HPV subtypes have direct stimulatory effects on proliferation by interaction with regulators of the cell cycle. E6 binds p53 with high affinity and causes p53 ubiquitinylation and the degradation of this essential regulator of DNA replication. This abrogates the proliferation control of mutated cells. E6 of HR-HPV causes degradation of the p63 isoform TAp63β through a UBE3A-independent mechanism. Since TAp63β activates cell adhesion and focal adhesion pathways, HP-HPV E6-mediated TAp63β degradation together with p53 degradation contributes to establishment of anchorage independent growth (Khalifa et al. 2011; McLaughlin-Drubin et al. 2012) and hence might be responsible for early metastasis of HPV-driven HNSCC and especially the higher frequency of local lymph node metastases observed even in small (T1 or T2) primary tumors. E7 by inactivating pRB causes release of E2F, a transcription factor required for cell-cycle progression and DNA synthesis. E7 additionally induces expression of the histone demethylases KDM6A and KDM6B. The latter demethylates the (trimethylated) lysine 27 of histon 3 (H3K27me3) triggering epigenetic changes at the $p16^{INK4a}$-ARF locus followed by increased expression of $p16^{INK4a}$ (McLaughlin-Drubin et al. 2011). However, $p16^{INKa}$ is unable to achieve cell-cycle arrest in HPV-driven HNSCC due to the E7-mediated pRB inactivation. Other effects of E6 and E7 from HPV16 are described, e.g, activation of Wnt signaling (Rampias et al. 2010), and reprogramming of the cellular metabolism including induction of the Warburg effect (Zwerschke et al. 1999).

3 HPV Subtypes Differ in Their Capability to Infect Epithelial Cells and Trigger Neoplastic Transformation

In HPV-driven cancer, the replication control of HPV-infected cells is disrupted by E6 and E7. Due to the different NSs of the HPV genome of various subtypes, they show also variability in the amino acid sequence (AAS) of their proteins. Especially, the different AAS of particular HR-HPV subtypes (HPV16, 18, 31, 33, 35, 39, 45, 51, 52, 56, 58, 59, 66) and low-risk (LR-) HPV subtypes (HPV6, 11) in regions of E6 and E7 involved in binding of p53 and RB, respectively, cause essential heterogeneity in the capabilities of E6 and E7 of HPV subtypes to trigger neoplastic transformation of epithelial cells and driving development of cancer. This means that differences in the AAS of the E6 and E7 proteins of various HPV subtypes could be responsible for a different oncogenic impact on infected epithelia and may explain differences in their involvement in either development of HNSCC or carcinoma of the uterine cervix. For instance, members of the A7 group have a special tropism for glandular tissue and HPV18 is the most frequently detected type in ADC of the cervix (Clifford et al. 2003). This means not that HPV18 exclusively triggers ADC, and a recent publication suggested that HPV18 has the same capability to trigger both of the histological types of cervical carcinoma, ADC as well as SCC, and earlier epidemiological findings may be attributable to small case numbers in prior investigations and different geographical distribution of HPV18 variants with differences in this regard (Chen et al. 2015). However, ADCs are rare in the head and neck (9 %; Canto and Devesa 2002) and even more so in the oropharynx. Therefore, it is no surprise that HPV18 only accounts for 1 % of HPV detected in the oropharynx, while larynx (3.9 %) and oral cancer (16.0 %) where more often infected by this subtype (Kreimer et al. 2005). HNSCC positive for HPV DNA is mostly infected by HPV16 or other members of the A9 subgroup (e.g, HPV31, HPV33, HPV35; Kreimer et al. 2005). The most often detected HPV subtype detected in HNSCC is HPV16 (Kreimer et al. 2005) arguing for higher potential of this subtype to infect squamous cell epithelia not only of the uterine cervix (where HPV16 is also the predominant subtype in SCC; Yamada et al. 1997; Lavezzo et al. 2016) but also of the tonsils where HPV16 accounts for about 90 % of HPV-DNA positive cases. Target cells for HPV16 in mucosa of the head and neck region are especially epithelial cells of the tonsillar crypts (Klussmann et al. 2009). Since E6 and E7 of the various HR-HPV subtypes share some but not all amino acids in their p53 and RB binding sites, they also differ in kind and strength of their biological effects.

4 Variance Within HPV Subtypes

Variance in the NS and AAS exists not only between but also within HPV subtypes. Since subtypes are defined by differing in L1 in about of 2–10 % of the NS they each summarize intratype variants varying up to 2 % of nucleobases in the L1 region (Bernard et al. 1994; Pande et al. 2008), and within the same subtype the variability in other genes can be even higher. Of particular interest appears to be the heterogeneity within the HPV16 subtype. Within HPV16, at least 4 variants are known: African (Af-1, Af-2), Asian-American (AA), and European (E) and sometimes even more classes are distinguished (Yamada et al. 1995, 1997). However, the existence of sub-lineages within these variants, e.g. of either the AA variant (AA1, AA2; Smith et al. 2011) and the E variant (Yamada et al. 1997) has been proposed.

The existence of variants (or so-called lineages) within the HPV16 subtype is known right from the early beginning of research on HPV. For instance, HPV16 variant lineages in United States populations were characterized by nucleotide sequence analysis of the E6, L2 and L1 coding segments and revealed huge heterogeneity (Yamada et al. 1995). The strongest contrast (highest distance) was observed in comparison of the variants E (most related to the German HPV16 isolate serving as reference) and the AA variant (Fig. 1; Yamada et al. 1995). There are lots of variants detected in the genes of regulatory relevance and in L1 and E6 (Fig. 2; Yamada et al. 1995). However, also E7 variants are common (Eschle et al. 1992). Altogether, variants of the HPV16 and potentially also of other HPV subtypes appear to be a product of co-evolution of HPV and human races further influenced by several factors including founder effects, varying transmissibility of the virus, human migration patterns and recombination (Yamada et al. 1997; Jiang et al. 2009). Thus, it is no surprise that sequence variation in the HPV16 genes L1, L2, E6, and E7 shows geographical dependence (Yamada et al. 1997). Nowadays, however, migration causes widespread distribution of the various HPV16 variants, and in particular in the United States, the infection with more than one variant was reported in about 20 % of cases with HPV16 detection in women with cervical intraepithelial neoplasia (CIN) grade 2 or higher (Emeny et al. 1999). Of special interest may be reports on recombination processes between different HPV subtypes (Jiang et al. 2009). After simultaneous infection of a woman with HPV6, HPV16 (E variant), HPV45, and HPV56 the follow-up sample was only found positive for

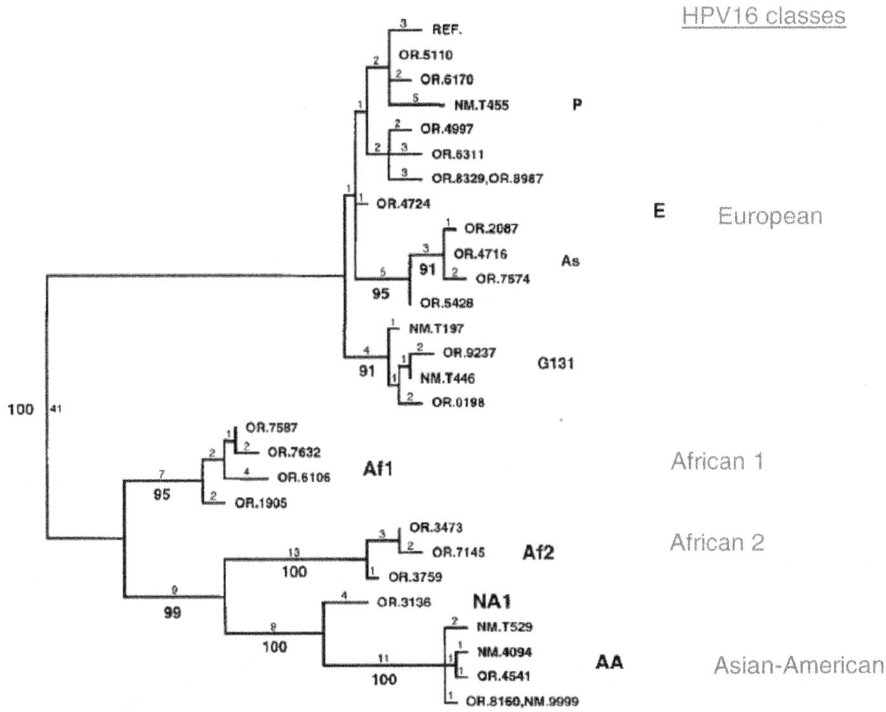

Fig. 1 Phylogenetic tree of the HPV16 variants identified by Yamada et al. (1995) in the United States within a sample of 30 HPV16 isolates based on parsimony analysis. Combined sequences from E6, L2, L1, and the LCR for 30 isolates (including the HPV16 reference [REF.] genome) yielded in their analyses an alignment of 129 variable positions. The single most parsimonious tree (157 steps) is shown. Small numbers above branches indicate numbers of steps (reconstructed point mutations) along the corresponding branch; the horizontal length of each branch is proportional to the number of steps, while vertical branch length is for layout only. Large numbers below branches indicate bootstrap values ≥ 90 %. On the right site, the HPV16 classes are indicated

HPV16 but due to recombination processes between HPV subtypes new HPV16 variants including HPV16 variants maintaining the E variant sequences in E6 but carrying Af2 in other genome regions emerged and led to simultaneous presence of 8 HPV16 variants (Jiang et al. 2009).

5 HPV16 Variants Have Variable Carcinogenic Potential

Most findings about variable carcinogenic potential of HPV16 variants come from research on cervix carcinoma. Women with non-E (including Af2 but predominantly AA) HPV16 variants have a 4.5 (95 % CI 1.2–16.8) times higher risk to develop CIN 2/3 lesions than women infected with HPV16 E variants (Xi et al. 1997).

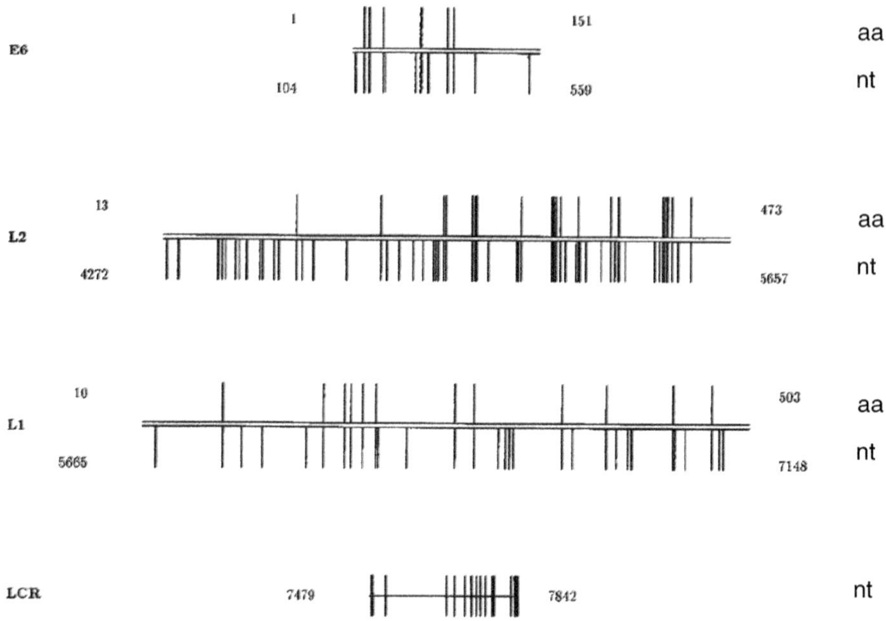

Fig. 2 Distribution of nucleotide (*nt*) and amino acid (*aa*) changes among HPV16 within *E6*, *L2*, and *L1* coding sequences and a segment of the *LCR*. For the coding regions, the beginning and ending nucleotide positions are indicated below the lines to the left and right, respectively; the beginning and ending residues of the predicted amino acid sequences are indicated above the lines. Vertical bars below the lines represent the positions of nucleotide substitutions, while vertical bars above the lines represent predicted amino acid changes. For the LCR, the beginning and ending nucleotide positions are indicated to the left and the right of the line, while bars through the line represent the positions of nucleotide substitutions (from Yamada et al. 1995, modified)

In a case-control study, the HPV16 AA variant has also been associated with a higher risk of cervical cancer than E variants; the risk of cervical cancer was eight times higher for patients with AA compared to E variants, when compared to a non-cancer control group (Berumen et al. 2001). Moreover, cancer patients with HPV16 AA were 7.7 years ($P = 0.004$) younger than patients with the E variant (Berumen et al. 2001). The AA variant was found being the most prevalent HPV16 variant (81.8 %) in Taiwan, and despite the probably expected co-evolution that might have led to adaptation processes, HPV16 AA was also associated with increased prevalence of histologically confirmed CIN grade 3 or worse in women from Taiwan (Chang et al. 2013). Compared to detection of HPV16 E the detection of HPV16 AA was accompanied by an age-adjusted increased odds ratio of 10.7 (1.62–451.05, $P = 0.0049$; Chang et al. 2013). The same increased risk associated with the AA HPV16 variant was detected in other investigations including prospective trials (Schiffman et al. 2010). However, different oncogenic potential of intra-subtype variants is not limited to HPV16 variants and significant also for other HR-HPV subtypes, e.g. HPV31, HPV35 and HPV51 (Schiffman et al. 2010).

Non-prototype HPV16 variants are associated with higher incidence of cervical neoplasia (Xi et al. 1997). Experimental findings revealed that HPV16 E6 amino acid 83 variants enhance E6-mediated MAPK and differentially regulate tumorigenesis by Notch signaling and oncogenic Ras (Chakrabarti et al. 2004). Related to extensive mutations in the E2 gene the copy number of AA variants per cell is higher than that of E variants (Casas et al. 1999), suggesting that AA variants replicate better than E variants. Since E2 is known to be a regulator of E6 and E7 transcription, this higher mutational level can also contribute to the more aggressive phenotype of AA variants. The European variant T350G, resulting in an amino acid change from leucine to valine at position 83 (L83V) in the E6 protein, is frequently found in cervical intraepithelial neoplasias and cancers and has been associated with progression to cervical cancer particularly in North European women (Zehbe et al. 1998). A recent study from Argentina about HPV16 variants in cervix carcinoma highlighted the most common mutation in the E6 sequences was T350G (L83V), detected in 67 % of the samples, to be associated with increased risk of persistent HPV16 infection (Mosmann et al. 2015). However, the strongest impact on oncogenic activity is caused of the HPV16 AA variant and triggered by their E6 that has some amino acid exchanges promoting cellular immortalization, undergoing transformation to resilient phenotypes, and promoting migration and invasiveness (Niccoli et al. 2012). The E6 protein of HPV16 AA alone is, as shown by in-vitro experiments utilizing keratinocytes solely transfected with the E6 protein of HPV16 AA (Jackson et al. 2014), able to deplete p53 and trigger $p16^{INK4A}$ expression, which is in sharp contrast to E6 from HPV16 E variant.

6 HPV16 Variants in HNSCC

There are only a few reports about HPV16 variants in HNSCC. In a study analyzing 21 HPV16 positive HNSCC from German patients (Hoffmann et al. 2004), only 6 of 21 (29 %) contained the HPV16 prototype sequence, while 8 of 21 (38 %) patients carried a T to G transversion at position 350 (T350G) in the E6 gene, and another 7 of 21 patients (33 %) carried the A131G (R10G in E6) variant together with the C712A mutation (H51N in E7). Since both E6 variants, R10G and L83V, have higher oncogenic potential than the prototype and were found enriched in this small cohort of HPV16-DNA positive HNSCC patients, HPV16 variants might also play an important role in head and neck carcinogenesis. Unfortunately, investigations on HPV16 variants in HNSCC, with the exception of the cited study from Markus Hoffmann and colleagues (Hoffmann et al. 2004), are missing. Nothing is known about their impact on development of HNSCC, treatment response and impact on outcome after treatment. Future investigations on HPV in HNSCC should no longer ignore the potentially very different oncogenic behavior of HPV16 variants that could be one cause for heterogeneity of HPV16 positive HNSCC in their clinical course. Due to geographically distinct patterns of HPV16 variants in cervical lesions (Yamada et al. 1997) and their well-known varying strength in biological effects they are causing, at least some of the differences observed also in the epidemiology of HPV16-driven HNSCC in various regions of the world could be explained. HPV16 positive HNSCC in Asia, Africa, South America and Europe might not be exactly the same as HPV16 positive HNSCC in the United States; they might not be caused by the same HPV16 variants. In the context of the different genetic background of the affected populations also the varying HPV16 variant patterns are expected to be strong modifiers of the respective immune responses to HPV16 infection. Vulnerability for infection with particular HPV16 variants depends on the genetic environment, and persistence of HPV-infection can increase the oncogenic effect of HPV16 and strongly influence the natural course of HPV-driven disease. This might at least partly explain some outcome differences observed in HPV-driven HNSCC. Therefore, investigations on the relevance of HPV16 variants in HNSCC are encouraged.

Acknowledgments Thanks to all my colleagues and collaborators in the Universities of Leipzig, Gießen, Poznan, Milano, and Heidelberg, the funders of our research, and especially all participating patients and their families.

References

Bernard HU, Chan SY, Manos MM, Ong CK, Villa LL, Delius H, Peyton CL, Bauer HM, Wheeler CM (1994) Identification and assessment of known and novel human papillomaviruses by polymerase chain reaction amplification, restriction fragment length polymorphisms, nucleotide sequence, and phylogenetic algorithms. J Infect Dis 170(5):1077–1085

Berumen J, Ordoñez RM, Lazcano E, Salmeron J, Galvan SC, Estrada RA, Yunes E, Garcia-Carranca A, Gonzalez-Lira G (2001) Madrigal-de la Campa A. Asian-American variants of human papillomavirus 16 and risk for cervical cancer: a case-control study. J Natl Cancer Inst 93(17):1325–1330

Canto MT, Devesa SS (2002) Oral cavity and pharynx cancer incidence rates in the United States, 1975-1998. Oral Oncol 38:610–617

Casas L, Galvan SC, Ordonez RM, Lopez N, Guido M, Berumen J (1999) Asian-American variants of human papillomavirus type 16 have extensive mutations in the E2 gene and are highly amplified in cervical carcinomas. Int J Cancer 83:449–455

Chakrabarti O, Veeraraghavalu K, Tergaonkar V, Liu Y, Androphy EJ, Stanley MA, Krishna S (2004) Human papillomavirus type 16 E6 amino acid 83 variants enhance E6-mediated MAPK signaling and differentially regulate tumorigenesis by notch signaling and oncogenic Ras. J Virol 78(11):5934–5945

Chang YJ, Chen HC, Pan MH, Lee BH, You SL, Lin CY, Chou YC, Hsieh CY, Cheng YJ, Liaw KL, Hsing AW, Schiffman M, Chen CJ, CBCSP-HPV Study Group (2013) Intratypic variants of human papillomavirus type 16 and risk of cervical neoplasia in Taiwan. J Med Virol 85(9):1567–1576. doi:10.1002/jmv.23651

Chen AA, Gheit T, Franceschi S, Tommasino M, Clifford GM; IARC HPV variant study group (2015) Human papillomavirus 18 genetic variation and cervical cancer risk worldwide. J Virol 89(20):10680–10687. doi:10.1128/JVI.01747-15

Clifford GM, Smith JS, Plummer M, Munoz N, Franceschi S (2003) Human papillomavirus types in invasive cervical cancer worldwide: a meta-analysis. Br J Cancer 88:63–73

Emeny RT, Herron JR, Xi LF, Koutsky LA, Kiviat NB, Wheeler CM (1999) Comparison of variant-specific hybridization and single-strand conformational polymorphism methods for

detection of mixed human papillomavirus type 16 variant infections. J Clin Microbiol 37 (11):3627–3633
Eschle D, Dürst M, ter Meulen J, Luande J, Eberhardt HC, Pawlita M, Gissmann L (1992) Geographical dependence of sequence variation in the E7 gene of human papillomavirus type 16. J Gen Virol 73(Pt7):1829–1832
Gillison ML, Koch WM, Capone RB et al (2000) Evidence for a causal association between human papillomavirus and a subset of head and neck cancers. J Natl Cancer Inst 92:709–720
Hoffmann M, Lohrey C, Hunziker A, Kahn T, Schwarz E (2004) Human papillomavirus type 16 E6 and E7 genotypes in -neck carcinomas. Oral Oncol 40(5):520–524
Jackson R, Togtema M, Lambert PF, Zehbe I (2014) Tumourigenesis driven by the human papillomavirus type 16 Asian-American E6 variant in a three-dimensional keratinocyte model. PLoS ONE 9(7):e101540. doi:10.1371/journal.pone.0101540
Jiang M, Xi LF, Edelstein ZR, Galloway DA, Olsem GJ, Lin WC, Kiviat NB (2009) Identification of recombinant human papillomavirus type 16 variants. Virology 394(1):8–11. doi:10.1016/j.virol.2009.08.040
Khalifa YB, Teissier S, Tan MK, Phan QT, Daynac M, Wong WQ, Thierry F (2011) The human papillomavirus E6 oncogene represses a cell adhesion pathway and disrupts focal adhesion through degradation of TAp63beta upon transformation. PLoS Pathog 7:e1002256. doi:10.1371/journal.ppat.1002256
Klussmann JP, Preuss SF, Speel EJ (2009) Human papillomavirus and cancer of the oropharynx. Molecular interaction and clinical implications. HNO 57(2):113–122. doi:10.1007/s00106-008-1867-y
Kreimer AR, Clifford GM, Boyle P, Franceschi S (2005) Human papillomavirus types in head and neck squamous cell carcinomas worldwide: a systematic review. Cancer Epidemiol Biomark Prev 14:467–475
Lavezzo E, Masi G, Toppo S, Franchin E, Gazzola V, Sinigaglia A, Masiero S, Trevisan M, Pagni S, Palù G, Barzon L (2016) Characterization of intra-type variants of oncogenic human papillomaviruses by next-generation deep sequencing of the E6/E7 region. Viruses 8(3). pii: E79. doi:10.3390/v8030079
McLaughlin-Drubin ME, Crum CP, Münger K (2011) Human papillomavirus E7 oncoprotein induces KDM6A and KDM6B histone demethylase expression and causes epigenetic reprogramming. Proc Natl Acad Sci USA 108(5):2130–2135. doi:10.1073/pnas.1009933108
McLaughlin-Drubin ME, Meyers J, Munger K (2012) Cancer associated human papillomaviruses. Curr Opin Virol 2(4):459–466. doi:10.1016/j.coviro.2012.05.004
Mosmann JP, Monetti MS, Frutos MC, Kiguen AX, Venezuela RF, Cuffini CG (2015) Mutation detection of E6 and LCR genes from HPV 16 associated with carcinogenesis. Asian Pac J Cancer Prev 16(3):1151–1157
Muñoz N, Bosch FX, de Sanjosé S, Herrero R, Castellsagué X, Shah KV, Snijders PJ, Meijer CJ (2003) International agency for research on cancer multicenter cervical cancer study group. Epidemiologic classification of human papillomavirus types associated with cervical cancer. N Engl J Med 348(6):518–527
Niccoli S, Abraham S, Richard C, Zehbe I (2012) The Asian-American E6 variant protein of human papillomavirus 16 alone is sufficient to promote immortalization, transformation, and migration of primary human foreskin keratinocytes. J Virol 86:12384–12396
Pande S, Jain N, Prusty BK, Bhambhani S, Gupta S, Sharma R, Batra S, Das BC (2008) Human Papillomavirus type 16 variant analysis of E6, E7, and L1 genes and long control region in biopsy samples from cervical cancer patients in north India. J Clin Microbiol 46(3):1060–1066. doi:10.1128/JCM.02202-07
Rampias T, Boutati E, Pectasides E, Sasaki C, Kountourakis P, Weinberger P, Psyrri A (2010) Activation of Wnt signaling pathway by human papillomavirus E6 and E7 oncogenes in HPV16-positive oropharyngeal squamous carcinoma cells. Mol Cancer Res 8(3):433–443. doi:10.1158/1541-7786.MCR-09-0345

Schiffman M, Rodriguez AC, Chen Z, Wacholder S, Herrero R, Hildesheim A, Desalle R, Befano B, Yu K, Safaeian M, Sherman ME, Morales J, Guillen D, Alfaro M, Hutchinson M, Solomon D, Castle PE, Burk RD (2010) A population-based prospective study of carcinogenic human papillomavirus variant lineages, viral persistence, and cervical neoplasia. Cancer Res 70(8):3159–3169. doi:10.1158/0008-5472.CAN-09-4179

Smith B, Chen Z, Reimers L, van Doorslaer K, Schiffman M, Desalle R, Herrero R, Yu K, Wacholder S, Wang T, Burk RD (2011) Sequence imputation of HPV16 genomes for genetic association studies. PLoS ONE 6(6):e21375. doi:10.1371/journal.pone.0021375

Xi LF, Koutsky LA, Galloway DA, Kuypers J, Hughes JP, Wheeler CM, Holmes KK, Kiviat NB (1997) Genomic variation of human papillomavirus type 16 and risk for high grade cervical intraepithelial neoplasia. J Natl Cancer Inst 89(11):796–802

Yamada T, Wheeler CM, Halpern AL, Stewart AC, Hildesheim A, Jenison SA (1995) Human papillomavirus type 16 variant lineages in United States populations characterized by nucleotide sequence analysis of the E6, L2, and L1 coding segments. J Virol 69(12): 7743–7753

Yamada T, Manos MM, Peto J, Greer CE, Munoz N, Bosch FX, Wheeler CM (1997) Human papillomavirus type 16 sequence variation in cervical cancers: a worldwide perspective. J Virol 71(3):2463–2472

Zehbe I, Wilander E, Delius H, Tommasino M (1998) Human papillomavirus 16 E6 variants are more prevalent in invasive cervical carcinoma than the prototype. Cancer Res 58(4):829–833

Zwerschke W, Mazurek S, Massimi P, Banks L, Eigenbrodt E, Jansen-Dürr P (1999) Modulation of type M2 pyruvate kinase activity by the human papillomavirus type 16 E7 oncoprotein. Proc Natl Acad Sci USA 96(4):1291–1296

Tumor Staging and HPV-Related Oropharyngeal Cancer

Claus Wittekindt and Jens Peter Klussmann

Abstract

The current TNM staging for oropharyngeal cancer (OSCC) was designed empirically for non-HPV-related disease. Emerging evidence suggests it is unsuited for Human papillomavirus (HPV)-related OSCC. Patients with HPV-positive tumors have improved prognosis, despite presenting at advanced stages. These shortcomings of the current staging system have been identified in single- and multi-institutional trials. Patients with HPV related OSCC typically present with advanced N-stages leading to higher stage groupings. A rarity of stages I and II therefore represents the nature of HPV-related OSCC. Concerning prognosis of the patients, N-category and extracapsular spread seem to be of minor importance, whereas advanced T-stages result in unfavourable outcome. Anatomical staging therefore has been implied into different proposals to prognostic risk classifications in HPV-related disease as an additive compound. Prognostic risk groupings are further enhanced by incorporating non-anatomical factors. To summarize, it can be suggested that the current TNM system alone has little prognostic value in HPV-related OSCC.

Keywords

Staging · Oropharyngeal Cancer · HPV · Prognosis · Risk Groupings

C. Wittekindt (✉) · J.P. Klussmann
Department of Otorhinolaryngology, Head and Neck Surgery, University of Giessen, Giessen, Germany
e-mail: claus.wittekindt@hno.med.uni-giessen.de

W. Golusiński et al. (eds.), *HPV Infection in Head and Neck Cancer*,
Recent Results in Cancer Research 206, DOI 10.1007/978-3-319-43580-0_9

1 Introduction

Staging is essential for successful management of head and neck cancer patients. It is the quintessence of diagnosis, treatment planning, application of therapeutics from a multidisciplinary approach, follow-up, and scientific investigation. The 7th edition of the TNM classification of the International Union Against Cancer (UICC) and the American Joint Committee on Cancer (AJCC) has been published in 2010 (Edge and Compton 2010). The system follows the tumor–node–metastasis (TNM) format (Table 1), and provides an overall disease stage from I to IV (Table 2), which helps treatment guidance and is able to predict prognosis. Historically, the most important staging component in terms of survival is the presence of nodal metastases at time of diagnosis, which is reported to reduce 5-year survival rates up to 50 % (Argiris et al. 2008). The incidence of carcinomas of the oropharynx (OSCC) has dramatically risen over the past decades, and is predicted to continue to rise. Risk factors include mainly tobacco and alcohol consumption, in the Western World both are reported to decline. OSCC driven by oncogenic human papilloma virus (HPV)-infections have been identified and are thought to be responsible for the dramatic increase of OSCC incidence rates in these last three

Table 1 TNM staging in OSCC

Primary tumor (T)	
TX	Primary tumor cannot be assessed
T0	No evidence of primary tumor
Tis	Carcinoma in situ
T1	Tumor = 2 cm in greatest dimension
T2	Tumor > 2 cm but not more than 4 cm in greatest dimension
T3	Tumor > 4 cm in greatest dimension or extension to lingual surface of the epiglottis
T4a	Tumor invades the larynx, deep/extrinsic muscle of the tongue, medial pterygoid, hard palate, or mandible
T4b	Tumor invades lateral pterygoid muscle, pterygoid plates, lateral nasopharynx, or skull base or encases the carotid artery
Regional lymph nodes (N)	
NX	Regional nodes cannot be assessed
N0	No regional lymph node metastasis
N1	Metastasis in a single ipsilateral lymph node = 3 cm in greatest dimension
N2a	Metastasis in a single ipsilateral lymph node > 3 cm but not more than 6 cm in greatest dimension
N2b	Metastasis in multiple ipsilateral lymph nodes, none > 6 cm in greatest dimension
N2c	Metastasis in bilateral or contralateral lymph nodes, none > 6 cm in greatest dimension
N3	Metastasis in a lymph node > 6 cm in greatest dimension
Distant metastasis (M)	
M0	No distant metastasis
M1	Distant metastasis

Table 2 Cancer stage grouping in OSCC

Stage	T	N	M
0	Tis	N0	M0
I	T1	N0	M0
II	T2	N0	M0
III	T3	N0	M0
	T1	N1	M0
	T2	N1	M0
	T3	N1	M0
IVA	T4a	N0	M0
	T4a	N1	M0
	T1	N2	M0
	T2	N2	M0
	T3	N2	M0
	T4a	N2	M0
IVB	T Any	N3	M0
	T4b	N Any	M0
IVC	T Any	N Any	M1

decades. The TNM staging system was established before HPV-driven OSCC has been identified as a distinct disease entity. HPV-positive OSCC typically presents at advanced TNM stages, because of early presence of nodal metastasis and therefore might be expected to result in unfavorable outcome. However, numerous studies reported survival rates for advanced stage OSCC cases that far exceed a 50 % survival rate, independent of treatment modality (Ang et al. 2010; Hong et al. 2010). Accordingly, only few published studies adress whether classical TNM staging accurately predicts survival in HPV-positive OSCC patients. This chapter describes the literature on the prognostic value of the current TNM staging system in the era of HPV-driven OSCC.

2 Clinical Differences in HPV-Related OSCC

In addition to molecular-genetic differences, different epidemiology and etiology, HPV relation in OSCC affects the clinical presentation of the patients. For example, secondary primary tumours are reported to be rare in patients with HPV-positive OSCC (Jain et al. 2013), possibly influencing the outcome and recommendations for screening and follow-up in this group of patients. In a retrospective work-up of 232 patients 64 % of toxicity and failure events occurred within the first 6 months of follow-up and the event incidence at each subsequent follow-up has been reported to be below 2 (Frakes et al. 2016). However, some differences reported between HPV- and non-HPV related cohorts are inconsistent. In some published series, patients with HPV-positive cancers were younger (Smith et al. 2004;

Klussmann et al. 2003), however, in other reports, the patients were older (Lindel et al. 2001). Summarized, patients with HPV positive OSCC probably are younger by approximately 5 years when compared with HPV negative patients. According to gender, men are reported to be at equal risk to women, however, slightly higher proportions of males or females in HPV-positive OSCC patients have both been reported. The majority of HPV-positive tumors usually arise from the lateral and anterior wall of oropharynx, compared with other anatomic subsites. Histopathologically, HPV-positive tumors tend to reveal a poorly differentiated, frequently basaloid and nonkeratinizing histology. The patients have commonly a shorter history of tobacco and alcohol consumption and usually have a better performance status compared to the HPV-negative patients.

3 TNM Staging: Clinical Presentation in HPV-Related OSCC

A common presentation of HPV-related OSCC is represented by a small primary tumor along with advanced nodal disease (Fig. 1). Nodal disease in HPV-related OSCC is often predominantly cystic on imaging (Goldenberg et al. 2008). However, HPV-positive OSCC have also been reported to have lower T-category (Porceddu et al. 2011) or to show no difference in size of the primary tumor (Hafkamp et al. 2009). Concerning regional metastases, most studies have noted higher nodal involvement in HPV-positive tumors but some authors have found no difference in N classification. In the majority of published papers HPV-related

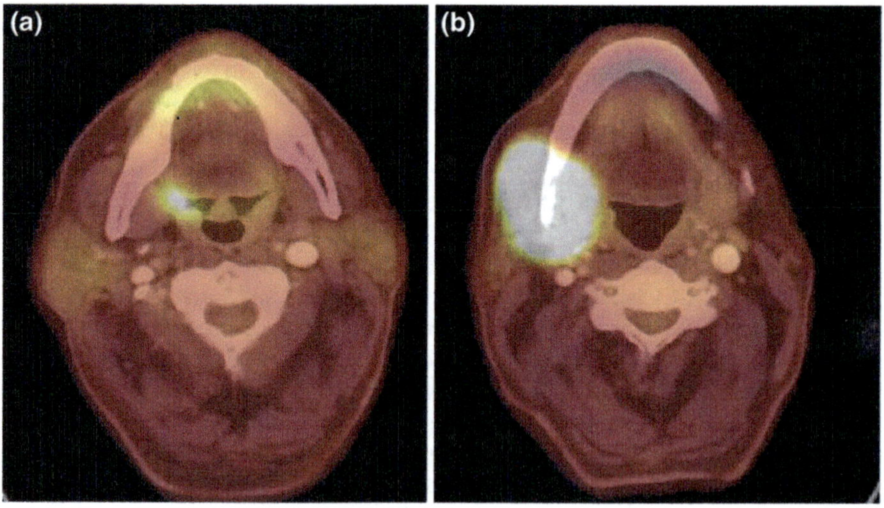

Fig. 1 Clinical presentaion of HPV-related OSCC typically includes a small primary tumor (**a**) in combination with advanced regional disease (**b**)

OSCC presents with a more advanced clinical stage, particularly with higher nodal involvement, when compared to non-HPV driven counterparts. According to this, HPV-related primary tumors may remain clinically occult, and often present with lymph node metastases only. For instance, tonsil SCCs are long known to present with early lymph node metastases (Thompson and Heffner 1998).

In our series of consecutive patients between 2000 and 2009, HPV-positive tumors had more often limited T-stages and advanced N- and M-stages (Table 3). In a further analysis of 266 patients, the differences of TNM staging according to HPV status has also been described. Patients with HPV-positive tumors were more likely to present with stage III/IV tumors (HPV-positive 93 % vs. HPV-negative 65 %; $p < 0.001$). A difference in T-classification was respectively not described, however, advanced stage HPV-positive OSCC were more likely to be either T1 or T2 than those that were HPV-negative (Ward et al. 2015). In agreement with both reports, the advanced stage in HPV-related OSCC is predominantly a result of nodal involvement. The study population of a large cohort treated with radiotherapy with or without chemotherapy consisted of 573 HPV-related OSCC yielding AJCC stages: I/n = 8; II/n = 25; III/n = 79; IV/n = 461). This fact later has been criticised, because only eight (1 %) patients had stage I disease and 25 (4 %) patients had stage II disease, which raised the question of whether the sample sizes for stages I and II were adequate. However, this rarity of stage I and II may particularly represent the nature of HPV-related OSCC. In a different analysis of almost 2000 OSCC patients, only 2 and 4 % were stage I and II, and stage I and II were also uncommon among >13,000 OSCCs in the SEER database (Setton et al. 2015; Keane et al. 2015).

Table 3 Tumor characteristics according to HPV-association (n = 396)

	All (N = 396)	HPV-unrelated (N = 305)		HPV-related (N = 75)		*p*-value*
		N	%	N	%	
T-stage						
T1-2	187 (47.2 %)	132	72.1	51	27.9	0.009
T3	88 (22.2 %)	76	87.4	11	12.6	
T4a/b	115 (29.0 %)	93	88.6	12	11.4	
Unknown	6 (1.5 %)					
N-stage						
N0	103 (26.0 %)	88	88.9	11	11.1	0.010
N+	283 (71.5 %)	209	76.8	63	23.2	
Unknown	10 (2.5 %)					
M-stage						
M0	341 (86.1 %)	268	81.5	61	18.5	0.203
M1	26 (6.6 %)	17	70.8	7	29.2	
Unknown	29 (7.3 %)					

4 TNM Staging as Prognosticator in HPV-Related OSCC

When describing classical prognostic factors in cohorts of OSCC patients, TNM classification, the number of involved nodes, and extracapsular spread, smoking, and performance show the most important influence on survival of the patients.

In a published series of 170 patients, Klozar et al. described that after adjustment for HPV, age, gender, smoking, alcohol consumption, and location of the tumor, only HPV and pT maintained statistical significance. After all, the authors concluded that none of the studied prognostic factors was significant in the group of patients with HPV-positive OSCC. According to this study, the characteristics of the extent of the disease in general and of regional lymph node metastasis in particular are probably not important for the outcome of HPV OSCC patients (Klozar et al. 2013). Particularly, for tonsil cancer patients, the N-stage has also been shown to be insignificant for the outcome in a series of 84 patients (Rahmati et al. 2015). In a cohort of 573 OSCC patients treated without surgery, Huang et al. reported lower 5-yOS in patients with higher TNM stages only in HPV-unrelated OSCC (stage I-70 % vs. Stage IV-30 %; P 0.004) but not for patients with HPV-related OSCC (stage I-88 % vs. Stage IV-74 %; P 0.56). Regarding only T-stages in HPV OSCC, the 5y OS rates only showed significant difference between T3 and T4 (74 % vs. 52 %). Survival rates also did not differ between N0 and N1, and N2a and N2b. The authors concluded that a recursive partitioning analysis may lead to new TNM stage groupings for HPV-related OSCC (Huang et al. 2015). In a published cohort of 211 patients with p16 positive OSCC that were all treated by surgery, pT4-stage was the strongest predictors of poor disease free-survival. Smoking, and multilevel node involvement were less important influencing factors for the outcome, in line with this, extracapsular spread, N stage, and involved margins did not reveal any prognostic significance (Haughey and Sinha 2012). In a further retrospective cohort of 266 patients treated with and without ablative surgery, TNM staging accordingly was only prognostic in HPV-negative OSCC. In HPV positive OSCC only T classification was prognostic. The Hazard ratio for death in this sample was 3.31 for T4 stage when compared to T3. Notably, there was no difference in survival of surgically treated patients according to whether they received adjuvant therapy and patients with HPV-positive OSCC had significantly better survival, regardless of treatment modality (Ward et al. 2015). According to this, the authors concluded that the current TNM system has little prognostic value in HPV-related OSCC.

When calculating the outcome in our own series of 379 patients acccording to AJCC stages, it turned out that also, regardless of HPV status, not all possible comparisons between stages turned out to deliver significant differences in survival. The groups were also clearly imbalanced and stage II turned out better than stage I. In HPV-related OSCC the AJCC stages showed no differences concerning survival even after merging close groups (Table 4). When calculating the outcome according to T- and N-categories we were able to show significant differences beween Kaplan Meier-curves. Dichotomizing the patients according to their

Table 4 Risk factors and survival in patients with HPV-related OSCC

		Patients with HPV-related OSCC (n = 75)			
		n	5-YOS (95 %)	Log-Rank	HR (95 %CI)
Age					
	Old (≥ 60)	37	61.1	0.006	1
	Young (< 60)	38	94.6		0.295
Comorbidity					
	(ECOG 2-4)	22	50.6	0.008	1
	(ECOG 0-1)	52	88.3		0.334
UICC-stages					
	Stage I-III	27	92.6	0.222	
	Stage IVa	35	76.4		
	Stage IVb-IVc	12	58.3		
	Stage I	4	100.0	0.159	
	Stage II	5	80.0		
	Stage III	18	94.4		
	Stage IVa	35	76.4		
	Stage IVb	5	80.0		
	Stage IVc	7	42.9		

T-stages into non-advanced (T1-2) and advanced (T3-4) local disease led to significant difference in survival (Fig. 2). Merging all possible groups of patients according to N-stage never led to significant differences. Best discriminative power was reached when comparing N0-2a with N2b-3, however, the log rank-test did not produce a significant difference. Extracapsular spread (ECS) is commonly used to justify adjuvant chemotherapy in patients with head and neck cancer. The role of ECS as a prognosticator and adjuvant therapy determinant in surgically resected, HPV-related OSCC has been determined in 152 patients that were treated with transoral laser microsurgery. After matched analyses, the presence of ECS or even soft tissue metastasis demonstrated no significant reduction in survival for the presence of ECS nor for the administration of adjuvant radiotherapy alone versus concurrent adjuvant chemoradiation in ECS-positive patients (Sinha et al. 2012).

Finally, the changing prognositc significance of tumor stage and nodal involvement has been shown in >13,000 patients who were diagnosed with OSCC from 1997 to 2008 in a population-based cohort with an increasing effect of the T stage and a declining effect of the N stage over time. The authors concluded that these changes reflect the increasing prevalence of HPV-related OSCC (Keane et al. 2015). In conclusion, it can be supposed that the current TNM system per se has reduced prognostic value in HPV-positive OSCC patients when compared to

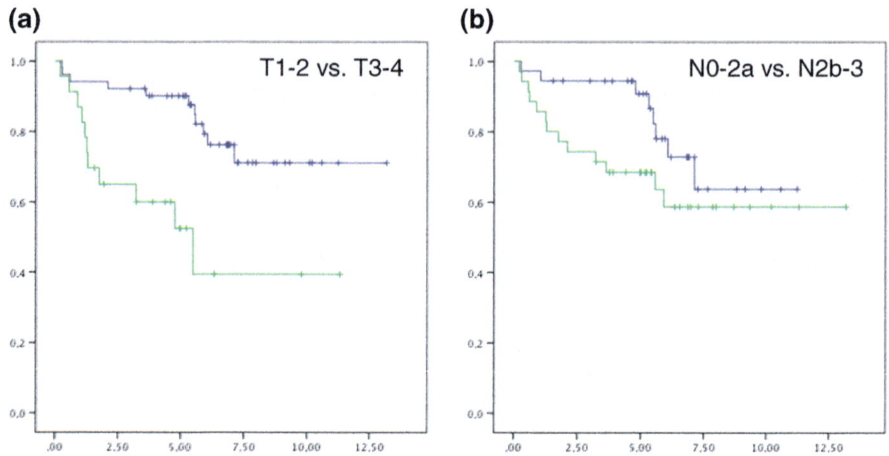

Fig. 2 Survival functions in HPV-related OSCC according to T-stage (**a**) and N-stage (**b**). Merging T1-2 and T3-4 led to significant diffferences. Best differences for N-categories was received after comparison of N0-2a versus N2b-3, however, the differences turned out to be not significant

non-HPV-related OSCC cases. There is mutual consent on (A) a lesser significance of N-stages and (B) a sustained significance of advanced T-stages for the outcome of the patients. Nevertheless, it is still important to perform reliable and accurate pretreatment clinical staging in patients with OSCC of both etiologies. The discriminatory power between the distinct TNM and UICC stages is yet reduced in HPV-OSCC.

5 TNM Staging in Risk Models

An increasing body of evidence suggests that specific information about HPV status and other patient characteristics including TNM stages have to be taken into account into tailored OSCC cancer therapies. Bevore the age of HPV defining the dominant risk factor in OSCC, different prognostic groups with regard to locoregional control were derived from recursive partitioning analysis (RPA) in 801 patients from the Netherlands. The authors final model resulted in three different risk groups: Class I (intermediate risk: <N3, free surgical margins, no ECS), Class II (high risk: N1 ECS +, T1, T2, or T4 tumors with close or positive surgical margins), or Class III (very high risk: N3 neck, >N2b ECS+, T3 with positive surgical margins). The 5-year local control rates were reported to be 88, 73 and 58 % (Langendijk et al. 2005). Later, in 2010, The publication of the RTOG 0129 study proposed a stratification algorithm, combining HPV, T-stage, N-stage and smoking history, to assign patients into different prognostic groups (Ang et al. 2010). This single-cohort based algorithm, based on patients treated within a randomized trial, including mainly patients with locally advanced tumors and with limited comorbidity was able to discriminate patients according to their risk of failure.

The phase III trial of the Radiation Therapy Oncology Group (RTOG 0129) revealed no differences in the OS between accelerated fractionation and standard fractionation when combined with concurrent high-dose cisplatin. In addition, the investigators were able to divide patients into categories of low, intermediate or high risk of death from RPA analysis. The RPA model consisted of HPV status, smoking history and TNM stages. Precisely, in patients with HPV-related OSCC, the number of pack-years of tobacco smoking (≤ 10 versus >10) and nodal stage (N0 to N2a versus N2b to N3) were additional determinants of OS rates (Ang et al. 2010). This model has later been validated by an Italian group. In 120 patients that were treated without surgery the 2y-OS estimates were 100, 86, and 70 %. A concordance index of 0.70 has been reported for both patient samples (Granata et al. 2012). However, the risk model according to Ang was primarily based on a clinical trial population, and patients with severe comorbidity were excluded. Moreover, cigarette smoking habits differ worldwide. We adopted the risk model according to Ang to our series of unselected patients and found heavily imbalanced group sizes and no discriminative power between the intermediate- and high-risk groups (unpublished data).

Unselected patients that were treated with radiotherapy or radiochemotherapy were evaluated to refine stages and prognostic groups in Canada and have been published in 2015 (Huang et al. 2015). For HPV related OSCC cases RPA analysis was performed with stages and nonanatomic factors. TNM stages led to RPA groups I (T1-3N0-2b), II (T1-3N2c), and III (T4 or N3) with 5y-OS rates of: 82, 76, and 54 %, respectively. A further RPA model including TNM stages, age, smoking derived the following four prognostic groups for survival: group I (T1-3N0-N2c_ 20 PY), group II (T1-3N0-N2c_ 20 PY), group III (T4 or N3_age 70), and group IVA (T4 or N3_age 70) with distinct survival rates. The authors conclude that new RPA-based TNM stage grouping can be proposed for HPV-related OSCC.

Series of unselected patients treated with different treatment modalities and with large heterogeneity in terms of stages, demographics and comorbidities were also published. An externally validated graphic normogramm has been published in 2014 with predictors for unfavorable outcomes being HPV-negativity, comorbidity, T3–T4 stage, N2b–N3 stage, male gender, lower hemoglobin levels and smoking history of more than 30 pack years. Hazard ratios for death were HPV > T3 > N2b-N3 > male gender > comorbidity > T4 in this series. Notably, Hazard ratios for smoking and alcohol consumption were nearly 1.0 The authors concluded that combining tumor HPV status with other important prognostic factors, including TNM were significantly better than those obtained with TNM alone or HPV status alone (Rios Velazquez E et al. 2014). Later, the validation of this model using a single-institutional cohort of 235 patients has been published with model variables including HPV, comorbidity and nodal stage. The 5-year OS estimates were approximately 85, 55 and 30 % in the low-, intermediate- and high-risk group (Rietbergen et al. 2015). The decision tree has been published in 2014, notably, in HPV-related OSCC only comorbidity stratifies patients into low or intermediate risk groups on not TNM stages (Rietbergen et al. 2013). In our own series of patients, the dominant risk factors for favorable outcome in OSCC were HPV and performance (ECOG 0-1). RPA modeling led to three risk groups in OSCC when adding information on T- and N-stages with high discriminative power in unselected patients treated with surgery or non-surgical therapy after shared decision making.

To conclude, a separate staging system is needed for HPV-related OSCC, because the cohorts are fundamentally different in the survival performance. New stage grouping schemes are proposed with help of RPA analyses. All published schemes that included nonanatomical information outperformed TNM stages.

6 Conclusions

Patients with HPV-related OSCC are fundamentally different concerning survival. The Literature data supports that the current anatomic staging system for OSCC patients has it's shortcommings for HPV-related OSCC as a prognostic tool. However, for HPV-related OSCC, advanced T stage still seems to be a useful prognostic marker. New stage grouping schemes that include anatomical TNM stages and non-anatomical markers are currently under investigation.

References

Ang KK et al (2010) Human papillomavirus and survival of patients with oropharyngeal cancer. N Engl J Med 363(1):24–35

Argiris A et al (2008) Head and neck cancer. Lancet 371(9625):1695–1709

Edge SB, Compton CC (2010) The American joint committee on cancer: the 7th edition of the AJCC cancer staging manual and the future of TNM. Ann Surg Oncol 17(6):1471–1474

Frakes JM et al (2016) Determining optimal follow-up in the management of human papillomavirus-positive oropharyngeal cancer. Cancer 122(4):634–641

Goldenberg D et al (2008) Cystic lymph node metastasis in patients with head and neck cancer: an HPV-associated phenomenon. Head Neck 30(7):898–903

Granata R et al (2012) Tumor stage, human papillomavirus and smoking status affect the survival of patients with oropharyngeal cancer: an Italian validation study. Ann Oncol 23(7):1832–1837

Hafkamp HC et al (2009) P21 Cip1/WAF1 expression is strongly associated with HPV-positive tonsillar carcinoma and a favorable prognosis. Mod Pathol 22(5):686–698

Haughey BH, Sinha P (2012) Prognostic factors and survival unique to surgically treated p16 + oropharyngeal cancer. Laryngoscope 122(Suppl 2):S13–S33

Hong AM et al (2010) Human papillomavirus predicts outcome in oropharyngeal cancer in patients treated primarily with surgery or radiation therapy. Br J Cancer 103(10):1510–1517

Huang SH et al (2015) Refining American joint committee on cancer/union for international cancer control TNM stage and prognostic groups for human papillomavirus-related oropharyngeal carcinomas. J Clin Oncol 33(8):836–845

Jain KS et al (2013) Synchronous cancers in patients with head and neck cancer: risks in the era of human papillomavirus-associated oropharyngeal cancer. Cancer 119(10):1832–1837

Keane FK et al (2015) Changing prognostic significance of tumor stage and nodal stage in patients with squamous cell carcinoma of the oropharynx in the human papillomavirus era. Cancer 121 (15):2594–2602

Klozar J et al (2013) Nodal status is not a prognostic factor in patients with HPV-positive oral/oropharyngeal tumors. J Surg Oncol 107(6):625–633

Klussmann JP et al (2003) Human papillomavirus-positive tonsillar carcinomas: a different tumor entity? Med Microbiol Immunol 192(3):129–132

Langendijk JA et al (2005) Risk-group definition by recursive partitioning analysis of patients with squamous cell head and neck carcinoma treated with surgery and postoperative radiotherapy. Cancer 104(7):1408–1417

Lindel K et al (2001) Human papillomavirus positive squamous cell carcinoma of the oropharynx: a radiosensitive subgroup of head and neck carcinoma. Cancer 92(4):805–813

Porceddu SV et al (2011) Results of a prospective study of positron emission tomography-directed management of residual nodal abnormalities in node-positive head and neck cancer after definitive radiotherapy with or without systemic therapy. Head Neck 33(12):1675–1682

Rahmati R et al (2015) Squamous cell carcinoma of the tonsil managed by conventional surgery and postoperative radiation. Head Neck 37(6):800–807

Rietbergen MM et al (2013) Human papillomavirus detection and comorbidity: critical issues in selection of patients with oropharyngeal cancer for treatment De-escalation trials. Ann Oncol 24(11):2740–2745

Rietbergen MM et al (2015) Different prognostic models for different patient populations: validation of a new prognostic model for patients with oropharyngeal cancer in Western Europe. Br J Cancer 112(11):1733–1736

Rios Velazquez E et al (2014) Externally validated HPV-based prognostic nomogram for oropharyngeal carcinoma patients yields more accurate predictions than TNM staging. Radiother Oncol 113(3):324–30

Setton J et al (2015) A multi-institution pooled analysis of gastrostomy tube dependence in patients with oropharyngeal cancer treated with definitive intensity-modulated radiotherapy. Cancer 121(2):294–301

Sinha P et al (2012) Extracapsular spread and adjuvant therapy in human papillomavirus-related, p16-positive oropharyngeal carcinoma. Cancer 118(14):3519–3530

Smith EM et al (2004) Age, sexual behavior and human papillomavirus infection in oral cavity and oropharyngeal cancers. Int J Cancer 108(5):766–772

Thompson LD, Heffner DK (1998) The clinical importance of cystic squamous cell carcinomas in the neck: a study of 136 cases. Cancer 82(5):944–956

Ward MJ et al (2015) Staging and treatment of oropharyngeal cancer in the human papillomavirus era. Head Neck 37(7):1002–1013

Part III
Non-Surgical Treatment of HPV Positive Tumours

Human Papillomavirus (HPV): A Criterion for Therapeutic Decision in Squamous Cell Carcinoma of the Head and Neck?

Jan B. Vermorken

Abstract

When deciding how to treat patients with squamous cell carcinoma of the head and neck (SCCHN), several factors have to be taken into account: disease factors, patient factors, treatment factors, and the wish of the patient. This symposium article is summarizing the information on HPV (p16) in the context of decision making in SCCHN patients with locoregionally advanced disease and those with recurrent/metastatic disease. The literature data suggest that HPV (p16) has prognostic significance, both in locoregionally advanced disease (in particular, in oropharynx cancer) and in recurrent/metastatic disease, while there are only limited data on its predictive significance. Results of HPV (p16) testing should not change management outside clinical trials.

Keywords

Decision making · Human papillomavirus · P16 · Prognostic factor · Predictive factor · Cetuximab · Panitumumab · Radiotherapy · Chemotherapy

1 Introduction

The traditional risk factors for squamous cell carcinoma of the head and neck (SCCHN) include, among others, tobacco use, alcohol use, and poor oral health. Recently, human papillomavirus (HPV) infection, in particular with HPV-16, has

J.B. Vermorken (✉)
Department of Medical Oncology, Antwerp University Hospital, Edegem, Belgium
e-mail: Jan.B.Vermorken@uza.be

W. Golusiński et al. (eds.), *HPV Infection in Head and Neck Cancer*, Recent Results in Cancer Research 206, DOI 10.1007/978-3-319-43580-0_10

emerged as a novel risk factor, and its prevalence in oropharyngeal carcinomas (OPCs) is growing in various countries, but with substantial geographic variation. Although HPV is found in SCCHN in many anatomical sites, HPV-16-induced carcinogenesis usually occurs in the oropharynx (Kreimer et al. 2005; D'Souza et al. 2007), which contains multiple structures that promote HPV-induced malignant transformation. HPV-associated OPCs have a different molecular profile (p16 overexpression, wild-type p53) compared to HPV-negative tumors (high burden of mutations, specifically p53 mutations, normal or suppressed p16) (Rampias et al. 2013). Patients with HPV+ (p16+) OPC have a different risk factor profile compared to their HPV-negative counterparts, and they tend to be younger, often have a different clinical presentation (early T stage with more extensive nodal involvement), but despite this they show a better prognosis, particularly in the locoregionally advanced disease setting (Ang et al. 2010; Rischin et al. 2010).

2 Decision Making

Diagnosis and treatment of SCCHN is a multidisciplinary challenge. It seems therefore self-evident that when a variety of professionals involved in the treatment of head and neck cancer patients sit together in multidisciplinary tumor boards, they will improve decision making and as results of that ultimately will improve patient management and outcome (Ruhstaller et al. 2006; Friedland et al. 2011). In that decision-making process, factors that need to be taken into account are as follows: (1) *disease factors*, such as disease site, stage of the disease, the biology of the disease (both HPV and the epidermal growth factor receptor [EGFR] are playing a role), and specific risk factors for locoregional relapse (such as deep invasion, soft tissue involvement, positive margins) or distant relapse (multiple lymph nodes involved and extracapsular extension [ECE]); (2) *patients factors*, such as age, sex, performance status, nutritional status, comorbid chronic disease, oral health, lifestyle habits, and socioeconomic status; (3) *treatment factors* (surgery, radiotherapy, chemotherapy, targeted therapy, and immunotherapy), each with their typical side effects; and (4) *what the patient wants* (it has become clear that survival is of paramount importance to the patient, overshadowing associated toxicities and potential dysfunction) (Gregoire et al. 2010; List et al. 2004). Also, the attitude of the patient in this decision making, being negative or positive, is extremely important. It has become increasingly apparent that patients need emotional support, not only to navigate through their cancer journey, but also to successfully integrate back into society and daily life (Reich et al. 2014). Acute toxicity, but even more late toxicity assessment, is becoming more and more of an issue, as well as quality of life of the survivors (Bentzen and Trotti 2007; Haddad and Shin 2008). This symposium article is summarizing the information on HPV (p16) in the context of decision making in SCCHN patients with locoregionally advanced disease and those with recurrent/metastatic disease.

3 Locoregionally Advanced SCCHN

Current data suggest that the HPV status is the strongest prognostic variable in locoregionally advanced (LA)-OPC. The prognostic significance of HPV is illustrated in Table 1, showing hazard ratios of survival in the range of 0.20–0.40 (a reduction in the risk of death of 60–80 %) when comparing HPV/p16 positive cohorts vs HPV/p16 negative cohorts in studies using different forms of treatment in OPC patients, and in some studies that also include other disease sites at the same time (Ang et al. 2010; Rischin et al. 2010; Gillison et al. 2000; Licitra et al. 2006; Fakhry et al. 2008; Lassen et al. 2010; Posner et al. 2011; Rosenthal 2014). The data from the Radiation Therapy Oncology Group (RTOG) 0129 trial have been instrumental and are most frequently quoted. Ang et al. reported that HPV (p16)-negative status, >10 pack-year tobacco exposure, T4, and N2b-N3 were adverse predictors for overall survival and progression-free survival for OPC in that study (Ang et al 2010). Further analysis revealed three groups of different outcome: a low risk group with a 3-year overall survival (OS) rate of 93.0 % (95 % confidence interval [CI], 88.3 to 97.7 %), an intermediate risk group with a 3-year OS rate of 70.8 % (95 % CI, 60.7 to 80.0 %), and a high-risk group with a 3-year OS rate of 46.2 % (95 % CI, 34.7 to 57.7 %). HPV (p16) positivity appeared to be associated with improved locoregional control (LRC), but not necessarily with improved distant control, suggesting that improved LRC is a major determinant of survival in HPV-positive LA-OPC (4). Also, as expected, there were significantly less second primary tumors in the HPV (p16)-positive patient cohort in that study, 5.9 % at 3 years versus 14.5 % in the HPV (p16)-negative cohort ($p = 0.02$).

The colleagues at the Princess Margaret Cancer Center in Toronto came to similar conclusions when performing a retrospective analysis of 624 stage III/IV OPC patients treated with radiotherapy alone or concurrent chemoradiotherapy (CCRT) in their institute for whom they had p16 data (Huang et al. 2013). Local control, regional control, and overall survival were all significantly improved in the p16-positive cases versus the p16-negative cases at 3 years ($p < 0.001$). In addition,

Table 1 Prognostic significance of HPV in locoregionally advanced SCCHN

Authors	Year	No.pts	Subsite	% HPV	Treatment	HR
Gillison et al.	2000	252	H&N	25	Surg a/o RT	0.40
Licitra et al.	2006	90	OPC	19	Surg ± RT	0.26
Fakhry et al.	2008	96	Lar/OPC	40	ICT → CCRT	0.36
Lassen et al.	2010	331	Lar/Phar*	25	RT ± Nimorazole	0.34
Rischin et al.	2010	185	H&N	57	CCRT ± TPZ	0.36
Ang et al.	2010	316	OPC	68	CCRT	0.33
Posner et al.	2011	111	OPC	50	ICT → CCRT	0.20
Rosenthal	2014	182	OPC	41	RT ± cetuximab	0.27

H&N all subsites included; *OPC* oropharyngeal cancer; *Lar* laryngeal cancer
Phar pharyngeal cancer; *Surg* surgery; *RT* radiotherapy; *ICT* induction chemotherapy; *CCRT* concurrent chemoradiotherapy; *74 patients with OPC (p16-positive in 32 %); *TPZ* tirapazamine

they focused their interest on the risk of developing distant metastases rather than survival outcome alone. Not only was the natural course of the distant metastases different, i.e., distant metastases in p16-positive OPC can occur later than what is usually seen in the p16-negative cases, but they also noticed that the occurrence of distant metastases was significantly associated with T4 category disease, the degree of nodal involvement, and, moreover, showing the same relationship with smoking history as observed in RTOG trial 0129, reported by Ang et al. (vide supra). The risk of distant metastases in T1-T3, N0-N2a disease seemed rather low both in heavy and light smokers, but a smoking history of >10 pack-years was important in N2b disease, while patients with N2c and N3 disease were at risk of distant metastases irrespective of smoking history (O'Sullivan et al. 2013). The colleagues from Princess Margaret Hospital also reported on differences in the type of distant metastases and the consequences thereof. In the p16-negative cases, distant failure is mostly seen in the lung, followed in frequency by metastases to bone and liver, and in general, these metastases are considered incurable. In the p16-positive cases, two types of distant metastases can be distinguished, i.e., the so-called *disseminating type*, occurring in multiple organs and in unusual sites, and the so-called *indolent phenotype*, which still might be cured with salvage procedures (surgery, chemotherapy, or radiation) (Huang et al. 2013).

Although the prognostic importance of HPV for OPC is irrefutable, the impact of the HPV status on treatment response is less established. Retrospective subanalyses in randomized trials are not conclusive on a specific benefit of one particular treatment over the other in HPV-positive OPC patients (Rischin et al. 2010; Lassen et al. 2010). In the DAHANCA 5 study, the benefit of nimorazole only seemed to be present in the p16-negative cohort, and in the TROG 02.02 phase III trial, there was only a trend favoring the tirapazamine arm for improved locoregional control in p16-negative patients. Because of these rather limited and unconfirmed data, the predictive significance of HPV status in patients with LA-OPC needs further study.

Therefore, it should be concluded that the HPV status does not currently alter the management of patients with LA-OPC. In fact, there are no guidelines for the treatment of HPV-positive OPC, neither in the USA nor in Europe. However, there are some proposed strategies, one of which is the use of induction chemotherapy (which had showed to be more efficacious in HPV-positive OPC than in HPV-negative OPC in a prospective trial (Fakhry et al. 2008) to select those patients who might need less intensive locoregional treatment afterward. This concept was studied in Eastern Cooperative Oncology Group (ECOG) trial 1308, originally presented at ASCO 2014, and more recently updated at ASCO 2015 (Cmelak 2015). ECOG 1308 allowed dose reduction of the intensity-modulated radiation therapy (IMRT: (54 Gy/27fx + cetuximab weekly) in HPV-positive resectable stage III or IV OPC patients if a complete clinical response were obtained to 3 cycles of induction chemotherapy, which consisted of cisplatin 75 mg/m^2 day 1, paclitaxel 90 mg/m^2 day 1, 8, and 15, and cetuximab 250 mg/m^2 day 1, 8, and 15, given at 3-week intervals. Those patients who achieved only a partial response or remained stable received full dose of bioradiotherapy (IMRT 69.3 Gy/33fx + cetuximab). The update reported on the symptom reduction observed in those patients, using the

Vanderbilt Head and Neck Symptom Survey version 2 [VHNSS V2] at 6 months and 12 months compared to baseline. Difference in difficulty swallowing solids (35 % vs 100 %) reached statistical significance ($p = 0.01$). A composite analysis evaluating moderate-to-severe symptoms at 12 months for any of the 3 clusters (difficulty swallowing solids, dry mouth, and taste/smell changes) was 70 % vs 100 %. The conclusion of the investigators was that a 15 Gy dose reduction seemed to be able to meaningfully reduce some late toxicities without compromising efficacy (Cmelak 2015). It should be mentioned that the observation time to make a final conclusion on efficacy is rather short to allow for a definitive conclusion. Another deintensification study that makes use of induction chemotherapy (ICT) is the Quarterback Trial. In this trial, stage III and IV HPVOPC patients receive 3 cycles of ICT with docetaxel, cisplatin, and 5-FU [TPF]; when CR/PR is achieved, then patients are randomized to receive 56 or 70 Gy, and when no response is obtained, patients receive standard CCRT. Another approach is using radiotherapy alone rather than CCRT, as done in the ADEPT trial. In this trial, patients with T1-4a, N + (ECE+) HPVOPC, and negative margins after transoral robotic surgery are randomized to receive RT alone vs CCRT with cisplatin. Finally, the use of bioradiation [BRT] instead of CCRT is investigated in order to study whether BRT leads to less acute and late toxicity. This latter approach is being studied in three studies around the world: RTOG 1016 in the USA, the DeESCALaTE study in UK, and the TROG 12.01 study in Australia. Most likely, the last three studies will be combined for specific analyses. However, again the efficacy outcome data will take many years. Future clinical trials in LA-OPC should at the very least stratify by HPV status. Ideally, HPV+ and HPV− groups should be evaluated in separate trials.

4 Recurrent/Metastatic SCCHN

Factors that should be considered when choosing a treatment option in patients with recurrent/metastatic (R/M)-SCCHN are as follows: the type of relapse (only local, only regional, local and regional, only distant metastases, or distant metastases with locoregionally recurrent disease), the time interval between the treatment of the primary disease and the relapse is detected, the type of treatment that the patient received in the curative setting, the performance status at the time of relapse, the presence of relevant comorbid disease, the patients preference, and the institute where the patient is going to be treated (Vermorken 2005). More recently, it became clear that also the HPV (p16) status might be of influence in the recurrent/metastatic disease setting.

Fakhry and colleagues reported on a retrospective analysis of the association between tumor p16 status and overall survival (OS) in stage III/IV OPC patients who progressed locally, regionally, and/or at distant sites after having been enrolled onto RTOG trials 0129 and 0522 and failing platinum-based CCRT. Tumor p16 expression was evaluated by immunohistochemistry (IHC), and p16 expression was scored as positive if strong and diffuse nuclear and cytoplasmic staining was present in at least 70 % of the tumor cells. After a median follow-up of 4.0 years after progression, patients with p16-positive OPC had significantly improved survival rates compared with p16-negative patients (2-year OS, 54.6 % vs. 27.6 %; median OS 2.6 vs. 0.8 years, $p < 0.001$). In multivariate analysis, factors independently associated with OS after disease progression included p16 status, tumor stage, cigarette pack-years at enrollment, distant versus locoregional progression, and salvage surgery (Fakhry et al. 2014). These data made the investigators conclude that HPV status should be used as a stratification factor for clinical trials for patients with recurrent or metastatic OPC.

Similar conclusions were expressed by Argiris and coworkers based on a pooled analysis of a relatively small set of patients with R/M-SCCHN derived from two ECOG trials, i.e., ECOG 1395, a phase III trial comparing cisplatin/5-FU (PF) versus cisplatin plus paclitaxel (PT), and ECOG 3301, a phase II study of irinotecan plus docetaxel (Argiris et al. 2014). Tumors were analyzed for HPV in 65 samples, whereby HPV DNA was detected by in situ hybridization [ISH] with a wide-spectrum probe, and slides were scored as positive for HPV ISH+ if a punctate signal specific to tumor cell nuclei was present. p16 was evaluated by IHC in 66 samples, and staining was considered positive if a strong and diffuse staining of more than 80 % of tumor cells was present and negative if absent or focal. According to these criteria, 11 (17 %) were HPV-positive and 12 (18 %) p16-positive, whereas 52 (80 %) were both HPV-negative and p16-negative. The objective response rate was 55 % for HPV-positive versus 19 % for HPV-negative patients ($p = 0.022$), and 50 % for p16-positive versus 19 % for p16-negative patients ($p = 0.057$). The median survival was 12.9 versus 6.7 months for HPV-positive versus HPV-negative patients ($p = 0.014$) and 11.9 versus 6.7 months for p16-positive versus p16-negative patients ($p = 0.027$) (see Table 2). Although the analysis had several limitations (retrospective, selection of a subset of the tumors from the original trials,

Table 2 Prognostic significance of HPV (p16) in patients with recurrent/metastatic SCCHN treated with cytotoxic chemotherapy (ECOG 1395 and 3301, control arms of the EXTREME and SPECTRUM trials)

Drugs	Median	Survival (months)/ [evaluable number of pts]		
	p16-pos	posp16-neg	HPV-pos	HPV-neg
PF vs PT; CPT-11 +docetaxel[1]	**11.9** [12]	**6.7***[53]	**12.9** [11]	**6.7**[§] [53]
Platinum/5-fluorouracil[2]	**9.6** [23]	**7.3** [162]	**7.1** [13]	**6.7** [152]
– Hazard ratio (95 % CI)	*0.83 (0.50–1.36)*			*0.92 (0.48–1.77)*
Platinum/5-fluorouracil[3]	**12.6** [42]	**8.6** [165]	–	–
– Hazard ratio (95 % CI)	*0.70 (0.47–1.04)*			

[1]Argiris et al. (reference 24; p16 by immunohistochemistry [IHC], HPV by in situ hybridization); [2]Vermorken et al. 2014 (p16 by IHC, HPV by Cervista 16/18, and Cervista HR assays) [3]Vermorken et al. 2013 (p16 by IHC)
*logrank test $p = 0.027$; [§]$p = 0.014$

small sample size), the magnitude of the effect illustrated that even a small number of HPV-positive R/M-SCCHN patients can impact the results of prospective therapeutic studies (Argiris et al. 2014).

Only recently the relationship between HPV (p16) and treatment outcomes has been evaluated in subanalyses of large randomized phase III trials in RM-SCCHN [not restricted to OPC], in which the role of anti-EGFR medication was tested. The incidence of HPV (p16) positivity has been remarkably low, in particular in the European trials. As an example, in the intention-to-treat population of the EXTREME trial, a phase III study comparing combination of chemotherapy with platinum/5-FU alone versus the same chemotherapy plus cetuximab, a chimeric monoclonal antibody against EGFR, 10 % of the patients were found p16-positive and 5 % HPV-positive. In the OPC subset of patients in this trial, these figures were 16 and 12 %, respectively. p16 expression was assessed by IHC. For this the CINtec®, p16INK4A assay was used and p16 expression was considered p16-positive if >70 % of tumor cells showed moderate or strong and diffuse nuclear staining (regardless of cytoplasmic staining intensity); low-intensity staining was classified as p16-negative; and heterogeneous moderate- to high-intensity staining (both cytoplasmic and nuclear) was considered inconclusive. HPV DNA was detected using oligonucleotide hybridization assays (the FDA approved Cervista® HPV 16/18 and Cervista® HPV HR assays). Overall, p16 positivity and HPV positivity were associated with a better survival compared to p16 negativity and HPV negativity in both the cetuximab and the control arms (Vermorken et al. 2014). The observations in the control arm are depicted in Table 2. The addition of cetuximab to chemotherapy improved the chances of achieving a response irrespective of the p16 and HPV status, and the same was true for the OS data, although the results were limited by the low number of patient, and significance was only reached in the HPV-negative subgroup (Table 3). The investigators concluded that the survival

Table 3 Predictive significance of HPV (p16) in R/M-SCCHN patients treated with platinum/5-fluorouracil with or without an anti-EGFR monoclonal antibody

Study	Ref.	Median survival (months) w/wo cetuximab or panitumumab			
		p16-positive	p16-negative	HPV-positive	HPV-negative
EXTREME[1]	25	**12.6** vs **9.6**	**9.7** vs **7.3**	**13.2** vs **7.1**	**9.7** vs **6.7**
– Number of pts		*18 vs 23*	*178 vs 16*	*11 vs 13*	*145 vs 152*
– Hazard ratio		*0.63*	*0.82*	*0.72*	*0.73*
–95 % CI		*0.30–1.34*	*0.65–1.04*	*0.28–1.83*	*0.56–0.94**
SPECTRUM[2]	27	**11.0** vs **12.6**	**11.7** vs **8.6**	–	–
–Number of pts		*57 vs 42*	*179 vs 165*		
–Hazard ratio		*1.00*	*0.73*		
–95 % CI		*0.62–1.61*	*0.58–0.93***		

[1]Vermorken et al. 2014 (EXTREME = platinum/5-FU w/wo cetuximab; p16 by IHC, HPV by Cervista 16/18 and Cervista HR assays)
[2]Vermorken et al. 2013. (SPECTRUM = cisplatin/5-FU w/wo panitumumab; p16 by IHC); *EGFR* epidermal growth factor receptor; *MoAb* monoclonal antibody; *CI* confidence interval

benefits of chemotherapy plus cetuximab over chemotherapy alone were independent of tumor p16 and HPV status (Vermorken et al. 2014). These observations are in line with the observations made in the retrospective analysis on the role of p16 in the "Bonner study" and reported by Rosenthal at ASCO 2014 (Rosenthal 2014, Table 1). The conclusion of that subgroup analysis in OPC patients suggested a more pronounced treatment effect of RT+ cetuximab vs RT alone in patients with p16-positive OPC across all endpoints (LRC, progression-free survival [PFS] and OS). Moreover, although the numbers of patients were small in the subgroups, the results suggested improved clinical outcome by RT+ cetuximab compared with RT alone regardless of p16 status (Rosenthal 2014).

The SPECTRUM trial is a phase III study randomizing R/M-SCCHN patients to receive first-line PF w/wo panitumumab, an anti-EGFR IgG_2 fully human monoclonal antibody. The addition of panitumumab to PF significantly improved response rate and PFS, but did not reach significance in OS, which was the primary endpoint. The results of this trial with respect to the prognostic effect and the predictive effect of p16 status on the addition of panitumumab are summarized in Tables 2 and 3. For p16 assessment, a validated IHC method was used, whereby samples were judged to be p16 positive when they had strong and diffuse nuclear and cytoplasmic staining in at least 10 % of tumor cells (Vermorken et al. 2013). Although these criteria differed from those used in the EXTREME trial, analysis using alternative cutoffs (between 10 and 70 %) demonstrated consistent outcomes (Vermorken et al. 2013). Of the patients in the control arm of the study, those who were p16-positive had numerically, but not statistically significantly longer survival than those who were p16-negative (Table 2). However, contrary to what was observed in the EXTREME trial, the p16 status was predictive for the effect of panitumumab, showing only benefit when panitumumab was added to PF in patients with p16-negative tumors (Table 3). It is unclear why the addition of panitumumab in p16-positive tumors is any different from the addition of cetuximab in p16-positive patients. It has been suggested that this might relate to the cetuximab-induced antibody-dependent cell-mediated cytotoxicity, which might enhance the antitumor effect against HPV-positive OPC, but this is merely speculative (Psyrri et al. 2014). Complicating issues in the comparisons in R/M-disease studies are the inclusion of disease sites other than OPC, the relatively small number of HPV (p16)-positive patients, and the variability in HPV assessment and differing criteria of what is called positivity.

Despite that, all three studies suggested that HPV (p16) is prognostic in R/M-SCCHN patients treated with chemotherapy. However, when anti-EGFR monoclonal antibodies are combined with chemotherapy, the predictive value of HPV (p16) is uncertain given the differing results in EXTREME and SPECTRUM. It is also unclear whether the role of HPV (p16) in its predictive capacity is any different in situations where anti-EGFR-targeted therapies are combined with DNA damaging agents (chemotherapy or RT) or not. Reasons for that are recent findings that suggest that single-agent anti-EGFR therapies are particularly active in HPV (p16)-negative patients (Fayette et al. 2014; Machiels et al. 2015). Therefore, it is important that further studies in that direction are being pursued. In conclusion, the present data in R/M-SCCHN suggest that HPV (p16) has prognostic but not predictive significance in R/M-SCCHN.

5 Summary

The following statements can be made with respect to HPV (p16) as a criterion for decision making in SCCHN:

Locoregionally advanced SCCHN

HPV (p16) has an established impact on prognosis, particularly for OPC patients.

There are only limited data on the predictive significance of HPV (p16).

Results of HPV (p16) testing should not change management outside clinical trials.

Recurrent/metastatic SCCHN

HPV (p16)-positive disease seems to have a more favorable outcome than HPV (p16)-negative disease, and stratification for HPV (p16) should be considered.

The predictive significance of HPV(p16) in R/M-SCCHN needs further study, and this is in particular the case for targeted therapies, whether given alone or in combination with DNA damaging agents.

References

Ang KK, Harris J, Wheeler R et al (2010) Human papillomavirus and survival of patients with oropharyngeal cancer. N Engl J Med 363:24–35

Argiris A, Li S, Ghebremichael M et al (2014) Prognostic significance of human papillomavirus in recurrent or metastatic head and neck cancer: an analysis of eastern cooperative oncology group trials. Ann Oncol 25:1410–1416

Bentzen SM, Trotti A (2007) Evaluation of early and late toxicities in chemoradiation trials. J Clin Oncol 25:4096–4103

Cmelak A (2015) Symprom reducrtion from IMRT dose deintensification: Resulkts from ECOG 1308 using the Vanderbilt Head and Neck Symptom Survey version 2 (VHNSS V2). J Clin Oncol 33 (suppl. Abstr 6021)

D'Souza G, Kreimer AR, Viscidi R et al (2007) Case-control study of human papillomavirus and oropharyngeal cancer. N Engl J Med 356:1944–1956

Fakhry C, Westra WH, Li S et al (2008) Improved survival of patients with human papillomavirus-positive head and neck squamous cell carcinoma in a prospective clinical trial. J Natl Cancer Inst 100:261–269

Fakhry C, Zhang Q, Nguyen-Tan PF et al (2014) Human papillomavirus and overall survival after progression of oropharyngeal squamous cell carcinoma. J Clin Oncol 32:3365–3373

Fayette J, Wirth LJ, Oprean C et al (2014) Randomized phase II study of MEHD7945A (MEHD) vs cetuximab (Cet) in >= 2nd-line recurrent/metastatic squamous cell Carcinoma of the head & neck (RMSCCHN) progressive on/after platinum-based chemotherapy (PtCT). Ann Oncol 25 (suppl 4): iv340, (Abstr # 986O)

Friedland PL, Bozic B, Dewar J, Kuan R, Meyer C, Phillips M (2011) Impact of multidisciplinary team management in head and neck cancer patients. Br J Cancer 104:1246–1248

Gillison ML, Koch WM, Capone RB et al (2000) Evidence for a causal association between human papillomvirus and a subset of head and neck cancers. J Natl Cancer Inst 92:709–720

Gregoire V, Lefebvre J-L, Licitra L, Felip E (2010) Squamous cell carcinoma of the head and neck: EHNS-ESMO-ESTRO cklinical practice Guidelines for diagnosis, treatment and follow-up. Ann Oncol 21(suppl. 5):v184–v186

Haddad RI, Shin DM (2008) Recent advances in head and neck cancer. N Engl J Med 359:1143–1154

Huang SH, Perez-Ordonez B, Weinreb I et al (2013) Natural course of distant metastases following radiotherapy or chemoradiotherapy in HPV-related oropharyngeal cancer. Oral Oncol 49:79–85

Kreimer AR, Clifford GM, Boyle P, Franceschi S (2005) Human papillomavirus types in head and neck squamous cell carcinomas worldwide: a systematic review. Cancer Epidemiol Biomarkers Prev 14:467–475

Lassen P, Eriksen JG, Hamilton-Dutoit S, Tramm T (2010) Alsner, Overgaard J. HPV-associated p16-expression and response to hypoxic modification of radiotherapy in head and neck cancer. Radiat Oncol 94:30–35

Licitra L, Perrone F, Bossi P et al (2006) High-risk human papillomavirus affect prognosis in patients with surgically treated oropharyngeal squamous cell carcinoma. J Clin Oncol 24:5630–5636

List MA, Rutherford JL, Strachs J et al (2004) Prioritizing treatment outcomes: head and neck cancer patients versus nonpatients. Head Neck 26:163–170

Machiels JP, Haddad RI, Fayette J et al (2015) LUX-H&N 1 investigators. Afatinib versus methotrexate as second-line treatment in patients with recurrent or metastatic squamous-cell carcinoma of the head and neck progressing on or after platinum-based therapy (LUX-Head & Neck 1): an open-label, randomised phase 3 trial. Lancet Oncol 16(5):583–594

O'Sullivan B, Huang SH, Siu LL et al (2013) Deintensification candidate subgroups in human papillomavirus–related oropharyngeal cancer according to minimal risk of distant metastasis. J Clin Oncol 31:543–550

Posner MR, Lorch JH, Goloubeva O et al (2011) Survival and human papillomavirus in oropharynx cancer in TAX 324: a subset analysis from an international phase III trial. Ann Oncol 22:1071–1077

Psyrri A, Rampias T, Vermorken JB (2014) The current and future impact of human papillomavirus on treatment of squamous cell carcinoma of the head and neck. Ann Oncol 25:2101–2115

Rampias T, Pectasides E, Prasad M et al (2013) Molecular profile of head and neck squamous cell carcinomas bearing p16 high phenotype. Ann Oncol 24:2124–2131

Reich M, Leemans CR, Vermorken JB, Bernier J, Licitra L, Parmar S, Golusinski W, Lefebvre JL (2014) Best practices in the management of the psycho-oncologic aspects of head and neck cancer patients: recommendations from the European head and neck cancer society make sense campaign. Ann Oncol 25:2115–2124

Rischin D, Young RJ, Fisher R et al (2010) Prognostic significance of p16INK4A and human papillomavirus in patients with oropharyngeal cancer treated on TROG 02.02 phase III trial. J Clin Oncol 28:4142–4148

Rosenthal DI (2014) Impact of p 16 status on the results of the phase III cetuximab (cet)/radiotherapy(RT). J Clin Oncol 32 (suppl. Abstr 6001)

Ruhstaller T, Roe H, Thürlimann B, Nicoll JJ (2006) The multidisciplinary meeting: an indispensable aid to communication between different specialties. Eur J Cancer 42:2459–2462

Vermorken JB (2005) Medical treatment in head and neck cancer. Ann Oncol 16 (suppl. 2): ii258–ii264

Vermorken JB, Stöhlmacher-Williams J, Davidenko I et al (2013) Cisplatin and fluorouracil with or without panitumumab in patients with recurrent or metastatoc squamous-cell carcinoma of the head and neck (SPECTRUM): an open-label phase 3 randomised trial. Lancet Oncol 14:697–710

Vermorken JB, Psyrri A, Mesia R et al (2014) Impact of tumor HPV status on outcome in patients with recurrent and/or metastatic squamous cell carcinoma of the head and neck receiving chemotherapy with or without cetxuyimab: retrospective analysis of the phase III EXTREME trial. Ann Oncol 25:801–807

Systemic Treatment in HPV-Induced Recurrent or Metastatic HNSCC

Damian T. Rieke and Ulrich Keilholz

Abstract

Recurrent or metastatic head and neck cancer describes tumor deposits that arise locally, regionally, or at distant sites after treatment or distant metastases at the time of primary diagnosis. Prognosis for R/M squamous cell carcinomas of the head and neck (HNSCC) is poor and treatment options are limited in this situation. Human papillomavirus (HPV) is an important risk factor for HNSCC. About 40 % of all HNSCC have been attributed to HPV in Europe. HPV positivity at initial diagnosis is the single best prognostic factor for survival. However, data for the prognostic and predictive value of HPV in the R/M situation are still scarce. Due to the rising incidence of HPV-associated cancers, the number of R/M HPV+ carcinomas is also expected to rise. This chapter therefore aims to give an overview of the current knowledge concerning the role of HPV as a prognostic and predictive marker in recurrent or metastatic HNSCC.

Keywords

HPV · R/M HNSCC · Predictive biomarker · Targeted therapy · Checkpoint inhibitor · Chemotherapy · EGFR inhibitor

D.T. Rieke · U. Keilholz (✉)
Charité Comprehensive Cancer Center, Charité – Universitätsmedizin Berlin, Berlin, Germany
e-mail: ulrich.keilholz@charite.de

W. Golusiński et al. (eds.), *HPV Infection in Head and Neck Cancer*,
Recent Results in Cancer Research 206, DOI 10.1007/978-3-319-43580-0_11

1 Prevalence and Prognostic Implications of HPV-Induced HNSCC in Recurrent or Metastatic Population

The incidence of HPV-associated HNSCC has risen dramatically over the last years in Northern America and Western Europe (Chaturvedi et al., J Clin Oncol. 2011; Mehanna et al., Head Neck 2013; Abogunrin et al., BMC Cancer 2014; Tinhofer et al., Eur J Cancer 2015). In a subset of these patients, locoregional or distant recurrence will eventually develop.

When looking at the rate and pattern of treatment failure in HPV+ HNSCC, data are largely missing because of several limitations: The diagnosis of HPV has not been standardized in clinical routine, and sensitivity and specificity vary between p16 immunohistochemistry (IHC), HPV IHC, or PCR. Additionally, prevalence and test performance vary between different anatomic sites. Because of better prognosis, fewer HPV+ patients will eventually reach the R/M situation. Additional risk factors (e.g., pack years, tumor stage) as well as the mutational profile contribute to the prognosis of HPV-positive carcinomas (Ang et al., N Engl J Med. 2010; Tinhofer et al. Eur J Cancer 2016). Furthermore, the rise in incidence results in different prevalences of HPV depending on the timing of recruitment into different cohorts and since HPV has only relatively recently been described as causal, older cohorts oftentimes lack information on HPV status.

We have identified several key questions regarding prevalence and prognostic implications.

1.1 What Is the Prevalence of HPV+ Carcinomas in the R/M Situation?

Several studies in R/M HNSCC patients have assessed either p16 (by immunohistochemistry, IHC) as a surrogate marker of HPV positivity or HPV directly (e.g., by in situ hybridization, ISH). In oropharyngeal cancers, both methods overlap well. Other cancer sites do show relevant differences because of a lower prevalence of HPV-associated non-oropharyngeal cancer and a lower sensitivity of the HPV and lower specificity of the p16 test. Therefore, results should be taken with caution. A false-positive rate for p16 IHC has been reported as high as 7 %, a false-negative rate for HPV ISH as high as 11 % (Jordan et al., Am J Surg Pathol. 2012). More accurate testing methods (e.g., HPV-DNA PCR) are rarely used in clinic and a standard for HPV testing is required. With these limitations, the rate of HPV+ recurrent or metastatic tumors, as estimated from studies in R/M squamous cell carcinomas of the head and neck, should be estimated somewhere between 10 and 20 % (Table 1). The observed differences between studies and testing methods can be explained not only by the different sensitivities and specificities of the testing methods but also by the anatomical site, the geographical location, and the time of study inclusion. When looking at clinical studies, a risk of selection bias has also to be taken into account. HPV-positive patients are slightly younger, have a better

Table 1 Prevalence of HPV or p16 positivity in patients in R/M cohorts

Study	Method	Tested	Positive (%)	Citation
SPECTRUM	P16	443	99 (22 %)	Vermorken et al., Lancet Oncol (2013)
EXTREME	P16	381	41 (12 %)	Vermorken et al., Ann Oncol (2014)
EXTREME	HPV	321	24 (8 %)	Vermorken et al., Ann Oncol (2014)
ADVANTAGE	P16	177	25 (14 %)	Vermorken et al., Ann Oncol (2014)
E1395 & E3301	HPV	64	11 (17 %)	Argiris et al., Ann Oncol (2014)
E1395 & E3301	P16	65	12 (18 %)	Argiris et al., Ann Oncol (2014)
LUX-H&N1	P16	257	49 (19 %)	Machiels et al., Lancet Oncol (2015)
PRISM	P16	30	6 (20 %)	Rischin et al., Head Neck (2016)
Seiwert et al.	P16	65	17 (26 %)	Seiwert et al., Ann Oncol (2014)
PARTNER	P16	66	19 (29 %)	Wirth et al., J Clin Oncol. 31, (2013) (suppl; abstr 6029)
Gilbert et al.	P16	44	9 (20 %)	Gilbert et al., Oral Oncol (2015)
Machiels et al.	HPV	21	1 (5 %)	Machiels et al., Canc Chemother Pharmacol (2015)
TEMHEAD	HPV	24	4 (17 %)	Grünwald et al., Ann Oncol (2015)
GORTEC	P16	12	3 (25 %)	Guigay et al., Ann Oncol (2015)

1540 patients total were tested for p16, 280 (18 %) are positive. 430 patients were tested for HPV, 40 (9 %) are positive.

prognosis, and might therefore be overrepresented. Accordingly, a small study has observed a trend towards a higher number of treatment interventions in HPV+ patients (Deeken et al., Head Neck 2015).

Another way of estimating the percentage of HPV-positive patients in the R/M population would be to look at the amount of failures in prospectively followed HPV-positive cohorts.

In a study by Posner et al. (Ann Oncol. 2011), 111 patients with oropharyngeal cancer (56 HPV+, 55 HPV− as assessed by E6/7 PCR) treated in the TAX324 study were followed for 5 years. In the HPV+ group, 27 % had disease progression in comparison with 71 % in the HPV- group.

In a study by Ang et al. (N Engl J Med. 2010), 323 patients were tested for HPV (HPV ISH, p16). After 3 years, 26.3 % of 206 HPV+ positive patients had progressive disease in comparison with 56.6 % of 117 HPV− patients.

Extrapolating these numbers to a general HNSCC population with 40 % HPV prevalence, 20–30 % of R/M patients would be expected to be HPV+. However, these numbers come from studies in advanced oropharyngeal carcinoma and are therefore not representative for a general HNSCC population.

1.2 What Is the Rate of Locoregional and/or Distant Recurrence?

The previous data show that treatment failures occur regularly in HPV+ HNSCC. Treatment failure can occur locoregionally or at distant sites. For clinical practice, it is important to look at differences in the clinical characteristics of these recurrences. This section therefore aims at identifying patterns of disease recurrence in the HPV + population and its differences compared to HPV− cancers.

In oropharyngeal carcinomas, the study by Ang et al. (N Engl J Med. 2010) is a retrospective analysis of stage III/IV oropharyngeal carcinoma (no significant difference in survival after treatment with accelerated fractionation RTx+ cisplatin or standard fractionation radiotherapy + cisplatin). 206 (63.8 %) of 323 patients with oropharyngeal carcinoma were HPV positive (HPV ISH & p16). After 3 years, the tumor had relapsed locoregionally significantly more often in HPV-negative than in HPV-positive patients (35.1 %, 95 %CI 26.4–43.8 vs. 13.6 %, 95 %CI 8.9–18.3). The frequency of distant metastases did not differ significantly between both groups.

A retrospective analysis by Rischin et al. (J Clin Oncol. 2010) identified 106 (57 %) of 185 stage III or IV oropharyngeal carcinomas (treated with radiotherapy and cisplatin ± tiranzapine) that were p16 positive. After 2 years, locoregional failures were observed more often in the HPV-negative group (14 % vs. 7 %, $p = 0.091$) with similar rates of distant failure in both groups.

The study by Posner et al. (Ann Oncol. 2011) identified 56 (50 %) HPV-positive (HPV PCR) carcinomas among 111 patients with locally advanced oropharyngeal carcinomas. After 5 years, local-regional failure was significantly less common in HPV positive than in negative carcinomas but no significant difference was seen in the rate of distant metastases.

The study by Huang et al. (Oral Oncol. 2013) identified 457 p16+ patients among 624 patients with oropharyngeal cancer treated with definite radiotherapy or chemoradiation. The median follow-up was longer in p16+ patients (4.2 vs. 3.3 years). 27 (6 %) p16+ patients had locoregional failure as compared to 35 (21 %) p16− patients. Distant metastases (with or without concurrent locoregional recurrence) were identified in 54 (12 %) p16+ and 25 (15 %) p16− patients.

Taken together, these results suggest that locoregional recurrences were less common in HPV+ carcinomas, whereas the rate of distant metastases was similar.

1.3 Do the Characteristics of Metastatic Spread Differ in HPV-Associated Tumors?

Since the rate of distant metastases seems to be similar between HPV-positive and HPV-negative patients, it is of interest to investigate potential differences in clinical presentation between these groups.

The study by Fakhry et al. (J Clin Oncol. 2014) did not report significant differences in the anatomic site of metastasis between p16+ and p16– oropharyngeal carcinoma. Lung (p16+ vs. p16−; 72.9 % vs. 69.7 %), bone (14.6 % vs. 15.2 %), and liver (16.7 % vs. 12.1 %) were the most common sites in 81 patients with distant metastases.

Huang et al. (Int J Radiat Oncol Biol Phys. 2012) observed 36 distant metastases after a median 3.3 years of follow-up. The overall incidence did not differ significantly between p16+ and negative patients (10 % vs. 16 %). In both groups, lung, liver, and bone metastases were common sites of recurrence but in HPV+ patients metastatic spread to the skin (7 patients), intra-abdominal lymph nodes (n = 5), brain (n = 4), duodenum (n = 1), paraspinal muscle (n = 1), and axillary lymph nodes (n = 1) were observed. Multiple distant metastases were seen in 11 patients with p16+ tumors compared to 0 in p16− patients. The median time to distant metastases was also significantly longer in p16+ cancer patients (1.6 years vs. 0.5 years).

A similar pattern of metastasis has also been described by other authors. In a cohort of 11 HNSCC patients with brain metastases, 5 patients were p16+ (Bulut et al., Eur Arch Otorhinolaryngol. 2014). A later presentation of brain metastases in the p16+ subgroup was also described in this study (45.6 vs. 26.4 months). A study by Ruzevick et al. (J Neurooncol. 2013) identified 7 brain metastases from head and neck primaries. 4 of these were HPV+ and the mean time between treatment and brain metastases was 45 months.

A disseminating metastatic phenotype has been described in another study by Huang et al. (Oral Oncol. 2013). In this study, 457 p16+ and 167 p16− oropharyngeal cancer patients were followed for a median of 3.9 years. 54 and 25 distant metastases were observed in p16+ and p16- groups, respectively. Metastases to more than two organs were observed in 18 p16+ (0 p16− patients) with 11 of these exhibiting what the authors call an "explosive" character with rapid deterioration and large metastases. Oligometastatic spread to the lung was associated with a relatively indolent course in HPV+ cancers.

Taken together, these information suggest that the most common pattern of metastatic spread is similar between HPV+ and HPV− patients with lung, bone, and liver metastases. A subgroup of HPV+ patients that might be as large as 30 % presents with relevant differences. Atypical sites (brain, skin, intra-abdominal lymph nodes) and rapid clinical deterioration are of concern in these patients. A longer interval to metastasis is also of clinical relevance, because of its impact on follow-up schedules. An increased exposition to X-ray-based imaging in follow-up is of concern in these patients, since they are younger on average (Misiukiewicz et al., Clin Adv Hem Onc 2014). Taken together, the reported differences reflect a poor-prognosis subgroup in the HPV+ population. Therefore, prognostic factors identifying patients at risk for these patterns are warranted. Additional cigarette smoking might be a risk factor but the unusual timing, site, and dissemination of HPV-associated distant metastases do not differ significantly between patients with > 10 pack years or patients with 10 pack years or less (Huang et al. Int J Rad Oncol Biol Physics 2012). A stratification into high-, medium-, or low-risk groups according to p16 status, pack years and T and N stage has been proposed but did not find a significant difference in regard to distant metastases (Fakhry et al., J Clin Oncol. 2014). Circulating tumor cells and additional molecular aberrations including Bcl2 or TP53 might help in the future to identify patients at risk for poor prognosis. (Tinhofer et al., Ann Oncol. 2014; Tinhofer et al., Eur J Cancer 2016; Nichols et al. Clin Canc Res. 2010; Morris et al., JAMA Oncol. 2016).

1.4 What Is the Specific Prognosis?

It has been shown that HPV is the strongest prognostic factor on initial presentation. Since metastatic spread is common in HPV+ patients and some of them show a rapid deterioration as described above, the overall prognosis of R/M HPV+ patients will be reviewed here.

With respect to distant metastases, the study by Huang et al. (Oral Oncol. 2013) shows a significantly longer survival after distant metastases in p16 positive oropharyngeal carcinomas. The poor-prognosis subgroup therefore appears not to be relevant for the overall better prognosis of HPV+ patients in the metastatic situation.

Only recently have studies explicitly addressed this question. Fakhry et al. (J Clin Oncol. 2014) could show that p16+ oropharyngeal tumors still had a reduced risk of death after disease progression. A pooled analysis from E1395 and E3301 also showed longer OS for HPV+ patients that was statistically significant (Argiris et al., Ann Oncol. 2014). Vermorken et al. (Ann Oncol. 2014) could reproduce this result in HPV+ HNSCC. Therefore, HPV positivity still remains an important prognostic factor in R/M HNSCC, but the magnitude of the impact in recurrent/metastatic disease is far smaller than in the primary disease setting.

2 Sensitivity of HPV-Induced HNSCC to Cytotoxic Drugs

Since many of the cited studies show a better OS and PFS for HPV+ tumors, data from these studies can also be queried for the predictive value of HPV status when comparing the treatment and control arms.

In the combined analysis of the E1395 and E3301 studies, 65 patients (12 p16 positive) were treated with cisplatin/5FU vs. cisplatin/paclitaxel or docetaxel/irinotecan, respectively. The objective response rate (ORR) was 50 % for p16+

compared to 19 % for p16- patients (p = 0.057), and significance was reached when the HPV status (ISH) was assessed (HPV+ vs. HPV−, 55–19 %, p = 0.022) (Argiris et. al., Ann Oncol. 2014).

In the EXTREME trial, patients were treated with platinum/5-FU with or without the addition of cetuximab (Vermorken et al., Ann Oncol. 2014; Vermorken et al., N Engl J Med 2008). In the chemotherapy alone arm, OS and ORR did not show significant differences between p16+ and – as well as HPV+ and – patients (ORR 22 vs. 17 %, p = 0.6 and 8 vs. 20 %, p = 0.27, respectively).

In the SPECTRUM trial, patients were randomized to receive cisplatin/5-FU with or without the addition of panitumumab (Vermorken et al., Lancet Oncol. 2013). In the chemotherapy alone arm, overall survival was nonsignificantly better in p16+ patients. PFS did not differ between both groups. (p16+ vs. p16−; PFS 5.5 months, 95 %CI 3.4-6.7 vs. 5.1 months, 95 %CI 4.1-5.5).

In the PARTNER trial, patients received docetaxel/cisplatin with or without panitumumab. In the chemotherapy alone arm, ORR were nonsignificantly higher in p16+ patients (54 %, 95 %CI 27-81 vs. 27 % 95 %CI 9-46) (Wirth et al., J Clin Oncol. Abstr 6029, 2013).

Taken together, these studies do not provide sufficient evidence to use HPV status as a predictive biomarker for cytotoxic chemotherapy. The slight benefits in overall survival, as reported in some studies might reflect the better prognosis of HPV+ patients. Some studies also suggest better response rates of HPV+ patients. This effect seems not to be limited to a specific type of chemotherapy used and is not consistent among studies.

3 Sensitivity of HPV-Induced HNSCC to EGFR Blockade

EGFR inhibition in addition to cytotoxic chemotherapy is standard of treatment in recurrent or metastatic squamous cell carcinoma of the head and neck. Efficacy of various inhibitors of EGFR had been shown, including cetuximab (Bonner et al., N Engl J Med. 2006; Vermorken et al., N Engl J Med. 2008), afatinib (Machiels et al., Lancet Oncol. 2015; Seiwert et al., Ann Oncol. 2014), or panitumumab (Vermorken et al., Lancet Oncol. 2013). An unplanned subgroup analysis of the SPECTRUM trial (Vermorken et al., Lancet 2013) suggested that a benefit from panitumumab addition to chemotherapy was limited to the p16 negative patients. A subgroup analysis of the PRISM trial also identified higher disease control rates with panitumumab in p16-negative patients but interpretation was limited because of the small sample size (30 patients with available p16 status) (Rischin et al., Head Neck 2016). In a biomarker analysis of the LUX-H&N1 study (Machiels et al., Lancet Oncol. 2015), a benefit of afatinib vs. methotrexate in R/M HNSCC was more pronounced in p16 negative tumors.

Taken together, most studies suggest that HPV-positive tumors have a smaller effect of the addition of EGFR inhibitors, but because of the retrospective nature of almost all analyses, this interpretation has to be viewed with caution. Further results are of interest in this context: The rate of EGFR aberrations in HPV-negative tumors as observed in genomic analyses was lower than in HPV positives (TCGA, Nature 2015; Seiwert et al., Clin Canc Res. 2015). Neither EGFR expression nor amplification has been reported as predictive for clinical outcome after EGFR blockade (Licitra et al., Eur J Cancer 2013; Licitra et al., Ann Oncol. 2011). In vivo and in vitro data could not show an effect of E6/E7 expression or HPV status on cetuximab efficacy (Pogorzelski et al., Cell Death Dis. 2014). Clinical data further contradict the hypothesis of HPV positivity as a biomarker for EGFR-inhibitor resistance:

In a retrospective analysis of the EXTREME trial in recurrent/metastatic disease, benefit of cetuximab therapy was independent of p16 status (Vermorken et al., Ann Oncol. 2014). Another small cohort of R/M patients treated with afatinib or cetuximab did also not find relevant differences according to p16 status (Seiwert et al., Ann Oncol. 2014). Preliminary results from the PARTNER study did also not identify differences in response to panitumumab treatment in R/M HNSCC according to p16-status (Wirth et al., J Clin Oncol 31, 2013 (suppl; abstr 6029)). The same was found for radiotherapy-based primary treatment with cetuximab of oropharyngeal carcinoma (Rosenthal et. al., JCO, 2016). Pogorzelski et al. did also not identify differences in a small cohort of HNSCC patients treated with cetuximab (Pogorzelski et al., Cell Death Dis. 2014).

How can these diverse results be reconciled? One possible explanation might be pharmacological differences of the used inhibitors. Afatinib is an irreversible tyrosine kinase inhibitor and might therefore be more active against somatic alterations as observed more frequently in HPV-negative tumors. Antibodies like cetuximab on the other hand have been proposed as more active against ligand-activated receptors (Arteaga et al., Cancer Cell 2014). Furthermore, the mechanism of EGFR inhibition in cancer is not limited to disruption of the relevant pathways. Antibody dependent cellular cytotoxicity describe the T-cell-mediated cytotoxicity mediated by antibody binding. Panitumumab, in contrast to cetuximab, has been proposed to not have this effect. This might also contribute to the observed differences in the predictive value of HPV status for EGFR-antibody-based treatment, as observed in the previously cited studies.

Another possible explanation for heterogeneity of results is the small sample sizes and limited data that are available. From the current data, HPV status should not be used as a biomarker for EGFR inhibition. Further trials with different types of EGFR inhibitors and stratification according to HPV status (as assessed by reliable methods, e.g., combined p16 IHC and HPV ISH) are warranted.

4 Sensitivity of HPV-Induced HNSCC to Immunotherapy

Immunotherapy and especially checkpoint blockade by PD-L1 inhibition has recently shown promising results in R/M HNSCC. Does HPV status provide predictive information regarding this treatment option? In the Keynote012 study, HPV+ and HPV- patients with PD-L1+ (>1 % PD-L1 expression of tumor cells or stroma by IHC) R/M HNSCC were recruited to receive the PD-1 inhibitor pembrolizumab (Seiwert et al., Lancet Oncol., 2016). 60 patients were enrolled and treated, of which 23 (38 %) were p16 positive. The overall response rate was nonsignificantly higher in the p16 positive group (p16+ ORR 25 %, 95 %CI 7-52 vs. p16- 14 %, 95 % CI 4-32). Another study did not find differences in the expression of PD-L1 between HPV-positive and HPV-negative patients (Kim et al., Canc Res Treat. 2016). As another potential marker of inflammation and response to checkpoint inhibition, infiltration by CD8 and CD3 positive cells is significantly more common in HPV+ patients (Balermpas et al., Int J Cancer 2016). Russell et al. (Head Neck Oncol. 2013) describe higher intratumoural CD8/Foxp3 T-cell ratios and CD20 expression in HPV+ compared to HPV− tumors. The expression of an inflamed signature has been proposed as predictive biomarker but does not necessarily encompass the above reported genes. A comparative analysis of gene expression in HNSCC identified a subset of HPV-positive tumors with an "inflamed" expression phenotype (Keck et. al., Clin Canc Res. 2015). However, the inflamed subgroup in HNSCC was not limited to HPV-positive tumors.

In conclusion, some studies suggest a higher degree of T-cell infiltration in HPV + HNSCC. The premature clinical data do not support a stratification of treatment with checkpoint inhibitors according to HPV status.

HPV testing is of utmost importance for all prospective clinical trials, and currently accruing specific trials will answer the key questions in the coming three to five years.

5 Conclusion

What are the consequences for clinical practice from these results? HPV-positive patients make up approximately 10–20 % of the R/M population. The difference to the prevalence at first presentation is explained by a lower rate of locoregional recurrence. Distant metastasis is similar between HPV-positive and HPV-negative patients, and HPV-positive patients might present with atypical metastatic patterns as defined by unusual anatomic site and later occurrences. Despite these differences, the better prognosis of patients with HPV + HNSCC is still applicable in the R/M situation, despite a subgroup with poor prognosis. The differences might be mediated by additional risk factors (mutational signature, pack years), and follow-up practices might be guided by these stratifiers in future.

The predictive value of HPV positivity in the R/M situation still remains to be defined. Current studies do not support a different treatment strategy of HPV+ R/M HNSCC.

References

Abogunrin S, Di Tanna GL, Keeping S et al. (2014) Prevalence of human papillomavirus in head and neck cancers in European populations: a meta-analysis. BMC Cancer 14:968

Ang KK, Harris J, Wheeler R et al. (2010) Human papillomavirus and survival of patients with oropharyngeal cancer. N Engl J Med 363:24–35

Argiris A, Li S, Ghebremichael M et al. (2014) Prognostic significance of human papillomavirus in recurrent or metastatic head and neck cancer: an analysis of Eastern Cooperative Oncology Group trials. Ann Oncol 25:1410–1416

Arteaga CL, Engelman JA (2014) ERBB receptors: from oncogene discovery to basic science to mechanism-based cancer therapeutics. Cancer Cell 25:282–303

Balermpas P, Rodel F, Rodel C et al. (2016) CD8+ tumour-infiltrating lymphocytes in relation to HPV status and clinical outcome in patients with head and neck cancer after postoperative chemoradiotherapy: A multicentre study of the German cancer consortium radiation oncology group (DKTK-ROG). Int J Cancer 138:171–181

Bonner JA, Harari PM, Giralt J et al. (2006) Radiotherapy plus cetuximab for squamous-cell carcinoma of the head and neck. N Engl J Med 354:567–578

Bulut OC, Lindel K, Hauswald H et al. (2014) Clinical and molecular characteristics of HNSCC patients with brain metastases: a retrospective study. Eur Arch Otorhinolaryngol 271:1715–1722

Cancer Genome Atlas N (2015) Comprehensive genomic characterization of head and neck squamous cell carcinomas. Nature 517:576–582

Chaturvedi AK, Engels EA, Pfeiffer RM et al. (2011) Human papillomavirus and rising oropharyngeal cancer incidence in the United States. J Clin Oncol 29:4294–4301

Deeken JF, Newkirk K, Harter KW et al. (2015) Effect of multimodality treatment on overall survival for patients with metastatic or recurrent HPV-positive head and neck squamous cell carcinoma. Head Neck 37:630–635

Fakhry C, Zhang Q, Nguyen-Tan PF et al. (2014) Human papillomavirus and overall survival after progression of oropharyngeal squamous cell carcinoma. J Clin Oncol 32:3365–3373

Gilbert J, Schell MJ, Zhao X et al. (2015) A randomized phase II efficacy and correlative studies of cetuximab with or without sorafenib in recurrent and/or metastatic head and neck squamous cell carcinoma. Oral Oncol 51:376–382

Grünwald V, Keilholz U, Boehm A et al. (2015) TEMHEAD: a single-arm multicentre phase II study of temsirolimus in platin- and cetuximab refractory recurrent and/or metastatic squamous cell carcinoma of the head and neck (SCCHN) of the German SCCHN Group (AIO). Ann Oncol 26:561-567

Guigay J, Fayette J, Dillies AF et al. (2015) Cetuximab, docetaxel, and cisplatin as first-line treatment in patients with recurrent or metastatic head and neck squamous cell carcinoma: a multicenter, phase II GORTEC study. Ann Oncol 26:1941–1947

Huang SH, Perez-Ordonez B, Liu FF et al. (2012) Atypical clinical behavior of p16-confirmed HPV-related oropharyngeal squamous cell carcinoma treated with radical radiotherapy. Int J Radiat Oncol Biol Phys 82:276–283

Huang SH, Perez-Ordonez B, Weinreb I et al. (2013) Natural course of distant metastases following radiotherapy or chemoradiotherapy in HPV-related oropharyngeal cancer. Oral Oncol 49:79–85

Jordan RC, Lingen MW, Perez-Ordonez B et al. (2012) Validation of methods for oropharyngeal cancer HPV status determination in US cooperative group trials. Am J Surg Pathol 36:945–954

Keck MK, Zuo Z, Khattri A et al. (2015) Integrative analysis of head and neck cancer identifies two biologically distinct HPV and three non-HPV subtypes. Clin Cancer Res 21:870–881

Kim HS, Lee JY, Lim SH et al. (2016) Association Between PD-L1 and HPV Status and the Prognostic Value of PD-L1 in Oropharyngeal Squamous Cell Carcinoma. Cancer Res Treat 48:527-536

Licitra L, Mesia R, Rivera F et al. (2011) Evaluation of EGFR gene copy number as a predictive biomarker for the efficacy of cetuximab in combination with chemotherapy in the first-line treatment of recurrent and/or metastatic squamous cell carcinoma of the head and neck: EXTREME study. Ann Oncol 22:1078–1087

Licitra L, Storkel S, Kerr KM et al. (2013) Predictive value of epidermal growth factor receptor expression for first-line chemotherapy plus cetuximab in patients with head and neck and colorectal cancer: analysis of data from the EXTREME and CRYSTAL studies. Eur J Cancer 49:1161–1168

Machiels JP, Haddad RI, Fayette J et al. (2015) Afatinib versus methotrexate as second-line treatment in patients with recurrent or metastatic squamous-cell carcinoma of the head and neck progressing on or after platinum-based therapy (LUX-Head & Neck 1): an open-label, randomised phase 3 trial. Lancet Oncol 16:583–594

Machiels JP, Specenier P, Krauss J et al. (2015) A proof of concept trial of the anti-EGFR antibody mixture Sym004 in patients with squamous cell carcinoma of the head and neck. Cancer Chemother Pharmacol 76:13–20

Mehanna H, Beech T, Nicholson T et al. (2013) Prevalence of human papillomavirus in oropharyngeal and nonoropharyngeal head and neck cancer–systematic review and meta-analysis of trends by time and region. Head Neck 35:747–755

Misiukiewicz K, Camille N, Gupta V et al. (2014) The role of HPV status in recurrent/metastatic squamous cell carcinoma of the head and neck. Clin Adv Hematol Oncol 12:812–819

Morris LG, Chandramohan R, West L et al. (2016) The Molecular Landscape of Recurrent and Metastatic Head and Neck Cancers: Insights From a Precision Oncology Sequencing Platform. JAMA Oncol

Nichols AC, Finkelstein DM, Faquin WC et al. (2010) Bcl2 and human papilloma virus 16 as predictors of outcome following concurrent chemoradiation for advanced oropharyngeal cancer. Clin Cancer Res 16:2138–2146

Pogorzelski M, Ting S, Gauler TC et al. (2014) Impact of human papilloma virus infection on the response of head and neck cancers to anti-epidermal growth factor receptor antibody therapy. Cell Death Dis 5:e1091

Posner MR, Lorch JH, Goloubeva O et al. (2011) Survival and human papillomavirus in oropharynx cancer in TAX 324: a subset analysis from an international phase III trial. Ann Oncol 22:1071–1077

Rischin D, Spigel DR, Adkins D et al. (2016) PRISM: Phase 2 trial with panitumumab monotherapy as second-line treatment in patients with recurrent or metastatic squamous cell carcinoma of the head and neck. Head Neck 38 Suppl 1:E1756–1761

Rischin D, Young RJ, Fisher R et al. (2010) Prognostic significance of p16INK4A and human papillomavirus in patients with oropharyngeal cancer treated on TROG 02.02 phase III trial. J Clin Oncol 28:4142–4148

Rosenthal DI, Harari PM, Giralt J et al. (2016) Association of Human Papillomavirus and p16 Status With Outcomes in the IMCL-9815 Phase III Registration Trial for Patients With Locoregionally Advanced Oropharyngeal Squamous Cell Carcinoma of the Head and Neck Treated With Radiotherapy With or Without Cetuximab. J Clin Oncol 34:1300–1308

Russell S, Angell T, Lechner M et al. (2013) Immune cell infiltration patterns and survival in head and neck squamous cell carcinoma. Head Neck Oncol 5:24

Ruzevick J, Olivi A, Westra WH (2013) Metastatic squamous cell carcinoma to the brain: an unrecognized pattern of distant spread in patients with HPV-related head and neck cancer. J Neurooncol 112:449–454

Seiwert TY, Burtness B, Mehra R et al. (2016) Safety and clinical activity of pembrolizumab for treatment of recurrent or metastatic squamous cell carcinoma of the head and neck (KEYNOTE-012): an open-label, multicentre, phase 1b trial. Lancet Oncol 17:956–965

Seiwert TY, Fayette J, Cupissol D et al. (2014) A randomized, phase II study of afatinib versus cetuximab in metastatic or recurrent squamous cell carcinoma of the head and neck. Ann Oncol 25:1813–1820

Seiwert TY, Zuo Z, Keck MK et al. (2015) Integrative and comparative genomic analysis of HPV-positive and HPV-negative head and neck squamous cell carcinomas. Clin Cancer Res 21:632–641

Tinhofer I, Budach V, Saki M et al. (2016) Targeted next-generation sequencing of locally advanced squamous cell carcinomas of the head and neck reveals druggable targets for improving adjuvant chemoradiation. Eur J Cancer 57:78–86

Tinhofer I, Johrens K, Keilholz U et al. (2015) Contribution of human papilloma virus to the incidence of squamous cell carcinoma of the head and neck in a European population with high smoking prevalence. Eur J Cancer 51:514–521

Tinhofer I, Konschak R, Stromberger C et al. (2014) Detection of circulating tumor cells for prediction of recurrence after adjuvant chemoradiation in locally advanced squamous cell carcinoma of the head and neck. Ann Oncol 25:2042–2047

Vermorken JB, Mesia R, Rivera F et al. (2008) Platinum-based chemotherapy plus cetuximab in head and neck cancer. N Engl J Med 359:1116–1127

Vermorken JB, Peyrade F, Krauss J et al. (2014) Cisplatin, 5-fluorouracil, and cetuximab (PFE) with or without cilengitide in recurrent/metastatic squamous cell carcinoma of the head and neck: results of the randomized phase I/II ADVANTAGE trial (phase II part). Ann Oncol 25:682–688

Vermorken JB, Psyrri A, Mesia R et al. (2014) Impact of tumor HPV status on outcome in patients with recurrent and/or metastatic squamous cell carcinoma of the head and neck receiving chemotherapy with or without cetuximab: retrospective analysis of the phase III EXTREME trial. Ann Oncol 25:801–807

Vermorken JB, Stohlmacher-Williams J, Davidenko I et al. (2013) Cisplatin and fluorouracil with or without panitumumab in patients with recurrent or metastatic squamous-cell carcinoma of the head and neck (SPECTRUM): an open-label phase 3 randomised trial. Lancet Oncol 14:697–710

Wirth LJ, Dakhil SR, Kornek G et al. PARTNER: A randomized phase II study of docetaxel/cisplatin (doc/cis) chemotherapy with or without panitumumab (pmab) as first-line treatment (tx) for recurrent or metastatic squamous cell carcinoma of the head and neck (R/M SCCHN). J Clin Oncol 31, 2013 (suppl; abstr 6029)

Further Reading

Misiukiewicz K et al (2014) The role of HPV status in recurrent/metastatic squamous cell carcinoma of the head and neck. Clin Adv Hematol Oncol 12(12):812–819

Psyrri A et al (2014) The current and future impact of human papillomavirus on treatment of squamous cell carcinoma of the head and neck. Ann Oncol

Spreafico A et al (2014) Demystifying the role of tumor HPV status in recurrent and/or metastatic squamous cell carcinoma of the head and neck. Ann Oncol 25(4):760–762

Vokes E et al (2015) HPV-associated head and neck cancer. J Natl Cancer Inst 107(12)

Optimizing Radiotherapy in HPV-Associated Oropharyngeal Cancer Patients

Johannes A. Langendijk and Roel J.H.M. Steenbakkers

Abstract

Concurrent chemoradiation is considered the golden standard in the treatment of locally advanced OPC. However, given the very high survival rates in favorable HPV-positive OPC and the high rates of acute and late treatment-related side effects, de-escalation strategies have to be considered. In this chapter, the potential benefit of a number of de-escalation strategies is described, including of replacement of concurrent chemotherapy by cetuximab, radiation dose de-escalation based on response to induction chemotherapy, radiotherapy alone without systemic treatment, and limiting elective nodal target volumes for radiation. In addition to de-escalation, modern radiation technologies like protons will offer increasing opportunities to decrease the dose to normal tissues in order to prevent radiation-induced toxicities. Initial analysis showed that radiation dose de-escalation based on response to induction chemotherapy in combination with intensity-modulated proton therapy (IMPT) has the highest potential to decrease acute and late toxicities.

Keywords

HPV-positive OPC · Radiotherapy · De-escalation · Proton therapy · Cetuximab · Chemoradiation · Toxicity

---

J.A. Langendijk (✉)
Department of Radiation Oncology, University Medical Center Groningen, Groningen, The Netherlands
e-mail: j.a.langendijk@rt.umcg.nl

R.J.H.M. Steenbakkers
University of Groningen, Groningen, The Netherlands

W. Golusiński et al. (eds.), *HPV Infection in Head and Neck Cancer*,
Recent Results in Cancer Research 206, DOI 10.1007/978-3-319-43580-0_12

1 Introduction

At present, concurrent chemoradiation (CRT) is considered the golden standard in the treatment of locally advanced (stages III–IV) oropharyngeal carcinoma (OPC). However, there are several reasons to consider de-escalation strategies in HPV-positive OPC.

First, excellent results have been obtained with CRT with overall survival rates of over 90 % in the most favorable patient groups (Ang et al. 2010; O'Sullivan et al. 2013). These excellent results have led to the assumption that favorable HPV-positive patients might be overtreated. This overtreatment might lead to unnecessary acute and late treatment-related side effects. Thus, for these patients, less intensive treatment regimens might give similar results with regard to locoregional tumor control and overall survival with fewer side effects.

Second, the cumulative incidence of severe late treatment-related side effects in head and neck cancer patients treated with CRT is 43 % after 5 years, mainly consisting of pharyngeal dysfunction, tube feeding dependence, and laryngeal dysfunction (Machtay et al. 2008). In addition, there are a number of studies indicating that even after 5 years, new severe late side effects may occur (Ward et al. 2016; Forastiere et al. 2013; Cooper et al. 2012). The long-term results of RTOG study 91-11 in which patients with laryngeal cancer were randomly assigned to receive either radiotherapy alone, sequential chemotherapy, and radiotherapy of concurrent CRT showed increased rates of non-cancer-related deaths in the CRT arm occurring after 7–8 years of follow up (Forastiere et al. 2013). Recently, Ward et al. (Ward et al. 2016) reported on a retrospective analysis in 84 laryngeal cancer patients treated with CRT for laryngeal cancer that would have met the eligibility criteria for the RTOG 91-11 and showed indeed that 60 % of aspiration admissions and 63 % of tube feeding insertions occurred beyond 5 years of follow up. In the postoperative setting, similar results were found in RTOG study 95-01 in which postoperative radiotherapy alone was compared to postoperative chemoradiation (Cooper et al. 2012). In that study, the cumulative 10-year incidence of grade 4 toxicity was nearly twice as high after CRT (7.3 % vs. 3.9 %). This is clinically relevant, as a number of studies showed that radiation-induced side effects have a major impact on the general dimensions of QoL (Langendijk et al. 2008; Jellema et al. 2007). Moreover, unpublished results from the department of Radiation Oncology of the University Medical Centre Groningen showed significantly higher rates of non-cancer-related death when higher rates of radiation induced dysphagia. Given the favorable outcome of HPV-positive patients, it is expected that the prevalence of long-term survivors who are at risk of late and very late radiation-induced side effects will dramatically increase in the next decades. Therefore, there is a strong need to consider how definitive organ-sparing treatment strategies can be further optimized in particular with regard to the prevention of late and very late side effects.

Third, recent studies showed that locoregional control after definitive radiotherapy or CRT in HPV-positive HNSCC is excellent ranging from 80 % in the intermediate-risk patients to over 90 % in the low-risk patients. Moreover, it appears that distant failure has become the predominant site of failure, while in the HPV-negative cases, locoregional failure is the most frequent site of failure (O'Sullivan et al. 2013). So far, concurrent CRT does not have shown any effect on the occurrence of distant metastases (Pignon et al. 2009).

There are numerous ways to de-escalate CRT in head and neck cancer. One of the strategies that are currently under investigation is the replacement of concurrent CRT by concurrent cetuximab (Bonner et al. 2010; Bonner et al. 2006), which is discussed by others in this chapter. In this sub-chapter, de-escalation and detoxification strategies of radiotherapy itself will be discussed.

2 Radiotherapy Alone

Besides replacing one concurrent systemic treatment modality by another (e.g., cetuximab instead of chemotherapy), de-escalation can also be achieved by applying radiotherapy as single modality. A number of authors reported on the results of radiotherapy alone in HPV-positive tumors.

Lassen et al. reported on the results of HPV-positive patients who were included in the DAHANCA 5 trial, a phase III trial in which patients were randomly assigned to receive radiotherapy alone or radiotherapy plus nimorazole, a hypoxia cell sensitizer (Lassen et al. 2010). The 5-year locoregional control rate in the 84 patients with p16-positive tumors was 61 %, which was significantly better as compared to that observed among p16-negative cases (35 %). In addition, these authors also reported on the results of p16-positive HNSCC treated with conventional or accelerated radiotherapy either or not in combination with hypoxic modification that included in the DAHANCA 5 and 7 trials, showing a 5-year local and locoregional control rate of 84 and 72 %, respectively (Lassen et al. 2013). In the multivariate analysis, p16 positivity was an independent and the strongest prognostic factor for all relevant endpoints.

A series of the Princess Margaret Hospital in Toronto showed good results in a retrospective analysis of HPV-positive patients treated with radiotherapy alone or CRT. Radiotherapy alone was standard for those with stage I–II disease and some stage III cases, while in stage III and IV, RT alone was reserved for patients deemed unfit for CRT, such as in case of high age, frailty, medical reasons, or patient refusal (O'Sullivan et al. 2012). In this series, better outcome in terms of overall survival, local control, and regional control was observed in all HPV-positive cases as compared to all HPV-negative cases, while no difference was noted with regard to the occurrence of distant metastases. Stage IV HPV-positive patients treated with CRT had significantly better overall survival than those treated with radiotherapy alone (89 % vs. 70 %), but no difference was noted with regard to local, regional, and distant disease control. In particular, in HPV-positive patients with stage IV and ≤ 10 pack-years, outcome was excellent with a 3-year overall survival, local and regional control rates of 85, 95 and 97 %, respectively.

Chen et al. reported on a retrospective series of 23 HPV-positive HNC patients treated with radiotherapy alone (median dose: 70 Gy). The decision not to use CRT was highly individualized and on discretion of the treating physician (Chen et al. 2013). Excellent 3-year overall survival and locoregional control rates were observed for stage I–II disease (100 and 100 %, respectively). For patients with more advanced stages, the corresponding rates were 81 and 88 %, respectively. Moreover, 3-year overall and locoregional control rates were also 100 and 100 %, respectively, in 18 the HPV-positive patients who were never smokers.

Recently, Rosenthal et al. reported on a retrospective analysis of the IMCL-9815 trial in which HNSCC patients were randomly assigned to receive radiotherapy alone or radiotherapy plus cetuximab (Rosenthal et al. 2016). This analysis only included the subset of patients with OPC of which 41 % were p16-positive. The 3-year overall survival rate among p16-positive cases treated with radiotherapy alone was significantly lower as compared to those treated with radiotherapy plus cetuximab (72 % vs. 88 %). Similar results were shown for locoregional control which was 65 % after radiotherapy alone versus 87 % after radiotherapy plus cetuximab.

Taking into account the results of these studies, it is clear that p16/HPV status is a consistent and strong prognostic factor for patients treated with radiotherapy alone with locoregional control rates varying from 65 to 100 % in the HPV-positive cases, indicating that not all HPV-positive HNSCCs have excellent results after radiotherapy alone. The subset analysis of the IMCL trial suggests that also in HPV-positive cases, results can be significantly improved by adding cetuximab to radiation. However, the key question remains which HPV-positive HNSCC patients have such high locoregional control rates (e.g., beyond 90 %) that systemic treatment can be safely omitted.

O'Sullivan et al. made an attempt to identify a subset of patients suitable for de-escalation according to the risk of distant metastases using recursive partitioning analysis (O'Sullivan et al. 2013). They showed a 3-year locoregional control rate of 95 % among HPV-positive OPC patients with T1–T3 and N0-N2c disease. The distant control rates for HPV-positive, low-risk N0-2a or less than 10 pack-year N2b patients were similar for RT alone and CRT, but significantly more distant metastases were observed in the N2c subset managed by RT alone. Based on these results, the authors concluded that HPV-positive T1-3N0-2c patients have a low risk of distant metastases and excellent locoregional control rates, but that N2c patients have a higher risk of distant metastases when treated with RT alone and thus seem less suited for de-escalation strategies that omit chemotherapy (O'Sullivan et al. 2013).

In summary, radiotherapy alone may give high locoregional control rates in well-selected patients, but cannot be considered the standard of care yet in locally advanced cases.

3 De-escalation and Detoxification of Radiotherapy

There are several ways to decrease acute and late side effects induced by radiotherapy. Two general strategies can be distinguished, including de-escalation and detoxification.

De-escalation refers to a conceptual change in treatment strategy, e.g., by decreasing the total dose of radiation to the therapeutic (area with macroscopic tumor) or prophylactic (elective nodal areas) target volume or by excluding parts of the prophylactic target volume (e.g., unilateral instead of bilateral elective nodal irradiation). In this way, radiation exposure to healthy surrounding tissues can be significantly reduced, but may lead to higher rates of local and/or regional failures in the high-risk regions due to lower target dose levels or in the elective nodal areas as a result of omitting (part of) the prophylactic target volume.

Detoxification refers to radiotherapy technology improvement that allows for a better dose conformation around the target volume in order to reduce dose exposure to the healthy tissues while target volumes and dose to the targets remain unchanged. Technologies that may result in a further detoxification of radiotherapy include swallowing-sparing intensity-modulated radiotherapy (IMRT) (Christianen et al. 2016), multicriteria optimization (MCO) (Kierkels et al. 2014, 2015), and intensity-modulated proton therapy (IMPT) (van Dijk et al. 2016; van der Laan et al. 2013; van de Water et al. 2011). Theoretically, this approach is safer as target volumes and target dose levels remain similar, but the possibilities to spare healthy tissues are generally considered less.

At present, a number of randomized controlled trials (RCTs) are running, investigating different de-escalation strategies in HPV-positive HNSCC. In general, two general approaches can be distinguished, including (1) replacement of concurrent CRT by radiotherapy plus cetuximab, and (2) induction chemotherapy followed by lower total dose of radiation to the target in case of a partial or complete response to induction chemotherapy.

3.1 Chemoradiation Versus Bioradiation Trials

There are three randomized studies investigating whether concurrent cisplatin-based CRT can be replaced by radiotherapy plus cetuximab. This approach is mainly based on the findings of the RCT comparing radiotherapy versus radiotherapy plus cetuximab (Bonner et al. 2006, 2010). This study showed significantly improved locoregional control and overall survival in the radiotherapy with cetuximab arm, without enhancing radiation-induced side effects.

In the RTOG 1016 phase III trial, patients with HPV-associated OPC (p16-positive) were randomly assigned to receive accelerated IMRT with concurrent high-dose cisplatin (2×100 mg/m^2) versus accelerated IMRT with cetuximab (loading dose 400 mg/m^2 + 6×250 mg/m^2) (NCT01302834). The trial was designed as a non-inferiority study with 5-year overall survival as primary endpoint (threshold difference: 9 %). The most important secondary endpoints are acute and late side effects. In total, 987 patients have been included, and the study has been closed to accrual (www.clinicaltrial.gov).

In the De-ESCALaTE HPV trial (NCT018741710), 304 patients with p16-positive OPC patients will be randomized between conventional CRT (70 Gy in 7 weeks + 3 × cisplatin 100 mg/m^2) and conventional radiotherapy with cetuximab (loading dose of 400 mg/m^2 + 7 × 250 mg/m^2). The primary endpoint in this study is severe acute and late grade 3–5 toxicity caused by cetuximab plus radiotherapy or cisplatin plus radiotherapy (www.clinicaltrial.gov). This study is still recruiting patients.

TROG 12.01 (NCT01855451) aims at finding the optimal treatment for HPV-associated OPC and actually has a similar design as the De-ESCALaTE HPV trial with similar primary endpoint (www.clinicaltrial.gov). Target patients' accrual is 200, and the study is still recruiting patients.

3.2 Induction Chemotherapy Followed by Dose De-escalation Trials

There are three clinical studies including HPV-associated OPC patients investigating whether the total dose of radiation can be reduced in case of good response after induction chemotherapy.

In the ECOG 1308 trial (NCT01084083), a phase II trial, HPV-associated stage III–IV resectable OPCs were first treated with induction chemotherapy (3 × paclitaxel 90 mg/m^2, 1 × cisplatin 75 mg/m^2, and cetuximab loading dose of 400 mg/m^2 and weekly cetuximab 250 mg/m^2). Patients with a clinical complete response received a total dose of 54 Gy with concurrent weekly cetuximab, while patients with less than complete response were treated with a total dose of 70 Gy plus cetuximab. The aim of this study was to estimate the 2-year progression-free survival in the low-dose arm (www.clinicaltrial.gov). Patient accrual has been completed (90 patients). Preliminary results revealed a complete response rate after induction chemotherapy of 71 %, and 61 patients were assigned to low-dose radiotherapy (Cmelak et al. 2014). The 2-year progression-free survival was 84 % in all these patients and was excellent (96 %) in the 27 patients with $\leq$10 pack-years, T1–T3 and N0-N2b disease. Secondary endpoints were acute and late side effects. In addition, less radiation-induced head and neck cancer symptoms were suggested among patients treated with the low-dose arm (Cmelak et al. 2015).

The University of Chicago is currently running a randomized phase II study including stage III–IV HPV-related OPC (NCT01133678). Patients are randomly assigned to receive induction chemotherapy with everolimus or placebo in combination with cisplatin, paclitaxel, and cetuximab. Patients with good clinical response are then randomly assigned to receive 70 Gy or 55 Gy at the therapeutic target volume. The primary endpoint in this study is the 2-year progression-free survival, while secondary endpoints include response rate, overall survival, and acute and late toxicities (www.clinicaltrial.gov).

Finally, in the Quarterback Trial, patients with locally advanced HPV-associated OPC are first treated with 3 cycles of TPF induction chemotherapy (NCT01706939). Patients with a partial or complete response after induction chemotherapy are then randomly assigned to receive standard dose radiation (70 Gy) with carboplatin or reduced-dose radiotherapy (56 Gy) and carboplatin. The primary endpoint in this study is 3-year progression-free survival. Secondary endpoints also include acute and late side effects. The aim is to include 365 patients, and patient recruitment is still ongoing.

3.3 Detoxification Studies

The MD Anderson Cancer Centre in Houston is currently running a randomized phase II–III study including HPV-positive OPC treated with concurrent CRT (NCT01893307) (www.clinicaltrial.gov). Patients are randomly allocated for either concurrent CRT using IMRT or concurrent CRT using IMPT. Conventional fractionation is used to a total dose of 70 Gy in combination with cisplatin (3 cycles of 100 mg/m^2). The primary endpoint here is late grade 3–5 toxicity from 90 days to 2 years after completion of treatment. The target number of patients to be included in this study is 360, and the study is still recruiting patients.

In conclusion, a number of clinical phase II and phase III trials are currently recruiting patients, using different strategies to reduce the dose to healthy tissues. No final results can be presented yet. Thus, the question is which approach is most promising to reduce side effects.

4 Expected Benefits of De-escalation and Detoxification Strategies

To investigate the potential benefit of the aforementioned strategies, we recently performed an in silico planning comparative (ISPCS), including 50 locally advanced (stage III–IV) oropharyngeal cancer patients who were treated at the Department of Radiation Oncology of the UMCG with concurrent chemoradiation or radiotherapy with cetuximab (unpublished data).

All patients underwent a planning CT scan with contrast enhancement in treatment position. In summary, the therapeutic clinical target volume (CTV1) consisted of the primary tumor and pathological lymph nodes plus a 1.0-cm margin. The prophylactic nodal areas on both sides of the neck were selected according to the guidelines reported by Gregoire et al. [Gregoire]. The CTV for the boost irradiation (CTV2) consisted of the primary tumor and pathological lymph nodes with a 0.5-cm margin. A 0.5-cm margin was the used for the planning target volumes (PTV1 and PTV2).

Four different strategies were mimicked including:

1. Current standard CRT with standard dose swallowing-sparing IMRT (SW-IMRT) using a simultaneous integrated boost (SIB) technique (Cmelak et al. 2015). The prophylactic PTV was treated with 35 fractions of 1.55 Gy up to a total dose of 54.25 Gy while the therapeutic PTV was treated with 35 fractions of 2 Gy up to a total dose of 70 Gy (CRT-70).
2. Same approach as 1 but with replacement of concurrent CRT by radiotherapy plus cetuximab (BioRT-70).
3. CRT with reduced-dose SW-IMRT using a total dose of 56 Gy to therapeutic PTV in 1.6 Gy per fraction while the prophylactic PTV was planned with 35 fractions of 1.55 Gy up to a total dose of 54.25 Gy (CRT-56), mimicking a reduced dose to the target after a complete response after induction chemotherapy.
4. Same approach as in 1 but then with IMPT (CPT-70) (van der Laan et al. 2013).
5. Same approach as in 2 but then with IMPT (BioPT-70).
6. Same approach as in 3 but then with IMPT (CPT-56).

To estimate the potential clinical benefit in terms of reduction in radiation-induced side effects, recently published normal tissue complication probability (NTCP) models (Beetz et al. 2012a, b; Christianen et al. 2012) were used to translate the dose distributions in the different organs at risk (OARs) into estimations of the risk of side effects (NTCP values).

For moderate-to-severe patient-rated xerostomia, the multivariable NTCP model of Beetz et al. (2012a) was used. The risk of this side effect depends on the mean dose to the contralateral parotid gland and the baseline score of xerostomia.

For grade II–IV dysphagia, the multivariable NTCP model of Christianen et al. (2012) was used. The risk of this side effect depends on the mean dose to the superior pharyngeal constrictor muscle and the mean dose to the supraglottic area.

For tube feeding dependence, the multivariable model of Wopken et al. (2014) was used. The risk of this side effect depends on T-stage, baseline weight loss, treatment modality, and four dosimetric factors, including the mean dose to the superior and inferior pharyngeal constrictor muscles, the cricopharyngeal muscle, and the mean dose to the contralateral parotid gland. In this analysis, patients treated with cetuximab and concurrent CRT had relative risks of 1.74 and 6.73 to remain tube feeding dependent at 6 months.

The results are summarized in Fig. 1. The results show that based on these models, limited effect on late radiation-induced toxicity is expected from replacing CRT by radiotherapy plus cetuximab, besides a lower risk of tube feeding dependence. Low-dose radiotherapy is expected to result in a reduction in the risk of all side effects. The use of proton therapy is expected to further reduce the risk of late radiation-induced side effects, in particular with regard to xerostomia and tube feeding dependence.

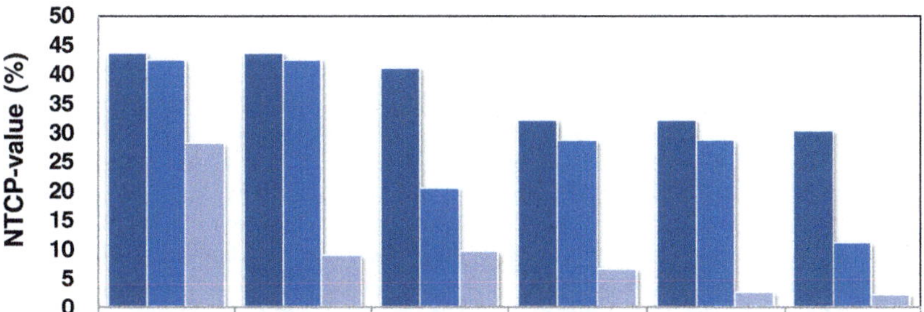

	CRT-70	BioRT-70	CRT-56	CPT-70	BioPT-70	CPT-56
Xerostomia	43,8	43,8	41,3	32,3	32,3	30,4
Dysphagia	42,7	42,7	20,6	28,8	28,8	11,2
Tube feeding	28,3	9,1	9,7	6,8	2,7	2,3

Fig. 1 NTCP values (risk on side effects) according to the 6 different approaches. *CRT-70* current standard chemoradiation; *BioRT-70* standard radiotherapy with cetuximab; *CRT-56* reduced radiation dose chemoradiation; *CPT-70* standard radiation dose concurrent IMPT; *BioPT* standard dose IMPT plus cetuximab; *CPT-56* reduced-dose concurrent IMPT

5 Conclusion

Radiotherapy alone for HPV-associated OPC provides high locoregional control rates in well-selected cases with favorable prognostic factors and can be applied in particular when CRT is considered too toxic. Radiation-induced toxicity in HPV-associated OPC can be reduced with different de-escalation and detoxification strategies. When patients are treated with IMRT, the most promising de-escalation approach is reduced-dose IMRT after good response to induction chemotherapy, but this may come at the cost of some loss in locoregional control. With IMPT, the risk of radiation-induced side effects can be further reduced and might be considered in the future for intermediate-risk patients in which de-escalation is less preferable.

References

Ang KK, Harris J, Wheeler R, Weber R, Rosenthal DI, Nguyen-Tân PF, Westra WH, Chung CH, Jordan RC, Lu C, Kim H, Axelrod R, Silverman CC, Redmond KP, Gillison ML (2010) Human papillomavirus and survival of patients with oropharyngeal cancer. N Engl J Med 363 (1):24–35

Beetz I, Schilstra C, Burlage FR, Koken PW, Doornaert P, Bijl HP, Chouvalova O, Leemans CR, de Bock GH, Christianen ME, van der Laan BF, Vissink A, Steenbakkers RJ, Langendijk JA (2012a) Development of NTCP models for head and neck cancer patients treated with three-dimensional conformal radiotherapy for xerostomia and sticky saliva: the role of dosimetric and clinical factors. Radiother Oncol 105(1):86–93

Beetz I, Schilstra C, van der Schaaf A, van den Heuvel ER, Doornaert P, van Luijk P, Vissink A, van der Laan BF, Leemans CR, Bijl HP, Christianen ME, Steenbakkers RJ, Langendijk JA

(2012b) NTCP models for patient-rated xerostomia and sticky saliva after treatment with intensity modulated radiotherapy for head and neck cancer: the role of dosimetric and clinical factors. Radiother Oncol 105(1):101–106

Bonner JA, Harari PM, Giralt J, Azarnia N, Shin DM, Cohen RB, Jones CU, Sur R, Raben D, Jassem J, Ove R, Kies MS, Baselga J, Youssoufian H, Amellal N, Rowinsky EK, Ang KK (2006) Radiotherapy plus cetuximab for squamous-cell carcinoma of the head and neck. N Engl J Med 354(6):567–578

Bonner JA, Harari PM, Giralt J, Cohen RB, Jones CU, Sur RK, Raben D, Baselga J, Spencer SA, Zhu J, Youssoufian H, Rowinsky EK, Ang KK (2010) Radiotherapy plus cetuximab for locoregionally advanced head and neck cancer: 5-year survival data from a phase 3 randomised trial, and relation between cetuximab-induced rash and survival. Lancet Oncol 11(1):21–28

Chen AM, Zahra T, Daly ME, Farwell DG, Luu Q, Gandour-Edwards R, Vaughan AT (2013) Definitive radiation therapy without chemotherapy for human papillomavirus-positive head and neck cancer. Head Neck 35(11):1652–1656

Christianen ME, Schilstra C, Beetz I, Muijs CT, Chouvalova O, Burlage FR, Doornaert P, Koken PW, Leemans CR, Rinkel RN, de Bruijn MJ, de Bock GH, Roodenburg JL, van der Laan BF, Slotman BJ, Verdonck-de Leeuw IM, Bijl HP, Langendijk JA (2012) Predictive modelling for swallowing dysfunction after primary (chemo)radiation: results of a prospective observational study. Radiother Oncol 105(1):107–114

Christianen ME, van der Schaaf A, van der Laan HP, Verdonck-de Leeuw IM, Doornaert P, Chouvalova O, Steenbakkers RJ, Leemans CR, Oosting SF, van der Laan BF, Roodenburg JL, Slotman BJ, Bijl HP, Langendijk JA (2016) Swallowing sparing intensity modulated radiotherapy (SW-IMRT) in head and neck cancer: clinical validation according to the model-based approach. Radiother Oncol 118(2):298–303

Cmelak A, Li S, Marur S et al (2014) E1308: reduced-dose IMRT in human papilloma virus (HPV)-associated resectable oropharyngeal squamous carcinomas (OPSCC) after clinical complete response (cCR) to induction chemotherapy (IC). J Clin Oncol 32(18) Supplement: S. Meeting Abstract: LBA6006

Cmelak A, Li S, Marur S et al (2015) Symptom reduction from IMRT dose deintensification: Results from ECOG 1308 using the vanderbilt head and neck symptom survey version 2 (VHNSS V2). J Clin Oncol 33(15) Supplement: S, Meeting Abstract: 6021

Cooper JS, Zhang Q, Pajak TF, Forastiere AA, Jacobs J, Saxman SB, Kish JA, Kim HE, Cmelak AJ, Rotman M, Lustig R, Ensley JF, Thorstad W, Schultz CJ, Yom SS, Ang KK (2012) Long-term follow-up of the RTOG 9501/intergroup phase III trial: postoperative concurrent radiation therapy and chemotherapy in high-risk squamous cell carcinoma of the head and neck. Int J Radiat Oncol Biol Phys 84(5):1198–1205

Forastiere AA, Zhang Q, Weber RS, Maor MH, Goepfert H, Pajak TF, Morrison W, Glisson B, Trotti A, Ridge JA, Thorstad W, Wagner H, Ensley JF, Cooper JS (2013) Long-term results of RTOG 91-11: a comparison of three nonsurgical treatment strategies to preserve the larynx in patients with locally advanced larynx cancer. J Clin Oncol 31(7):845–852

Jellema AP, Slotman BJ, Doornaert P, Leemans CR, Langendijk JA (2007) Impact of radiation-induced xerostomia on quality of life after primary radiotherapy among patients with head and neck cancer. Int J Radiat Oncol Biol Phys 69(3):751–760

Kierkels RG, Korevaar EW, Steenbakkers RJ, Janssen T, van't Veld AA, Langendijk JA, Schilstra C, van der Schaaf A (2014) Direct use of multivariable normal tissue complication probability models in treatment plan optimisation for individualised head and neck cancer radiotherapy produces clinically acceptable treatment plans. Radiother Oncol 112(3):430–436

Kierkels RG, Visser R, Bijl HP, Langendijk JA, van't Veld AA, Steenbakkers RJ, Korevaar EW (2015) Multicriteria optimization enables less experienced planners to efficiently produce high quality treatment plans in head and neck cancer radiotherapy. Radiat Oncol 10:87

Langendijk JA, Doornaert P, Verdonck-de Leeuw IM, Leemans CR, Aaronson NK, Slotman BJ (2008) Impact of late treatment-related toxicity on quality of life among patients with head and neck cancer treated with radiotherapy. J Clin Oncol 26(22):3770–3776

Lassen P, Eriksen JG, Hamilton-Dutoit S, Tramm T, Alsner J, Overgaard J, Danish Head and Neck Cancer Group (DAHANCA) (2010) HPV-associated p16-expression and response to hypoxic modification of radiotherapy in head and neck cancer. Radiother Oncol 94(1):30–35

Lassen P, Overgaard J, Eriksen JG (2013) Expression of EGFR and HPV-associated p16 in oropharyngeal carcinoma: correlation and influence on prognosis after radiotherapy in the randomized DAHANCA 5 and 7 trials. Radiother Oncol 108(3):489–494

Machtay M, Moughan J, Trotti A, Garden AS, Weber RS, Cooper JS, Forastiere A, Ang KK (2008) Factors associated with severe late toxicity after concurrent chemoradiation for locally advanced head and neck cancer: an RTOG analysis. J Clin Oncol 26(21):3582–3589

O'Sullivan B, Huang SH, Perez-Ordonez B, Massey C, Siu LL, Weinreb I, Hope A, Kim J, Bayley AJ, Cummings B, Ringash J, Dawson LA, Cho BC, Chen E, Irish J, Gilbert RW, Hui A, Liu FF, Zhao H, Waldron JN, Xu W (2012) Outcomes of HPV-related oropharyngeal cancer patients treated by radiotherapy alone using altered fractionation. Radiother Oncol 103 (1):49–56

O'Sullivan B, Huang SH, Siu LL, Waldron J, Zhao H, Perez-Ordonez B, Weinreb I, Kim J, Ringash J, Bayley A, Dawson LA, Hope A, Cho J, Irish J, Gilbert R, Gullane P, Hui A, Liu FF, Chen E, Xu W (2013) Deintensification candidate subgroups in human papillomavirus-related oropharyngeal cancer according to minimal risk of distant metastasis. J Clin Oncol 31(5): 543–550

Pignon JP, le Maître A, Maillard E, Bourhis J, MACH-NC Collaborative Group (2009) Meta-analysis of chemotherapy in head and neck cancer (MACH-NC): an update on 93 randomised trials and 17,346 patients. Radiother Oncol 92(1):4–14

Rosenthal DI, Harari PM, Giralt J, Bell D, Raben D, Liu J, Schulten J, Ang KK, Bonner JA (2016) Association of human papillomavirus and p16 status with outcomes in the IMCL-9815 phase III registration trial for patients with locoregionally advanced oropharyngeal squamous cell carcinoma of the head and neck treated with radiotherapy with or without cetuximab. J Clin Oncol 34(12):1300–1308

van de Water TA, Bijl HP, Schilstra C, Pijls-Johannesma M, Langendijk JA (2011) The potential benefit of radiotherapy with protons in head and neck cancer with respect to normal tissue sparing: a systematic review of literature. Oncologist 16(3):366–377

van der Laan HP, van de Water TA, van Herpt HE, Christianen ME, Bijl HP, Korevaar EW, Rasch CR, van't Veld AA, van der Schaaf A, Schilstra C, Langendijk JA, Rococo cooperative group (2013) The potential of intensity-modulated proton radiotherapy to reduce swallowing dysfunction in the treatment of head and neck cancer: a planning comparative study. Acta Oncol 52(3):561–569

van Dijk LV, Steenbakkers RJ, Ten Haken B, van der Laan HP, van't Veld AA, Langendijk JA, Korevaar EW (2016) Robust intensity modulated proton therapy (IMPT) increases estimated clinical benefit in head and neck cancer patients. PLoS One 11(3):e0152477

Ward MC, Adelstein DJ, Bhateja P, Nwizu TI, Scharpf J, Houston N, Lamarre ED, Lorenz R, Burkey BB, Greskovich JF, Koyfman SA (2016) Severe late dysphagia and cause of death after concurrent chemoradiation for larynx cancer in patients eligible for RTOG 91-11. Oral Oncol 57:21–26

Wopken K, Bijl HP, van der Schaaf A, van der Laan HP, Chouvalova O, Steenbakkers RJ, Doornaert P, Slotman BJ, Oosting SF, Christianen ME, van der Laan BF, Roodenburg JL, Leemans CR, Verdonck-de Leeuw IM, Langendijk JA (2014) Development of a multivariable normal tissue complication probability (NTCP) model for tube feeding dependence after curative radiotherapy/chemo-radiotherapy in head and neck cancer. Radiother Oncol 113(1): 95–101

Should We De-escalate the Treatment for HPV-Positive Tumors?

Andreas Dietz, Gunnar Wichmann and Susanne Wiegand

Abstract

De-escalation or de-intensification of therapy is discussed since many retrospective analyses of former trials demonstrated significantly better outcome for patients suffering from p16/HPV16-positive oropharyngeal squamous cell carcinoma of head and neck (OHNSCC). These observations are comprehensively addressed, but the reader has to keep in mind that none of the currently discussed data result from prospective controlled trials addressing the HPV-discrimination in the primary endpoint design. Identification of the true HPV16-related tumors is still challenging and in addition with different clinical reports and lack of data of prospective trials not mature for routine clinical decision making in 2016. Independent of the currently lacking evidence for HPV-dependent treatment de-escalation, there are some relevant arguments to address this question in ongoing and future trials.

Keywords

De-escalation · De-intensification · HPV-related treatment stratification · Transoral surgery · Late toxicity · Functional outcome · Quality of life (QoL) · Survival

De-escalation or de-intensification of therapy is discussed since many retrospective analyses of former trials demonstrated significantly better outcome for patients

A. Dietz (✉) · G. Wichmann · S. Wiegand
Klinik und Poliklinik für Hals-, Nasen-, Ohrenheilkunde, Department Kopf- und Zahnmedizin, Universitätsklinikum Leipzig, Leipzig, Germany
e-mail: Andreas.Dietz@medizin.uni-leipzig.de

A. Dietz · G. Wichmann · S. Wiegand
Clinic of Otolaryngology, Head and Neck Surgery, Department of Head Medicine and Oral Health, University of Leipzig, Leipzig, Germany

W. Golusiński et al. (eds.), *HPV Infection in Head and Neck Cancer*,
Recent Results in Cancer Research 206, DOI 10.1007/978-3-319-43580-0_13

suffering from p16/HPV16-positive oropharyngeal squamous cell carcinoma of head and neck (OHNSCC). These observations are comprehensively addressed in this book, but the reader has to keep in mind that none of the currently discussed data result from prospective controlled trials addressing the HPV-discrimination in the primary endpoint design. Currently, a comprehensive body of trials is on the way in many countries and within the next years many new (perhaps praxis changing) data are awaited (Masterson et al. 2014; Mirghani et al. 2015). These favorable outcomes in retrospective analysis are independent of treatment choice so far, mentioning the remarkable differences in outcome depending on p16-positive staining in the RTOG 0129 (Ang et al. 2010) primary radiotherapy trial or the observation of Haughey et al. (2011) regarding significantly better outcome after transoral laser microsurgery (TLM) in p16-positive OHNSCC. Interestingly, the current debate is misbalanced suggesting that p16-positive OHNSCC is more benefiting from primary radiation as from primary surgery due to the lack of surgical trials. This misbalance of treatment trials in head and neck cancer is demonstrated in meta-analysis showing clear outcome benefits in favor of HPV16/p16 positivity based on majority of radiotherapy trials (O'Rorke et al. 2012). Nevertheless, results of prospective trials are lacking and therefore recommendations for change of routine treatment in OHNSCC are difficult to be fixed in guidelines today.

Independent of currently lacking evidence for HPV-dependent treatment de-escalation, there are some relevant arguments to address this question in ongoing and future trials. Given that these patients are generally young and have a high likelihood of surviving their disease, post-treatment quality of life becomes of paramount importance. Indeed, a significant number of patients will experience severe toxicities including xerostomia, swallowing disorders, pain and stiffness of the neck and ototoxicity. Since Machtay et al. (2008) focused on severe late toxicity outcome problems after primary chemoradiation a brought international growing awareness of late toxicity and late functional outcome disorders in head and neck cancer treatment could be observed. This awareness influenced thinking toward better functional outcome in radiation oncology [constrictor-sparing delineation in IMRT, reducing the dose in adjuvant treatment after R0-resection (Quon et al. 2011a, b)] and primary surgery (minimally invasive transoral laser and robotic surgery, TORS, TLM to reduce morbidity by avoiding external approaches). The goal of treatment de-intensification should be to maintain good cure rates while minimizing long-term morbidity. Currently, different approaches to achieve this reduction of treatment-related morbidity are being pursued: limiting radiation dose; cisplatin alternatives given concurrently with radiation; modulation of radiation dose according to induction chemotherapy response; integrating minimally invasive surgery.

These strategies are interesting but raise many questions as de-escalation needs to be achieved without jeopardizing the good survival results of HPV+ patients. The risk of metastatic relapse in this patient subgroup has to be taken into account. How to define precisely a HPV-induced cancer? What is new with "minimally invasive surgery" in the context of HPV? Treatment of the neck seems to meet different risk situations. What is the patient's preference? Is there a place for de-escalation in routine treatment outside of trials?

1 What Is the Patient's Preference?

In head and neck cancer and other cancer sites, studies suggest that patients highly value survival and are willing to accept added toxicities to maximize their chances to survive. Understanding the patient´s perspective in the context of a de-intensification study is critical in planning a multi-institutional trial, because patients with HPV-positive oropharyngeal SCC must potentially risk reduction of their higher survival probability with standard CRT in favor of reduced toxicity potentially achieved with the experimental arm. Brotherston et al. (2013) conducted an investigation to answer this specific question for patient´s preference regarding acceptable expense for de-escalating cancer treatment. Fifty-one patients with oropharyngeal SCC (post-CRT) underwent semi-structured interviews contrasting toxicities of radiotherapy (RT) alone and CRT. Patients were asked what potential difference in cancer survival was acceptable to prefer RT over CRT. Initially, survival rate was the same for both treatments, then the RT rate was reduced until the preference switched. Ninety percent of patients initially selected RT, but 69 % switched to CRT after 0 to 5 % reduction in survival. Patients that rated their treatment experience as mild would accept lower survival versus severe treatment (p. 0.02). Eighty-one percent of patients (33 of 40) indicated they preferred reduced chemotherapy in CRT. The study shows that the primary concern of patients is survival, with 35 % of patients surveyed unwilling to risk any drop in survival probability to switch to RT over CRT, and a further 34 % willing to accept a 5 % or less reduction in probability of survival. In conclusion, with the limited data available currently, the majority of patients with oropharyngeal SCC are willing to take little or no risk of a survival decrease to receive RT alone as a de-intensification strategy.

2 How to Define Precisely a HPV-Induced Cancer?

Nevertheless, head and neck cancers are categorized by HPV16 status, because the presence of the virus tends to correlate with better survival. But the presence of HPV16 DNA in the tumor may not influence the disease characteristics if that DNA is not expressed. The detection of E6/E7 mRNA is considered as the definitive proof of viral involvement; but, it is often not feasible on a routine daily praxis. Therefore, p16-staining was established as easy to detect surrogate parameter in many centers worldwide. Indeed, several authors have reported that approximately 15–20 % of p16-positive OPSCCs are HPV16-negative by polymerase chain reaction and in situ hybridization (Robinson et al. 2012; Smeets et al. 2007; Lewis 2012; Rischin et al. 2010; Wasylyk et al. 2013; Adelstein et al. 2009). Stratification of head and neck squamous cell carcinomas (HNSCC) based on HPV16 DNA and RNA status, gene expression patterns, and mutated candidate genes may facilitate patient treatment decision. Recently our group could in concordance with other consortial research groups show that DNA-positive and RNA-positive OHNSCC have to be distinguished precisely regarding real HPV16 involvement and correlating typical biological tumor behavior (Wichmann et al. 2015). We characterized OHNSCC with different HPV16 DNA and RNA (E6*I) status from 290 consecutively recruited patients by gene expression profiling and targeted sequencing of 50 genes. We showed that tumors with transcriptionally inactive HPV16 (DNA+ RNA-) are similar to HPV-negative (DNA-) tumors regarding gene expression and frequency of *TP53* mutations (47 %, 8/17 and 43 %, 72/167, respectively). We also found that an immune response-related gene expression cluster is associated with lymph node metastasis, independent of HPV16 status.

In line with our observations, Holzinger et al. (2013) pointed out that at present, detection of HPV16-specific viral RNA patterns in snap-frozen biopsies is best suited to identify OHNSCC patients with biologically active HPV in their tumors and improved prognosis. Tumor samples of 188 OHNSCC patients with known HPV16 DNA and RNA status were included. High p16^{INK4a}, but also low pRb, low Cyclin D1 and normal p53 protein levels were strongly associated with OHNSCCs harboring biologically active HPV. However, p16^{INK4a} alone had only limited prognostic value and unsatisfactory power to predict RNA+ tumors in this patient cohort. It conferred significantly longer survival in univariate Kaplan–Meier analysis, but lost significant survival advantage after adjusting for gender, age, clinical stage, therapy status and alcohol and tobacco consumption. Kostareli et al. (2013) additional could describe a HPV16-specific methylation signatures which correlated in three independent well-characterized patient cohorts (Chicago, Heidelberg, Leipzig) with significant better overall survival, but interestingly also correlated with better survival if HPV16 was negative. In this study, the CpG island methylome of 15 OHNSCC tumors (5 HPV DNA-, 5 DNA+ RNA-, 5 DNA+ RNA+) revealed specific methylation signatures (5-gene [ALDH1A2, OSR2, GATA4, GRIA4, IRX4] promoter-methylation signature score) screened in 220 OHNSCC. It could be demonstrated that, in addition to genetic aberrations, epigenetic alterations critically contribute to histopathological and clinical differences between HPV-driven and non-HPV-driven tumors.

In summary, isolated p16 screening is not sufficient to detect the real HPV16-driven OHNSCC. To determine an accepted clear-cut diagnostic procedure which can be recommended for clinical routine praxis is still under progress.

3 What Is New with "Minimally Invasive Surgery?"

Today's main guidelines for treatment of HNSCC are still based on phase-III trials and comprehensive meta-analyses (Pignon et al. 2009), with excess of radiation or chemoradiation studies at the expense of surgical trials. As stated by Higgins and Wang (2008), clinical recommendations for HNSCC treatment based on evidences are difficult due to a disproportion of surgical and non-surgical trials. This conflict is augmented by the fact that instruments for evaluating best surgical practice are different from methodological standards in non-surgical phase-II or phase-III trials. But, going back to clinical routine, well-established and proven standards in surgery of HNSCC are defined as state-of-the-art tumor resection procedures and reconstruction, following consented resection criteria like clear margins (R0 resection) (Shah and Patel 2003). In general, as recently proposed by Wittekind et al. (2009), the inclusion of the minimal distance between tumor tissue and resection margins into the current R-classification would be useful. In HNSCC, a distance of 5 mm in minimum (except tumors of the glottis fold) is highly recommended. Also standardized neck dissection (Robbins et al. 2008) should be included into the tumor stage-related surgical concept. Altogether, primary surgery and additional adjuvant treatment of HNSCC is ever recommended if R0 resection is possible (also consequently ignoring molecular biological tumor configurations in today's clinical routine). Therefore, the choice of either surgery or multimodality treatment is mainly based on clinical experience and medical culture since there is still a high degree of haziness in view of the best biology-based treatment.

Triggered by some key note publications regarding transoral micro-laser (TLM: Canis et al. 2013a, b, 2015; Sinha et al. 2014) and robotic surgery (TORS: Hockstein et al. 2005; Gross et al. 2016; Kaczmar et al. 2016) in strong coincidence with recognition of the prognostic impact of HPV for OHNSCC, de-escalation in surgery also was raised as a strong topic in treatment of oropharyngeal cancer. As already mentioned, also TLM in OHNSCC provided significant better outcome in p16+ tumors (Haughey et al. 2011). TLM and TORS produce minimal comorbidities depending on the surgical approach since external comprehensive destructive opening of the oral cavity and pharyngeal structures can be avoided by transoral surgery. Both techniques are well described and can be performed in trained hands without compromising quality of oncologic surgery providing R0-resection. Using the term de-escalation of surgery, transoral approaches are definitely less aggressive regarding damage by external conventional classic approaches (i.e., mandibular split). Moreover, treatment de-escalation trials including non-surgical and surgical treatment are on the way implicating minimally invasive surgical techniques (TLM, TORS) as acceptable choices to minimize functional deficits in HPV16-positive disease.

Comparing outcomes of both transoral and open approaches in head and neck surgery demonstrates equality with definitive better functional late outcome for transoral approaches in limited disease. This observation is HPV independent as standards in correct oncological resection are not changing by using transoral approaches. But remarkably, HPV pushed the field of developments in transoral surgery in the US and established there those techniques which were common standard by using TLM in Europe many years before the HPV-debate started. Recently, TORS has been approved for small (T1, T2) oropharyngeal lesions and is used in routine treatment for lesions of the tonsillar region and base of tongue in many North American centers with good results. In Europe, TORS is in strong competition to TLM that has limitations especially in base of tongue lesions but is highly sufficient in well trained hands in most regions of the upper aero-digestive tract. Since TORS is still new and neither evidence for superiority toward TLM does exist nor reimbursements in Europe cover the terrific costs, this technique is not recommended for first choice routine treatment.

Another view is raised by comparing larger extent of surgery with need for reconstruction by flaps and primary radiochemotherapy in OHNSCC. Tschiesner et al. (2012) performed a highlighted cross-sectional, multi-institutional study, to compare functional outcome in patients with advanced head and neck cancer (oral cavity + oropharynx) treated by surgical resection and reconstruction with microvascular free flaps followed by adjuvant radiochemotherapy versus primary radiochemotherapy (RCT) on the basis of the International Classification of Functioning, Disability and Health (ICF) from WHO. Global quality of life scores suggested a slightly superior functional outcome for the surgical approach. The majority of ICF categories (81/93, 87 %) did not show a difference in functional outcome between the two treatment approaches. In the remaining 12 ICF categories, n = 3 body structures were more affected in the surgical group, while n = 3 body functions, and n = 6 activities/participations were more problematic in the RCT group. This included oral swallowing and weight maintenance functions as well as social relationships, acquiring a job, and economic self-sufficiency. This functional analysis shows clearly that avoiding surgery per se does not mean that a suggestively less harming therapy like RCT in advanced OHNSCC could be called de-escalation. Comparing late functional outcome, platinum-based RCT is recognized as highly toxic and definitely not less destructive than newer techniques of free-flap reconstruction in advanced OHNSCC. Keeping this in mind, Quon et al. (2010) raised some highly relevant questions regarding late functional outcome and better treatment planning in radiation oncology. As these minimally invasive surgical techniques gain popularity, there exist many unanswered questions such as how postoperative radiation (PORT) and chemotherapy should be integrated into the management for patients undergoing primary surgery for oropharyngeal carcinomas. Questions regarding the risks and benefits of a potential trimodality therapy are also important questions to address as these surgical techniques become integrated into traditional therapeutic paradigms. Constrictor-sparing radiation techniques using IMRT and customized reduction in cisplatin have to be discussed. Further thinking should be focused on radiation dose reduction after R0-resection in the primary tumor field in cases requiring adjuvant treatment. All these questions have to be addressed in prospective clinical trials to work out specific HPV-related effects by treating OHNSCC patients more precisely. It may be that we learn to move on into direction of precise surgical concepts achieving improved outcome with reduced late toxicity independent of any prognostic factors like HPV.

4 Conclusion

De-escalation in HPV-related OHNSCC is a highly relevant topic in clinical research to improve quality of therapy and outcome for our patients. Identification of the true HPV16-related tumors is still challenging and in addition with different clinical reports and lack of data of prospective trials, de-escalation strategies are not mature for integration into routine clinical decision making in 2016. Nevertheless, the HPV-driven developments of less destructive transoral approaches like TLM and TORS in OHNSCC pushed a wonderful clinical scientific debate and returned some neglected advantages of precise surgery in head and neck cancer to higher recognition.

References

Adelstein DJ, Ridge JA, Gillison ML, Chaturvedi AK, D'Souza G, Gravitt PE, Westra W, Psyrri A, Kast WM, Koutsky LA, Giuliano A, Krosnick S, Trotti A, Schuller DE, Forastiere A, Ullmann CD (2009) Head and neck squamous cell cancer and the human papillomavirus: summary of a National Cancer Institute State of the Science Meeting, November 9–10, 2008, Washington, D.C. Head Neck 31(11):1393–1422

Ang KK, Harris J, Wheeler R, Weber R, Rosenthal DI, Nguyen-Tân PF, Westra WH, Chung CH, Jordan RC, Lu C, Kim H, Axelrod R, Silverman CC, Redmond KP, Gillison ML (2010) Human papillomavirus and survival of patients with oropharyngeal cancer. N Engl J Med 363(1):24–35

Brotherston DC, Poon I, Le T, Leung M, Kiss A, Ringash J, Balogh J, Lee J, Wright JR (2013) Patient preferences for oropharyngeal cancer treatment de-escalation. Head Neck 35(2): 151–159

Canis M, Martin A, Kron M, Konstantinou A, Ihler F, Wolff HA, Matthias C, Steiner W (2013a) Results of transoral laser microsurgery in 102 patients with squamous cell carcinoma of the tonsil. Eur Arch Otorhinolaryngol 270(8):2299–2306

Canis M, Ihler F, Wolff HA, Christiansen H, Matthias C, Steiner W (2013b) Oncologic and functional results after transoral laser microsurgery of tongue base carcinoma. Eur Arch Otorhinolaryngol 270(3):1075–1083

Canis M, Wolff HA, Ihler F, Matthias C, Steiner W (2015) Oncologic results of transoral laser microsurgery for squamous cell carcinoma of the posterior pharyngeal wall. Head Neck 37(2):156–161

Gross ND, Holsinger FC, Magnuson JS, Duvvuri U, Genden EM, Ghanem TA, Yaremchuk KL, Goldenberg D, Miller MC, Moore EJ, Morris LG, Netterville J, Weinstein GS, Richmon J (2016) Robotics in otolaryngology and head and neck surgery: recommendations for training and credentialing: a report of the 2015 AHNS Education Committee, AAO-HNS Robotic Task Force and AAO-HNS Sleep Disorders Committee. Head Neck (Epub ahead of print)

Haughey BH, Hinni ML, Salassa JR, Hayden RE, Grant DG, Rich JT, Milov S, Lewis JS Jr, Krishna M (2011) Transoral laser microsurgery as primary treatment for advanced-stage oropharyngeal cancer: a United States multicenter study. Head Neck 33(12):1683–1694

Higgins KM, Wang JR (2008) State of head and neck surgical oncology research–a review and critical appraisal of landmark studies. Head Neck 30(12):1636–1642

Hockstein NG, Nolan JP, O'Malley BW Jr, Woo YJ (2005) Robot-assisted pharyngeal and laryngeal microsurgery: results of robotic cadaver dissections. Laryngoscope 115(6): 1003–1008

Holzinger D, Flechtenmacher C, Henfling N, Kaden I, Grabe N, Lahrmann B, Schmitt M, Hess J, Pawlita M, Bosch FX (2013) Identification of oropharyngeal squamous cell carcinomas with active HPV16 involvement by immunohistochemical analysis of the retinoblastoma protein pathway. Int J Cancer 133(6):1389–1399

Kaczmar JM, Tan KS, Heitjan DF, Lin A, Ahn PH, Newman JG, Rassekh CH, Chalian AA, O'Malley BW Jr, Cohen RB, Weinstein GS (2016) HPV-related oropharyngeal cancer: risk factors for treatment failure in patients managed with primary transoral robotic surgery. Head Neck 38(1):59–65

Kostareli E, Holzinger D, Bogatyrova O, Hielscher T, Wichmann G, Keck M, Lahrmann B, Grabe N, Flechtenmacher C, Schmidt CR, Seiwert T, Dyckhoff G, Dietz A, Höfler D,

Pawlita M, Benner A, Bosch FX, Plinkert P, Plass C, Weichenhan D, Hess J (2013) HPV-related methylation signature predicts survival in oropharyngeal squamous cell carcinomas. J Clin Invest 123(6):2488–2501

Lewis JS Jr (2012) p16 immunohistochemistry as a standalone test for risk stratification in oropharyngeal squamous cell carcinoma. Head Neck Pathol 6(Suppl 1):S75–S82

Machtay M, Moughan J, Trotti A, Garden AS, Weber RS, Cooper JS, Forastiere A, Ang KK (2008) Factors associated with severe late toxicity after concurrent chemoradiation for locally advanced head and neck cancer: an RTOG analysis. J Clin Oncol 26(21):3582–3589 (Epub 2008 Jun 16)

Masterson L, Moualed D, Liu ZW, Howard JE, Dwivedi RC, Tysome JR, Benson R, Sterling JC, Sudhoff H, Jani P, Goon PK (2014) De-escalation treatment protocols for human papillomavirus-associated oropharyngeal squamous cell carcinoma: a systematic review and meta-analysis of current clinical trials. Eur J Cancer 50(15):2636–2648

Mirghani H, Amen F, Blanchard P, Moreau F, Guigay J, Hartl DM, Lacau St Guily J (2015) Treatment de-escalation in HPV-positive oropharyngeal carcinoma: ongoing trials, critical issues and perspectives. Int J Cancer 136(7):1494–1503

O'Rorke MA, Ellison MV, Murray LJ, Moran M, James J, Anderson LA (2012) Human papillomavirus related head and neck cancer survival: a systematic review and meta-analysis. Oral Oncol 48(12):1191–1201

Pignon JP, le Maître A, Maillard E, Bourhis J, MACH-NC Collaborative Group (2009) Meta-analysis of chemotherapy in head and neck cancer (MACH-NC): an update on 93 randomised trials and 17,346 patients. Radiother Oncol 92(1):4–14 (Epub 2009 May 14)

Quon H, O'Malley BW Jr, Weinstein GS (2011) Postoperative adjuvant therapy after transoral robotic resection for oropharyngeal carcinomas: rationale and current treatment approach. ORL J Otorhinolaryngol Relat Spec 73(3):121–130 (Epub 2011 Mar 10. Review)

Quon H, O'Malley BW Jr, Weinstein GS (2011b) Postoperative adjuvant therapy after transoral robotic resection for oropharyngeal carcinomas: rationale and current treatment approach. ORL J Otorhinolaryngol Relat Spec 73(3):121–130

Rischin D, Young RJ, Fisher R, Fox SB, Le QT, Peters LJ, Solomon B, Choi J, O'Sullivan B, Kenny LM, McArthur GA (2010) Prognostic significance of p 16INK4A and human papillomavirus in patients with oropharyngeal cancer treated on TROG 02.02 phase III trial. J Clin Oncol 28(27):4142–4148

Robbins KT, Shaha AR, Medina JE, Califano JA, Wolf GT, Ferlito A, Som PM, Day TA, Committee for Neck Dissection Classification, American Head and Neck Society (2008) Consensus statement on the classification and terminology of neck dissection. Arch Otolaryngol Head Neck Surg 134(5):536–538

Robinson M, Schache A, Sloan P, Thavaraj S (2012) HPV specific testing: a requirement for oropharyngeal squamous cell carcinoma patients. Head Neck Pathol 6(Suppl 1):S83–S90

Shah JP, Patel SG (eds) (2003) Head and neck surgery and oncology, Mosby Ltd. ISBN: 0723432236

Sinha P, Hackman T, Nussenbaum B, Wu N, Lewis JS Jr, Haughey BH (2014) Transoral laser microsurgery for oral squamous cell carcinoma: oncologic outcomes and prognostic factors. Head Neck 36(3):340–351

Smeets SJ, Hesselink AT, Speel EJ, Haesevoets A, Snijders PJ, Pawlita M, Meijer CJ, Braakhuis BJ, Leemans CR, Brakenhoff RH (2007) A novel algorithm for reliable detection of human papillomavirus in paraffin embedded head and neck cancer specimen. Int J Cancer 121(11):2465–2472

Tschiesner U, Schuster L, Strieth S, Harréus U (2012) Functional outcome in patients with advanced head and neck cancer: surgery and reconstruction with free flaps versus primary radiochemotherapy. Eur Arch Otorhinolaryngol 269(2):629–638

Wasylyk B, Abecassis J, Jung AC (2013) Identification of clinically relevant HPV-related HNSCC: in p16 should we trust? Oral Oncol 49(10):e33–e37

Wichmann G, Rosolowski M, Krohn K, Kreuz M, Boehm A, Reiche A, Scharrer U, Halama D, Bertolini J, Bauer U, Holzinger D, Pawlita M, Hess J, Engel C, Hasenclever D, Scholz M, Ahnert P, Kirsten H, Hemprich A, Wittekind C, Herbarth O, Horn F, Dietz A, Loeffler M, Leipzig Head and Neck Group (LHNG) (2015) The role of HPV RNA transcription, immune response-related gene expression and disruptive TP53 mutations in diagnostic and prognostic profiling of head and neck cancer. Int J Cancer 137(12):2846–2857

Wittekind C, Compton C, Quirke P, Nagtegaal I, Merkel S, Hermanek P, Sobin LH (2009) A uniform residual tumor (R) classification: integration of the R classification and the circumferential margin status. Cancer 115(15):3483–3488

Part IV
Surgical Treatment of HPV Positive Tumours

The Role of Conventional Surgery in Oropharyngeal Cancer

Wojciech Golusinski

Abstract

Anatomically, the oropharynx can be divided into four subsites: the soft palate, pharyngeal wall, base of tongue, and the tonsillar complex. Surgical access to these tumours is often challenging due to the anatomic localization. For this reason, such tumours were traditionally managed with open surgical techniques, usually involving a mandibulotomy, to provide better visualization and access to the oropharynx, followed by free-flap reconstruction of the oropharyngeal defect. However, the invasiveness of this approach could lead to significant morbidity, including speech, swallowing, and airway dysfunction, in addition to poor cosmetic outcomes. In response, less invasive approaches (Mercante et al. 2013) have been developed including minimally invasive surgical approaches (chiefly transoral surgery) as well as non-surgical methods, primarily radiotherapy, and chemotherapy (Mercante et al. 2013).

Keywords

Oropharyngeal cancer · Open surgical approaches · Minimally invasive surgical approaches

W. Golusinski (✉)
Department of Head and Neck Surgery, The Greater Poland Cancer Centre,
Poznan University of Medical Sciences, Poznań, Poland
e-mail: wgolus@ump.edu.pl

W. Golusiński et al. (eds.), *HPV Infection in Head and Neck Cancer*,
Recent Results in Cancer Research 206, DOI 10.1007/978-3-319-43580-0_14

1 Introduction

Oropharyngeal cancer (OPC) is a relatively rare cancer of the head and neck region. Histologically, most OPCs ($\approx$90 %) are squamous cell carcinomas (SCC). Anatomically, the oropharynx can be divided into four subsites: the soft palate, pharyngeal wall, base of tongue, and the tonsillar complex. Surgical access to these tumours is often challenging due to the anatomic localization. For this reason, such tumours were traditionally managed with open surgical techniques, usually involving a mandibulotomy, to provide better visualization and access to the oropharynx, followed by free-flap reconstruction of the oropharyngeal defect. However, the invasiveness of this approach could lead to significant morbidity, including speech, swallowing, and airway dysfunction, in addition to poor cosmetic outcomes. In response, less invasive approaches (Mercante et al. 2013) have been developed including minimally invasive surgical approaches (chiefly transoral surgery) as well as non-surgical methods, primarily radiotherapy and chemotherapy (Mercante et al. 2013).

Trials carried out in the late 1980s/early 1990s showed that concurrent chemoradiotherapy could achieve survival rates that were equivalent to open surgical approaches with significantly less morbidity (Dowthwaite et al. 2012). As a result, this approach began to replace surgery in many centres, particularly for early-stage disease (Yeh et al. 2015). Despite the popularity of these non-surgical approaches, no randomized trials have been conducted to compare chemoradiotherapy to surgery plus post-operative radiotherapy (PORT). Moreover, high-dose regimens can induce significant treatment-related toxicity, particularly acute mucositis and severe dysphagia, which often requires insertion of a gastrostomy tube (Blanchard et al. 2011; Machtay et al. 2008; Caudell et al. 2009). For this reason, a significant number of centres with strong surgical traditions continue to manage these cancers surgically followed by PORT or post-operative chemoradiotherapy in cases with adverse histopathological features.

Due to the continuous improvements in both surgical and non-surgical techniques, decision-making with regard to treatment has become ever more complex, and both techniques can often be used. At present, conventional surgery, defined as open surgery, transoral surgery with traditional instrumentation, or transoral laser microsurgery (TLM), is primarily—but not solely—used for advanced cancers (stage III or IV) or for salvage surgery following recurrence. However, conventional surgery is also used in many early-stage tumours (stage I or II).

In this subchapter, we briefly describe the surgical approaches currently used in OPC and their role in managing this disease.

2 General Principles: Management of Oropharyngeal Cancers

The standard treatment for OPCs at present is mainly dependent on the disease stage, anatomical location, and patient and clinician preferences. Because survival outcomes are often comparable between surgical and non-surgical approaches,

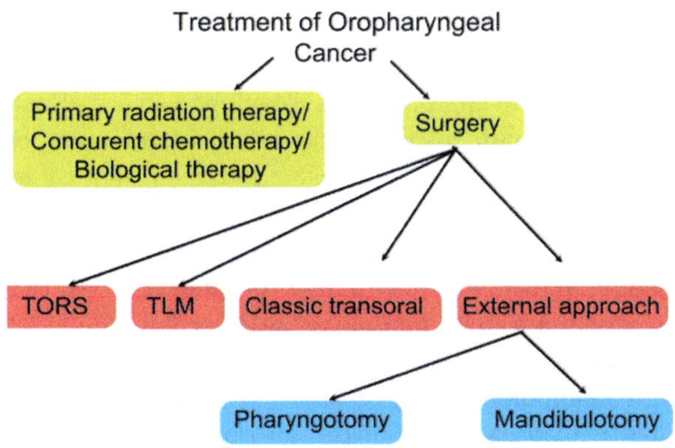

Fig. 1 Treatment options of oropharyngeal cancer

clinician preferences play an important role in the treatment decision. Figure 1 depicts the treatment options for OPCs. The first decision is to select the appropriate treatment modality, generally either surgery or radiotherapy, both of which yield similar rates of local control and survival in retrospective studies. Importantly, randomized trials comparing the two approaches are not available. In addition, treatment-related morbidity can be an important factor in selecting the treatment. As Fig. 1 makes clear, there are numerous surgical options.

An important concept in selecting a surgical approach is to develop a clear "concept of operation". This means that the surgeon selects the most appropriate operation type according to the results of diagnostic procedures and staging. By selecting the appropriate operation concept, it is possible to achieve the initial aims of the surgery without unnecessary complications. Based on the overall treatment concept, the surgeon chooses the optimal access route, the extent of resection, and the type of reconstruction. Communication between surgeons and other specialists is crucial for the success of the intervention. Numerous factors affect the choice of treatment, including patient characteristics such as age, occupation, general health and co-morbid conditions, lifestyle issues (e.g. refusal to stop smoking), distance from the hospital, and family status. The patient's opinion and preference for a particular treatment should also be considered. In addition, the expertise of both the centre and the surgeon can also play a role in decision-making. Finally, tumour-related factors (Fig. 2) are an important component of the decision-making process.

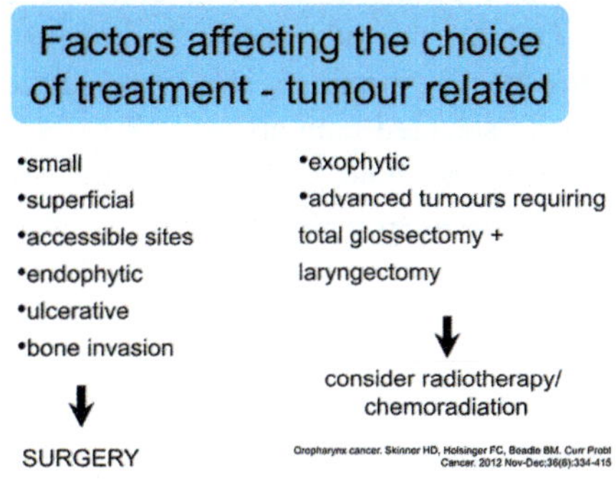

Fig. 2 Tumour-related factors in selecting treatment

3 Transoral Surgery

The transoral approach was developed in an attempt to minimize the morbidity associated with open surgery while maintaining oncologic outcomes. Transoral surgery is a minimally invasive treatment that offers many advantages over open techniques, including less damage to the musculature, the major neurovascular structures, and normal tissues (Tateya et al. 2016). Similarly, due to its less invasive nature, transoral surgery allows for quicker recovery and reduced hospital stay, both of which are important advantages for the patient and the hospital (Arens 2012).

Classic transoral approaches are limited to tumours that can be observed directly and manipulated with standard instrumentation and lighting (Dowthwaite et al. 2012). Consequently, in certain oropharyngeal tumour localizations, such as the back of tongue or the tonsillar complex, the classic transoral approach is not feasible due to lack of visualization and access. Magnification and finer instrumentation are needed to access deeper structures in the oropharynx, which is what led to the emergence of TLM in the mid-1990s. TLM, in which an endoscope provides visualization of the pharynx through the mouth while a laser is used to excise the tumour, overcame many of the barriers associated with classic transoral surgery, thus providing an organ preservation strategy that offers excellent local control rates with preservation of vocal and swallowing function (Dowthwaite et al. 2012). Compared to conventional open surgery, TLM minimizes the risk of fistula, flap failure, abscess, and osteoradionecrosis and is associated with a shorter hospital stay. However, TLM is not without drawbacks, the most important being the rigid equipment and the narrow-field view of the laryngoscopes, which make it challenging to manoeuver within the complex anatomy of the oropharynx.

Due in part to technical difficulties with TLM, a newer technique—transoral robotic surgery (TORS)—has been gaining ground in recent years, particularly in tonsillar cancer (Weinstein et al. 2007). TORS overcomes the restricted surgical access and limited view of the oropharynx associated with non-robotic transoral approaches. However, despite the apparent advantages of TORS (smaller incisions, decreased hospital stays, better optics, and improved range of motion of the surgical arms), longer term outcomes are not yet available and the body of evidence, though growing, is still small. Crucially, TORS requires expensive robotic equipment and extensive training, thus making it cost-prohibitive for many centres. For these reasons, among others, conventional approaches are still widely used in OPC.

Overall, the evidence for routine use of transoral endoscopic surgery is based on retrospective findings. However, studies are underway. The available results show that in selected patients as well as in the hands of experienced surgeons, transoral approaches, both endoscopic and classic, are a good alternative to both open organ-preserving surgery with reconstruction by microvascular anastomosed flaps and chemoradiotherapy (Arens 2012).

4 Early-Stage Oropharyngeal Cancer

At many centres, radiotherapy plus concurrent chemotherapy has largely replaced surgery in the treatment of early-stage (T1-2 N0-1) OPC (Lacocourreye 2011). However, it is important to consider the long-term consequences of chemoradiotherapy, which are not insignificant due to the possibility of treatment-related toxicities and the negative impact of failed radiotherapy on subsequent salvage surgery (Machtay et al. 2008). In this sense, an important advantage of surgery is that the excised tissue provides valuable staging information that may obviate the need for additional chemoradiotherapy, thus avoiding unnecessary toxicity. Moreover, survival rates are virtually identical, regardless of whether the primary treatment is surgery or radiotherapy: two-year survival rates for stage T1 patients range from 93 to 95 % for radiotherapy versus 92–100 % for surgery. For T2 tumours, the corresponding rates are 91–93 % for radiotherapy versus 91–94 % for surgery (Daly et al. 2010).

Transoral surgery with elective neck dissection (ipsilateral or bilateral, as appropriate) is generally the surgical treatment of choice in early-stage oropharyngeal tumours, except for the base of tongue tumours, in which definitive radiation therapy ± brachytherapy is preferred. A variety of transoral modalities can be utilized, including TLM, TORS, or even the classic transoral approach depending on the centre's preferences, experience, equipment availability, and tumour location. Although TLM and now TORS have largely displaced conventional transoral surgery, several studies have demonstrated excellent results with this approach, indicating that, for experienced centres with limited resources, laser and/or robotic systems are not essential to achieving good outcomes (Lacocourreye 2011; Shah et al. 2014).

In cases of recurrence, salvage surgery is the treatment of choice. Indeed, another argument in favour of primary surgery versus primary radiotherapy is that salvage treatment for local recurrence is not always possible after primary radiotherapy; in addition, even when salvage surgery is feasible, it is always associated with a significantly higher rate of post-operative complications. Finally, curative and function-sparing treatment options for metachronous second primary tumours in the upper aerodigestive tract are severely limited if the primary tumour was treated with radiotherapy.

4.1 Nodal Disease and Neck Metastases

The risk of occult neck metastasis is high, even when the neck is clinically negative for nodal involvement. For this reason, elective neck dissection, which may be ipsilateral (in lateralized tonsil primaries) or bilateral (midline tumours), is usually performed.

4.2 Soft Palate

Although most patients with early-stage OPC of the soft palate are treated with radiotherapy, both surgery and radiotherapy achieve comparable rates of survival and locoregional control. For T2NO tumours, a transoral approach with TLM can be used, with wound healing by secondary intention or reconstruction with split thickness skin graft.

4.3 Base of Tongue

Tumours in this location are usually more aggressive than other localizations. In most cases, radiotherapy plus brachytherapy is used for this localization (NCCN guidelines file, n.d). Since occult nodal metastasis is common, lymph node dissection is recommended in patients who undergo surgery. In carefully selected patients, TLM may improve local control and functional results (Steiner et al. 2003).

4.4 Tonsillar Complex

Outcomes with primary surgery or radiotherapy are essentially equivalent. For small tumours (T1N0) confined to the tonsil, simple tonsillectomy using the transoral approach with electrocautery is sufficient. However, more extensive resection may be needed if the tumour extends beyond the tonsil and may require an anterior approach with mandibulotomy and a transhyoid approach, or, alternatively, TLM, or TORS.

5 Advanced Oropharyngeal Cancers

In advanced cancers (T3-4a, N0-N1), both chemoradiotherapy and conventional surgery can be used, depending on the localization and expertise of the hospital. The surgical approach typically consists of conventional surgery followed by PORT or CRT. In patients with advanced disease, surgery offers a notable survival advantage over radiotherapy (Díaz-Molina et al. 2012): at five years, rates of overall survival and disease-specific survival (DSS) are 24–58 % and 33–63 % for radiotherapy plus chemotherapy compared to 38–56 % and 52–73 % for surgery plus PORT. Surgery requires an extensive resection of the visible or palpable tumour. A 2-cm margin should be applied, if feasible, with frozen section analysis performed to assess the surgical margins. The specific surgical approach depends in large measure on the tumour localization, and adequate visualization is essential. For this reason, an open approach with lip-splitting mandibulotomy is often required. For tumours of the tonsillar complex or base of tongue tumours, mandibulotomy is the treatment of choice, although lateral pharyngotomy may also be considered for the tonsillar complex. In some cases, partial mandibular resection may be used. Reconstruction options include primary closure, pedicle or free flaps, and skin grafts.

In most cases, radical neck dissection is mandatory due to local spread. Neck dissection depends on the nodal status. Patient with N0 status usually undergoes prophylactic selective neck dissection, either unilateral or bilateral (midline lesions). In clinical N1 disease, selective neck dissection (including levels I–IV) is recommended. Finally, in patients with more advanced nodal disease (clinical N2/N3), a modified radical neck dissection is necessary.

As with early-stage tumours, the only viable treatment option in case of recurrence is salvage surgery.

5.1 Soft Palate Tumour

Stage T3N2b soft palate tumours are managed by transoral resection with radical neck dissection reconstruction and radial forearm free flap (RFFF).

5.2 Base of Tongue

Advanced stage (T3-N2B) base of tongue tumours is usually reseacted with anterior mandibulotomy and radical neck dissection. Stage T4aN2B tumours are treated with hemiglossectomy with radical neck dissection and reconstruction with an anterolateral thigh flap.

5.3 Tonsillar Complex

Stage T3N2b tonsillar tumours are managed similar to that described above for soft palate tumours (i.e. transoral resection with radical neck dissection reconstruction and radial forearm free flap). Stage T2N2B tumours are also managed with the transoral approach and radical neck dissection. For more extensive tonsillar complex tumours with invasion of the buccal mucosa (T4A N2B), an anterior mandibulotomy with radical neck dissection and reconstruction with RFFF are required.

6 Human PapillomaVirus (Hpv)-Associated OPC

The incidence of HPV-positive SCC has doubled in the last decade, and by the year 2030, half of all head and neck tumours will be HPV+ (Pytynia et al. 2014). The rise of HPV+ tumours has changed the patient profile in OPC. HPV+ patients tend to be younger, more highly educated, white males with smaller primary tumours but with more advanced nodal stage (cystic in nature). Studies have shown that patients with HPV+ OPC have better outcomes than patients with HPV-negative tumours, regardless of whether they are treated surgically or by concurrent chemoradiotherapy. The increasing incidence of HPV positivity has important implications for the treatment because HPV-associated tumours are more susceptible to radiotherapy and survival rates in these patients are better than non-HPV tumours (Ang et al. 2010). In the radiation therapy oncology group (RTOG) trial 0129, HPV status was shown to be an independent prognostic factor for survival (Ang et al. 2010; Lim et al. 2015): in that study, 3-year locoregional failure was 21 % lower in patients with HPV-positive tumours. However, despite the benefits of radiotherapy in this subset of patients, the relatively young age of disease onset means that the patients may be at risk for the long-term side effects of radiotherapy, including osteonecrosis and radiation-induced secondary malignancies. This presents an important dilemma for physicians. However, one solution is to use minimally invasive surgical techniques to achieve local tumour control while reserving radiotherapy for future use if the patient develops either a local recurrence or a second primary tumour. Interestingly, HPV positivity confers a similar survival advantage, regardless of whether patients are treated surgically or with chemoradiation (Licitra et al. 2006; Fakhry et al. 2008). Indeed, one study compared survival outcomes in HPV+ patients treated with either surgery or chemoradiation, finding that the cohort that underwent primary surgery had the best outcomes (Fischer et al. 2010).

From a treatment selection perspective, the longer survival of HPV+ patient increases the risk of late-onset treatment-related effects, including osteoradionecrosis, fibrosis, trismus, dental issues, xerostomia, and dysphagia. At present, there are no level 1 data comparing primary surgery to radiation or chemoradiotherapy in HPV+ OPC (Mydlarz et al. 2015). However, this question may be resolved once the results of the ongoing ECOG 3311 trial are reported.

In summary, HPV positivity does not imply that radiotherapy should be preferred to surgery as the primary treatment modality given that the survival benefit applies to both groups. Moreover, considering the importance of patient age and health status, transoral approaches such as TLM or TORS followed by PORT may offer the optimal approach to selected HPV+ patients because this may allow the use of lower doses of radiation therapy, better functional outcomes, and improved survival.

7 Salvage Treatment

As described above, the role of surgery has undergone significant changes in the last 20–30 years, and in many centres, combined chemoradiotherapy has replaced surgery, even in advanced tumours. In recurrent OPC, surgery is the only feasible option in the vast majority of cases. However, in patients who suffer a recurrence after primary treatment with combined chemoradiotherapy, there are many issues that complicate the salvage surgery. For instance, the presence of tissue oedema, necrosis, and chondritis often make it difficult to locate the recurrence. Moreover, recurrence is often multifocal, widely dispersed, and located in many instances below an intact mucosa. In addition, complication rates are significantly increased in this patient population and wound healing is complicated by poor tissue quality in the surgical site. Finally, tumours that managed to survive chemoradiation therapy are usually more aggressive and more resistant to other treatment modalities.

8 Conclusions

Despite the shift from surgery to chemoradiotherapy in the treatment of OPC, there is no conclusive evidence to demonstrate the superiority of either approach. In most cases, as shown by the RTOG 73-03 trial (Kramer et al. 1987), survival is equivalent. Improvements in minimally invasive surgical techniques, together with the rising incidence of HPV-associated cancers, have given new momentum towards the use of surgery as the primary therapy in OPC, with radiotherapy and/or chemoradiotherapy given as adjuvant treatments (Chan et al. 2015).

The treatment options for an individual patient rely on multiple factors, including the tumour location and size, features of the tumour, and patient comorbidities. The continued study of these techniques is important to match the patient with the most appropriate treatment (Helman et al. 2015). Based on current data, transoral resection competes with primary chemoradiotherapy in terms of cure rates and functional outcomes, and for this reason, the main controversy in the treatment of patients with resectable OPC is whether to use definitive chemoradiotherapy or primary transoral surgery with appropriate adjuvant therapy (Samuels et al. 2015). It is hoped that ongoing and future studies will help to resolve these dilemmas and help us to better understand the optimal treatment approach, whether surgical or non-surgical, based on patient and tumour characteristics.

References

Ang KK, Harris J, Wheeler R, Weber R, Rosenthal DI, Nguyen-Tân PF et al (2010) Human papillomavirus and survival of patients with oropharyngeal cancer. N Engl J Med 363:24–35. doi:10.1056/NEJMoa0912217

Arens C (2012) Transoral treatment strategies for head and neck tumors. GMS Curr Top Otorhinolaryngol Head Neck Surg 11:Doc05. doi:10.3205/cto000087

Blanchard P, Baujat B, Holostenco V, Bourredjem A, Baey C, Bourhis J et al (2011) Meta-analysis of chemotherapy in head and neck cancer (MACH-NC): a comprehensive analysis by tumour site. Radiother Oncol 100:33–40. doi:10.1016/j.radonc.2011.05.036

Caudell JJ, Schaner PE, Meredith RF, Locher JL, Nabell LM, Carroll WR et al (2009) Factors associated with long-term dysphagia after definitive radiotherapy for locally advanced head-and-neck cancer. Int J Radiat Oncol Biol Phys 73:410–415. doi:10.1016/j.ijrobp.2008.04.048

Chan KKW, Glenny AM, Weldon JC, Furness S, Worthington HV, Wakeford H (2015) Interventions for the treatment of oral and oropharyngeal cancers: targeted therapy and immunotherapy. Cochrane Database Syst Rev 12:CD010341. doi:10.1002/14651858.CD010341.pub2

Daly ME, Le Q-T, Maxim PG, Loo BW, Kaplan MJ, Fischbein NJ et al (2010) Intensity-modulated radiotherapy in the treatment of oropharyngeal cancer: clinical outcomes and patterns of failure. Int J Radiat Oncol Biol Phys 76:1339–1346. doi:10.1016/j.ijrobp.2009.04.006

Díaz-Molina JP, Rodrigo JP, Alvarez-Marcos C, Blay P, de la Rúa A, Estrada E, et al (2012) Functional and oncological results of non-surgical vs surgical treatment in squamous cell carcinomas of the oropharynx. Acta Otorrinolaringológica Española 63:348–54. doi:10.1016/j.otorri.2012.02.005

Dowthwaite S, Franklin JH, Palma D, Fung K, Yoo J, Nichols AC (2012) The role of transoral robotic surgery in the management of oropharyngeal cancer: a review of the literature. ISRN Oncol 2012:1–14. doi:10.5402/2012/945162

Fakhry C, Westra WH, Li S, Cmelak A, Ridge JA, Pinto H et al (2008) Improved survival of patients with human papillomavirus-positive head and neck squamous cell carcinoma in a prospective clinical trial. J Natl Cancer Inst 100:261–269. doi:10.1093/jnci/djn011

Fischer CA, Zlobec I, Green E, Probst S, Storck C, Lugli A et al (2010) Is the improved prognosis of p16 positive oropharyngeal squamous cell carcinoma dependent of the treatment modality? Int J Cancer 126:1256–1262. doi:10.1002/ijc.24842

Helman SN, Schwedhelm T, Kadakia S, Wang Y, Schiff BA, Smith RV (2015) Transoral robotic surgery in oropharyngeal carcinoma. Arch Pathol Lab Med 139:1389–1397. doi:10.5858/arpa.2014-0573-RA

Kramer S, Gelber RD, Snow JB, Marcial VA, Lowry LD, Davis LW et al (1987) Combined radiation therapy and surgery in the management of advanced head and neck cancer: final report of study 73–03 of the radiation therapy oncology group. Head Neck Surg 10:19–30. doi:10.1002/hed.2890100105

Lacocourreye O (2011) Transoral lateral oropharyngectomy for squamous cell carcinoma of the tonsillar region, vol 131, pp 592–599

Licitra L, Perrone F, Bossi P, Suardi S, Mariani L, Artusi R et al (2006) High-risk human papillomavirus affects prognosis in patients with surgically treated oropharyngeal squamous cell carcinoma. J Clin Oncol 24:5630–5636. doi:10.1200/JCO.2005.04.6136

Lim GC, Holsinger FC, Li RJ (2015) Transoral endoscopic head and neck surgery: the contemporary treatment of head and neck cancer. Hematol Oncol Clin North Am 29:1075–1092. doi:10.1016/j.hoc.2015.08.001

Machtay M, Moughan J, Trotti A, Garden AS, Weber RS, Cooper JS et al (2008) Factors associated with severe late toxicity after concurrent chemoradiation for locally advanced head and neck cancer: an RTOG analysis. J Clin Oncol 26:3582–3589. doi:10.1200/JCO.2007.14.8841

Mercante G, Ruscito P, Pellini R, Cristalli G, Spriano G (2013) Transoral robotic surgery (TORS) for tongue base tumours. Acta Otorhinolaryngol Ital Organo Uff Della Soc Ital Di Otorinolaringol E Chir Cerv-Facc 33:230–235

Mydlarz WK, Chan JYK, Richmon JD (2015) The role of surgery for HPV-associated head and neck cancer. Oral Oncol 51:305–313. doi:10.1016/j.oraloncology.2014.10.005

Pytynia KB, Dahlstrom KR, Sturgis EM (2014) Epidemiology of HPV-associated oropharyngeal cancer. Oral Oncol 50:380–386. doi:10.1016/j.oraloncology.2013.12.019

Samuels SE, Eisbruch A, Beitler JJ, Corry J, Bradford CR, Saba NF et al (2015) Management of locally advanced HPV-related oropharyngeal squamous cell carcinoma: where are we? Eur Arch Otorhinolaryngol. doi:10.1007/s00405-015-3771-x

Shah J, Vyas A, Vyas D (2014) The history of robotics in surgical specialties. Am J Robot Surg 1:12–20. doi:10.1166/ajrs.2014.1006

Steiner W, Fierek O, Ambrosch P, Hommerich CP, Kron M (2003) Transoral laser microsurgery for squamous cell carcinoma of the base of the tongue. Arch Otolaryngol Head Neck Surg 129:36–43

Tateya I, Shiotani A, Satou Y, Tomifuji M, Morita S, Muto M et al (2016) Transoral surgery for laryngo-pharyngeal cancer—the paradigm shift of the head and cancer treatment. Auris Nasus Larynx 43:21–32. doi:10.1016/j.anl.2015.06.013

Weinstein GS, O'Malley BW, Snyder W, Sherman E, Quon H (2007) Transoral robotic surgery: radical tonsillectomy. Arch Otolaryngol Head Neck Surg 133:1220–1226. doi:10.1001/archotol.133.12.1220

NCCN guidelines file (n.d) www.nccn.org/professionals/physician_gls/f_guidelines.asp#site

Yeh DH, Tam S, Fung K, MacNeil SD, Yoo J, Winquist E et al (2015) Transoral robotic surgery vs. radiotherapy for management of oropharyngeal squamous cell carcinoma—a systematic review of the literature. Eur J Surg Oncol 41:1603–1614. doi:10.1016/j.ejso.2015.09.007

The Role of Surgery in the Management of Recurrent Oropharyngeal Cancer

Neil D. Gross and Ehab Y. Hanna

Abstract

The incidence of oropharyngeal squamous cell carcinoma (OPSCC) continues to rise worldwide at a dramatic pace, buoyed by the predominance of human papilloma virus (HPV) driven disease (Panwar et al. 2014). While the outcomes of patients with HPV-positive OPSCC are dramatically improved compared to HPV-negative OPSCC, treatment failures do occur. The result is an inevitable rise in the incidence of recurrent OPSCC. Since the majority of incident OPSCC cases are treated with some form of radiation therapy (primary or adjuvant), surgery remains the backbone of treatment for recurrent OPSCC. This section will focus on options for surgical management of recurrent OPSCC.

Keywords

TORS · Transoral robotic surgery · Oropharynx · HPV negative · Squamous cell carcinoma of the oropharynx

1 Introduction

The incidence of oropharyngeal squamous cell carcinoma (OPSCC) continues to rise worldwide at a dramatic pace, buoyed by the predominance of human papilloma virus (HPV) driven disease (Panwar et al. 2014). While the outcomes of patients with HPV-positive OPSCC are dramatically improved compared to

N.D. Gross (✉) · E.Y. Hanna
Department Head and Neck Surgery, University of Texas MD Anderson Cancer Center, 1400 Pressler Street, Unit 1445, Houston, TX 77030, USA
e-mail: NGross@MDAnderson.org

W. Golusiński et al. (eds.), *HPV Infection in Head and Neck Cancer*, Recent Results in Cancer Research 206, DOI 10.1007/978-3-319-43580-0_15

HPV-negative OPSCC, treatment failures do occur. The result is an inevitable rise in the incidence of recurrent OPSCC. Since the majority of incident OPSCC cases are treated with some form of radiation therapy (primary or adjuvant), surgery remains the backbone of treatment for recurrent OPSCC. This section will focus on options for surgical management of recurrent OPSCC.

It is important to recognize that while surgery is paramount for the treatment of recurrent OPSCC, a multidisciplinary approach remains important for this complex and lethal disease. Patient with recurrent OPSCC, often HPV-negative, face an overall dismal prognosis (Agra et al. 2006). Innovative treatment strategies are warranted utilizing all contemporary medical resources including: biologic therapies, immunotherapies, induction approaches and or adjuvant re-irradiation. In this manner, surgery for recurrent OPSCC rarely occurs in a vacuum and each case requires a careful examination of the pathology and patient's potential tolerance of treatment.

2 Challenges with Surgery for Recurrent OPSCC

Treatment of OPSCC is challenging given the proximity of pathology to structures critical for breathing, deglutition and speech. Surgery, in particular, for recurrent OPSCC can be exceptionally challenging and should only be considered by experienced head and neck oncologic surgeons. Recurrent OPSCC is often poorly circumscribed with a propensity for insidious submucosal spread. Of course, access to the oropharynx is more difficult than for many other subsites of the head and neck. Decreased exposure and limited ability to palpate the extent of disease contribute to the challenge of surgery for recurrent OPSCC. Perhaps most importantly, the sequelae of prior treatments can make surgery for recurrent OPSCC particularly difficult via altered anatomy and or accessibility. For example, prior radiation therapy often yields soft tissue fibrosis and induration that can hinder identification and preservation of normal structures and obscure the clear delineation of pathology. Prior radiation for OPSCC invariably causes some degree of restriction in jaw opening. Even a moderate degree of trismus can negatively impact the workup and treatment for recurrent OPSCC. Combined, these factors can make all aspects of management of recurrent OPSCC more difficult including diagnosis, workup and treatment.

The diagnosis of recurrence of head and neck cancer if often delayed. For patients with recurrent OPSCC, in particular, signs or symptoms of disease typically manifest late. Therefore, routine surveillance imaging is recommended to help facilitate earlier diagnosis of recurrence (National Comprehensive Cancer Network (NCCN) 2015). A biopsy to confirm the diagnosis of recurrent OPSCC often requires examination under anesthesia which can occasionally present a challenge in management of the airway. Even pathologic confirmation of recurrence can be difficult given prior therapies.

The workup of recurrent OPSCC requires careful imaging. The goals of imaging are to assess resectability, to evaluate regional lymphatics and to rule out distant metastases. There is no single optimal imaging study for evaluating recurrent OPSCC, and the decision regarding choice of imaging is specific to the patient, pathology and surgeon preference. Contrast-enhanced computed tomography (CT) imaging is usually sufficient for evaluation of the primary site and regional lymph nodes. Magnetic resonance (MR) imaging may be useful for evaluation of perineural spread and better delineation of soft tissue involvement. Positron emission tomography (PET)/CT imaging can also be useful in assessing regional adenopathy and ruling out distant metastases.

3 Surgical Approaches and Patient Selection

Given the complex anatomy and functional importance of the oropharynx, a variety of surgical approaches have been explored. OPSCC was historically treated via an open surgical approach, requiring mandibulotomy, mandibulectomy and/or pharyngotomy. Each of these approaches has a significant potential for morbidity including prolonged hospital stay, cosmetic deformity, gastrostomy tube and tracheostomy dependence. Recent technological advances including transoral laser microsurgery (TLM) and transoral robotic surgery (TORS) have afforded improved access to pathology and the opportunity for decreased treatment-related morbidity. However, it is artificial to consider surgery for recurrent OPSCC as limited to the extreme options: open versus endoscopic. In fact, many patients with recurrent OPSCC may benefit from a hybrid approach that incorporates both open and endoscopic techniques. In this manner, surgical approaches for recurrent OPSCC can be considered as a continuum (Fig. 1).

Patient selection is critical to the successful application of surgery for recurrent OPSCC. Patient selection goes beyond simply identifying which patients may benefit from surgery. Rather, in the context of recurrent OPSCC, it also involves selecting which surgical approach is best suited for the disease. The broad surgical options for recurrent OPSCC include transmandibular, transcervical and transoral approaches.

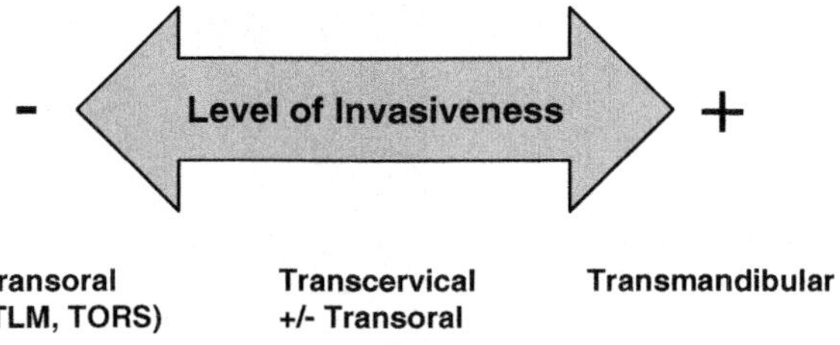

Fig. 1 Range of surgical approaches to recurrent oropharyngeal squamous cell carcinoma (OPSCC). *TLM* Transoral laser microsurgery. *TORS* Transoral robotic surgery

3.1 Transmandibular Approaches

The mandible can represent a barrier to exposure for resection of recurrent OPSCC. Mandibulotomy or mandibulectomy may need to be considered depending on the extent of disease. A common scenario requiring mandibulectomy is direct tumor involvement of the pterygoid musculature with resulting severe trismus. Resection of the ascending ramus of the mandible may be necessary in such cases to afford exposure and an adequate lateral margin. For deeply invasive lateral pharyngeal cancers, the mandible may even be directly involved (Fig. 2). In other cases, a mandibulotomy may be useful for facilitating resection and reconstruction. This approach is most applicable to bulky recurrent OPSCC involving the base of tongue. Utilizing either a visor flap or a lip-splitting approach, the mandible may be divided and retracted laterally to allow broad access to the oropharynx (Fig. 3). Internal fixation is utilized to restore the mandibular arch at completion of the procedure. While these approaches greatly expand the scope of tumors that may be resected and reconstructed, they also entail significant additional morbidity. Complications from mandibulotomy or mandibulectomy include difficulty with speech, swallowing, malocclusion, temporomandibular joint pain and cosmetic deformity (Babin and Calcaterra 1976; Sessions 1983).

3.2 Transcervical Approaches

As an alternative to mandibulotomy or mandibulectomy, recurrent OPSCC of the tongue base, inferior tonsillar fossae or pharyngeal wall may be approached via a transcervical approach. Depending on the location of the cancer and the extent of exposure needed, a lateral pharyngotomy, transhyoid pharyngotomy and or suprahyoid pharyngotomy can be utilized. Acceptable oncologic outcomes have

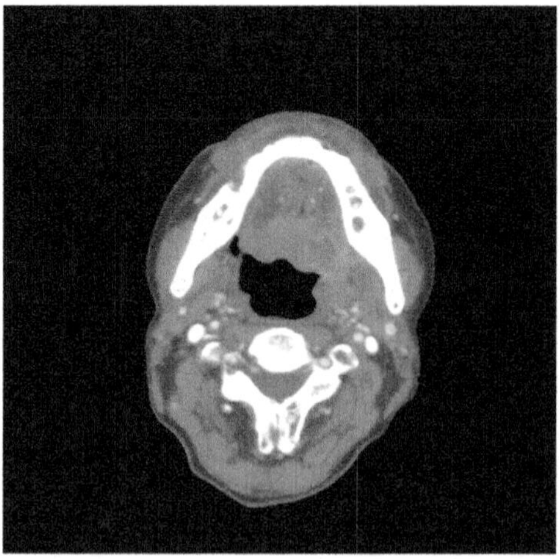

Fig. 2 Computed tomography (CT) neck with contrast demonstrating direct involvement of the mandible from recurrent left base of tongue oropharyngeal squamous cell carcinoma (OPSCC)

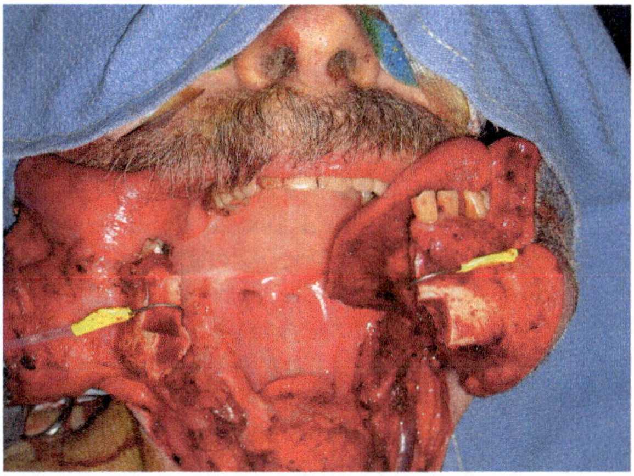

Fig. 3 Transmandibular approach for resection of recurrent right base of tongue oropharyngeal squamous cell carcinoma (OPSCC)

been reported using each of these approaches (Nasri et al. 1996; Zeitels et al. 1991). While transcervical approaches avoid many of the complications inherent in transmandibular surgery, the access afforded is substantially more limited. In addition, patients undergoing pharyngotomy are at increased risk of pharyngocutaneous fistula formation and long-term dysphagia.

Trancervical approaches to recurrent OPSCC also require considerable skill for proper execution. This is because a transcervical approach requires an "inside-out" understanding of the anatomy whereby at least some of the mucosal cuts are completed last. A transcervical approach is made even more challenging in the recurrent setting given fibrosis, induration and potential changes to the anatomy from prior therapies. For these reasons, transcervical approaches to recurrent OPSCC are infrequently reported.

3.3 Transoral Approaches

A transoral approach offers the quickest and most direct route to the oropharynx with the least potential for morbidity. The primary disadvantage of a transoral approach can be related to exposure. While the tonsil can often be adequately visualized directly, OPSCC involving the inferior tonsil, glossotonsillar sulcus or base of tongue may be difficult or impossible to reach through the mouth without specialized techniques and or instrumentation. Patient factors (trismus, kyphosis and dental obstruction) and tumor characteristics (tumor size and location) can limit direct visualization of the oropharynx, thereby preventing a direct transoral approach from being used.

Advancements in endoscopic surgery have led to the development of minimally invasive techniques that enable transoral surgery as an alternative to transmandibular and or transcervical approaches. TLM was the first minimally invasive technique to be applied to OPSCC (Moore and Hinni 2013). High-volume TLM surgeons have reported favorable oncologic outcomes using TLM for OPSCC. However, the technical challenges of this method have limited widespread adoption outside of select large academic centers. More recently, TORS has been applied to the management of OPSCC (Weinstein et al. 2012). Unlike TLM, TORS allows for *en bloc* resection of pathology and is not limited by line-of-site access. So the learning curve for TORS appears shorter than for TLM (White et al. 2013a). TORS using the da Vinci Surgical System (Intuitive Surgical, Inc. Sunnyvale, CA) was cleared by the Food and Drug Administration (FDA) in the United States in 2009. Since then, there has been a rapid rise in the use of TORS to treat OPSCC. In 2015, another robotic platform, the Flex Robotic System (MedRobotics Corp., Raynham, MA), was also approved for transoral surgery by the FDA. TORS has also been investigated for recurrent OPSCC.

In previously untreated patients with OPSCC, transoral approaches are most appropriate for addressing small-volume disease. In these cases, TLM or TORS is often being used with the intent of treatment de-intensification. For example, patients with early stage HPV-associated OPSCC (T1-2, N0-1) treated with TORS have the potential of single-modality therapy and avoiding radiation therapy (Brickman and Gross 2014). More advanced stage OPSCC can also be managed with TORS and de-intensified adjuvant therapies with the goal of potentially avoiding chemotherapy and limiting potential late toxicities (Weinstein et al. 2010). However, the utility of a transoral approach diminishes in patients with large volume or high tumor (T) classification primaries due to the challenges of obtaining negative surgical margins and the expected increased functional morbidity, without obviating the need for intensive adjuvant therapies.

The goal of a transoral approach is different in patients with recurrent OPSCC. In these cases, surgery may be the only available means of treatment or a method for treatment intensification. Small-volume recurrent OPSCC can be amenable to a transoral approach without reconstruction (Fig. 4). However, given the impact of prior radiation on wound healing and the risk of life threatening complications (e.g., bleeding) after transoral surgery, large-volume recurrent OPSCC may require simultaneous microvascular reconstruction. This is particularly important if re-irradiation is contemplated.

3.4 Hybrid Approaches

It is a fallacy to consider surgical approaches to recurrent OPSCC as mutually exclusive, and there are many instances when a hybrid approach is warranted. For example, a transoral approach may augment a transcervical approach by facilitating clearance of the pharyngeal mucosal margins and providing medial access to the lateral parapharyngeal space in recurrent OPSCC involving the tonsil. TORS-assisted resection of recurrent OPSCC is possible but should only be considered by experienced TORS surgeons. Many of these cases will require simultaneous microvascular reconstruction (Fig. 5). TORS-assisted microvascular

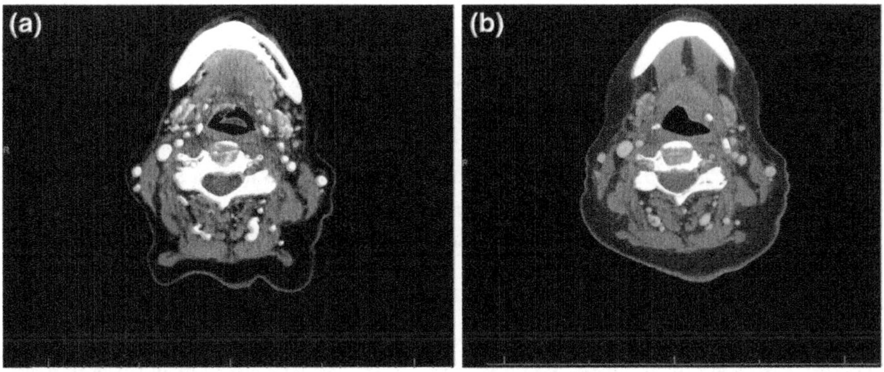

Fig. 4 Computed tomography (CT) neck with contrast of small, superficial recurrent right base of tongue oropharyngeal squamous cell carcinoma (OPSCC) before (**a**) and after (**b**) transoral robotic surgery (TORS)

reconstruction has been shown to be feasible and safe (de Almeida et al. 2014; Selber et al. 2014).

4 Outcomes

The oncologic and functional results of surgery for recurrent OPSCC are difficult to generalize. While the results of TORS are favorable for well-selected cases of previously untreated OPSCC (Moore et al. 2012), for recurrent OPSCC the outcome of surgery is less predictable. This is likely, in part, a reflection of the more aggressive biology of disease in recurrent OPSCC. One retrospective study of surgery for OPSCC noted improved survival at one, two and three years, respectively, for TORS (94, 91 89 %) compared to open surgery (85, 75, 73 %) (Ford

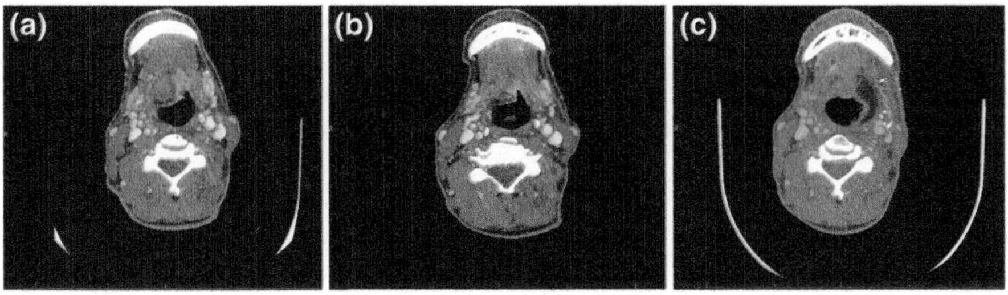

Fig. 5 Computed tomography (CT) neck with contrast of deeply infiltrative recurrent left base of tongue oropharyngeal squamous cell carcinoma (OPSCC) before (**a**) and after (**b**) neoadjuvant chemotherapy followed by a hybrid transoral robotic surgery (TORS)-assisted approach with microvascular free flap reconstruction (**c**)

et al. 2014). The oncologic outcome of TORS has also been investigated for recurrent OPSCC. In a study comparing TORS to open surgery for recurrent OPSCC, patients treated with TORS had improved two-year recurrence-free survival (74 % vs. 43 %, $p = 0.01$), decreased tracheostomy use (23 % vs. 82 %, $p < 0.001$), decreased feeding tube use (38 % vs. 79 %, $p < 0.001$) and shorter overall hospital stay (3.8 days vs. 8.0 days, $p < 0.001$) (White et al. 2013b). In this study, patients selected for TORS were more likely to have undergone microvascular reconstruction despite a similar distribution of primary tumor classification, suggesting other significant baseline differences between groups. Ultimately, comparing transoral approaches such as TORS to transmandibular and transcervical approaches is problematic as patients selected for TORS tend to have more favorable prognostic features. Regardless, a less invasive surgical approach would be expected to yield superior functional outcomes assuming the oncologic outcomes are similar. Unfortunately, functional data are lacking for patients treated surgically for recurrent OPSCC.

Experience is paramount to achieving a successful outcome after surgery for OPSCC (Chia et al. 2013). This is particularly true for recurrent OPSCC. Even in skilled hands, patient expectations regarding outcomes after surgery for recurrent OPSCC should be tempered. The prognosis for recurrent OPSCC remains relatively poor. Patients who survive still face a substantial risk of second primary malignancy and the long-term sequelae of treatment including variable degrees of permanent speech changes, disfigurement and or dysphagia. Less invasive surgical approaches to recurrent OPSCC, including TORS, offer the possibility for decreased treatment-related morbidity but cannot compensate for the cumulative negative impact of recurrent cancer and repeated treatments.

5 Summary

Recurrent OPSCC presents a therapeutic challenge given the likelihood of HPV-negative disease and the limiting effects of prior therapies. Surgery is often the most effective option for recurrent OPSCC but should be considered in the context of additional treatment if feasible given the overall poor prognosis. A variety of surgical approaches are possible for treating recurrent OPSCC including hybrid approaches. Investigation of novel treatment strategies and correlative biomarker studies should be promoted to improve the options for future patients with recurrent OPSCC.

Potential Conflict(s) of Interest Gross: Scientific advisor (unpaid), MedRobotics
Gross: Scientific advisor (unpaid), Intuitive Surgical, Inc.

References

Agra IM, Carvalho AL, Ulbrich FS et al (2006) Prognostic factors in salvage surgery for recurrent oral and oropharyngeal cancer. Head Neck 28:107–113

Babin R, Calcaterra TC (1976) The lip-splitting approach to resection of oropharyngeal cancer. J Surg Oncol 8:433–436

Brickman D, Gross ND (2014) Robotic approaches to the pharynx: tonsil cancer. Otolaryngol Clin North Am 47:359–372

Chia SH, Gross ND, Richmon JD (2013) Surgeon experience and complications with transoral robotic surgery (tors). Otolaryngol Head Neck Surg 149:885–892

de Almeida JR, Park RC, Villanueva NL, Miles BA, Teng MS, Genden EM (2014) Reconstructive algorithm and classification system for transoral oropharyngeal defects. Head Neck 36:934–941

Ford SE, Brandwein-Gensler M, Carroll WR, Rosenthal EL, Magnuson JS (2014) Transoral robotic versus open surgical approaches to oropharyngeal squamous cell carcinoma by human papillomavirus status. Otolaryngol Head Neck Surg 151:606–611

Moore EJ, Hinni ML (2013) Critical review: transoral laser microsurgery and robotic-assisted surgery for oropharynx cancer including human papillomavirus-related cancer. Int J Radiat Oncol Biol Phys 85:1163–1167

Moore EJ, Olsen SM, Laborde RR et al (2012) Long-term functional and oncologic results of transoral robotic surgery for oropharyngeal squamous cell carcinoma. Mayo Clin Proc 87:219–225

Nasri S, Oh Y, Calcaterra TC (1996) Transpharyngeal approach to base of tongue tumors: a comparative study. Laryngoscope 106:945–950

National Comprehensive Cancer Network (NCCN) (2015) Guidelines Head and Neck Cancers Version 1.2015. 5-12-2015. Ref Type: Online Source

Panwar A, Batra R, Lydiatt WM, Ganti AK (2014) Human papilloma virus positive oropharyngeal squamous cell carcinoma: a growing epidemic. Cancer Treat Rev 40:215–219

Selber JC, Sarhane KA, Ibrahim AE, Holsinger FC (2014) Transoral robotic reconstructive surgery. Semin Plast Surg 28:35–38

Sessions DG (1983) Surgical resection and reconstruction for cancer of the base of the tongue. Otolaryngol Clin North Am 16:309–329

Weinstein GS, Quon H, O'Malley BW Jr, Kim GG, Cohen MA (2010) Selective neck dissection and deintensified postoperative radiation and chemotherapy for oropharyngeal cancer: a subset analysis of the University of Pennsylvania transoral robotic surgery trial. Laryngoscope 120:1749–1755

Weinstein GS, O'Malley BW, Magnuson JS et al (2012) Transoral robotic surgery: a multicenter study to assess feasibility, safety, and surgical margins. The Laryngoscope 122:1701–1707

White HN, Frederick J, Zimmerman T, Carroll WR, Magnuson JS (2013a) Learning curve for transoral robotic surgery: a 4-year analysis. JAMA Otolaryngol Head Neck Surg 139:564–567

White H, Ford S, Bush B et al (2013b) Salvage surgery for recurrent cancers of the oropharynx: comparing TORS with standard open surgical approaches. JAMA Otolaryngol Head Neck Surg 139:773–778

Zeitels SM, Vaughan CW, Ruh S (1991) Suprahyoid pharyngotomy for oropharynx cancer including the tongue base. Arch Otolaryngol Head Neck Surg 117:757–760

TORS in HPV-Positive Tumors—The New Standard?

S. Lang, S. Mattheis and B. Kansy

Abstract

In this chapter, we discuss implications of tumor site and tumor microenvironment properties of human papilloma virus (HPV)-associated cancer formation with special emphasis on the therapeutic modality of transoral robotic surgery (TORS). Over the past years, the development of robotic systems has improved, and therefore, its use in the surgical treatment of HNSCC has become a relevant treatment modality for many patients. Yet, there are limitations. Especially for endolaryngeal TORS procedures, additional technical development is mandatory, particularly with respect to visualization and manipulation. The Flex System has provided new additions that need to be further evaluated. TORS systems are going to improve technical issues and therefore reduce patient morbidity, surgical handling and treatment costs. The developed systems have to be tested and evaluated in prospective trials in order to be able to identify benefits and disadvantages in patient care. With respect to HPV-related OPSCC, TORS has become a valuable surgical alternative for an increasing number of patients.

Keywords

Transoral robotic surgery · TORS · Visualization · Manipulation · Oropharynx · da Vinci · Flex System

S. Lang (✉) · S. Mattheis · B. Kansy
Department of Otorhinolaryngology, Head and Neck Surgery, University Hospital Essen, University Duisburg-Essen, Essen, Germany
e-mail: stephan.lang@uk-essen.de

W. Golusiński et al. (eds.), *HPV Infection in Head and Neck Cancer*,
Recent Results in Cancer Research 206, DOI 10.1007/978-3-319-43580-0_16

1 Introduction

During the past few decades, the incidence of oropharyngeal squamous cell carcinoma (OPSCC) has increased significantly (Tinhofer et al. 2015). This is mainly due to the rise in the incidence of human papilloma virus (HPV)-associated cancer formation in the oropharynx. Reasons for that have been widely discussed and commonly allocated to a change in sexual behavior, increased sexual promiscuity, and an earlier onset of sexual activities (Pytynia et al. 2014).

In the oropharynx, the reticulated squamous epithelium of the tonsillar tissue is characterized by a disrupted basilar membrane in order to facilitate the movement of lymphocytes and other cellular components of the immune system. These areas of physiological discontinuity of the basilar membrane have been proposed to be predilection sites for the entry of HPV (Best et al. 2012). Additionally, it has recently been shown that immune checkpoint ligands such as programmed death ligand-1 (PD-L1), which suppress overstimulation of immune responses, are overexpressed in the tonsillar crypts (Lyford-Pike et al. 2013; Pai 2013). Therefore, the crypts of the palatine and lingual tonsils in the oropharynx are considered to be the primary sites of HPV infection.

These unique tumor microenvironment properties, together with the location of the tumor site, i.e., oropharynx, have implications for both prognosis and therefore therapy of patients with OPSCC. In this chapter, we would like to discuss these implications with special emphasis on the therapeutic modality of transoral robotic surgery (TORS).

2 Anatomy of the Oropharynx and Implications for Surgical Approaches

The majority of HPV-associated head and neck squamous cell carcinoma (HNSCC) is located in the oropharynx. Anatomically, the oropharynx extends superiorly from the level of the hard and soft palate and inferiorly to the level of the hyoid bone, including anteriorly the base of tongue, vallecula, lingual surface of the epiglottis and posteriorly the pharyngeal wall comprising the superior and middle constrictor muscles and the buccopharyngeal fascia. The anterior and posterior pillars of the soft palate as well as the palatine tonsils represent the lateral limitations. The accessibility of the above structures differs intra- and inter-individually.

Therefore, surgical approaches depend not only on the tumor size, but also on the tumor location with important consequences for the following general aspects that have to be taken into consideration:

1. Complete tumor resection
2. Preservation of function
3. Minimization of cosmetic deformity
4. Plainness of technique

5. Cost-effectiveness

Usually, priorities decrease in the above-presented order, but have to be adjusted individually with respect to the patient's wishes and needs. These factors are dependent from an important surgical aspect: adequate exposure. Exposure of the oropharyngeal region can be achieved either by transoral (true transoral, pull-through, mandibulotomy) or by transcervical (pharyngotomy, laryngotomy and laryngectomy) approaches. Yet, for most oropharyngeal tumors (true) transoral approaches are the gold standard of surgery due to above-mentioned aspects. In the past decades, the transoral approaches have been augmented by the introduction of robot-assisted techniques, providing new modalities of tumor exposure and removal.

3 History of TORS

The use of robotics for surgical procedures started in 1985. The modified robotic device PUMA 200, originally from industrial background, was utilized to perform cerebral biopsies (Kwoh et al. 1988). Consequentially, the first medical robotic device for hip replacement surgery was developed, being able to drill the hip implant recess (Paul et al. 1992). This development led to a broadened use of robotic systems in surgery. Nowadays, there are two major systems that have been investigated and approved for the use in head and neck surgery (Remacle et al. 2015; O'Malley et al. 2006): The da Vinci® system (Intuitive Surgical Inc., Sunny vale, CA, USA) and the Flex® Robotic System (Medrobotics Corporation, Raynham, MA, USA). The da Vinci system was developed with the support of a research program at the Stanford University, California, in conjunction with the American Armed Forces. The goal was to establish a device that was able to perform remote-controlled surgery. A different company, Computer Motion Inc., initially developed two other robot types: Aesop and Zeus. Subsequently, both companies merged under the lead of Intuitive Surgical Inc. In 1997, a laparoscopic splenectomy was the first abdominal surgery assisted by the da Vinci system. Very soon, different procedures followed, such as gastrectomies, esophagectomies and prostatectomies. Altogether, the clinical feasibility was supported with positive reports concerning three-dimensional vision and surgical manipulation. Negative reports focused the missing tactile feedback and poor cost-effectiveness. In 2000, the FDA approved the da Vinci robot for human use (Himpens et al. 1998). The first study to describe the use of the da Vinci system in the cervical region in an animal model was performed by Haus and colleagues in 2003 (Haus et al. 2003). Ensuingly, Hockstein and Weinstein established a proof of feasibility in animal and human anatomical models at the University of Pennsylvania (Hockstein et al. 2005). This working group also established the term of transoral robotic surgery (TORS). The first-in-man study in the head and neck region was reported in 2005 by McLeod and Melder (2005). In the following years, the scope of application increased as the indications for TORS could be expanded. In the past years, a new robotic system, i.e., the Flex® Robotic System, was developed in order to enhance the spectrum of TORS and to overcome existing limitations. This system is specifically tailored to the needs of head and neck surgeons. In the head and neck region, the first resection of a benign tumor was reported by Remacle et al. (2015) and the first resection of a carcinoma by our team (Mattheis and Lang 2015; Mattheis et al. 2015). Both groups stated a safe and better access in comparison with the da Vinci device in more difficult to reach areas of the upper aerodigestive tract (Hasskamp et al. 2015).

4 Different TORS Systems

The current and most frequently in HNSCC resections used da Vinci Si® system allows the surgeon to operate robotic arms through a steering console. The system is based on the console for the surgeon, separated from a unit with three robotic arms and a unit with an interactive monitor (Fig. 1). One of the robotic arms is equipped with a 3D HD endoscope camera (either 0° or 30°) in order to visualize the surgical field while the other two arms carry the surgical instruments (EndoWrist®, Intuitive Surgical Inc., Sunnyvale, CA, USA) (Fig. 2). These instruments offer a three-dimensional movement capacity and can be manipulated using a remote control connected to the surgeon's hands in the surgeon console (Fig. 3). Usually, one hand is steering the tissue retraction, while the other hand is responsible for cutting or further manipulation. The new da Vinci Xi® system presented in 2014 offers an enhanced mobility of the robotic arms and a more sophisticated HD camera, although the instrument diameter increased from 5 to 8 mm, thus making the access in the head and neck region difficult. Due to the fact that this system was originally developed for large cavity surgery, there has been no FDA approval for HNSCC yet.

With the Flex® Robotic System—developed specifically for transoral head and neck resections—the surgeon is able to insert a flexible endoscope into the pharynx. The endoscope can be advanced and steered in a sequential manner, alternating between a flexible and rigid state. Thus, the surgeon can define a path of approach that is not limited by line-of-sight access. Ultimately, the surgeon creates a self-supporting, stable platform from which he or she may visualize and operate (Fig. 4). An HD camera can transmit the pictures on a touch screen and on an external monitor. The surgeon controls the motion of the endoscope with a joystick on the Flex® Console which allows the surgeon to reposition or stabilize the endoscope anytime during the surgery (Fig. 5). There are two different, non-crossing, flexible working channels aside the endoscope for direct manipulation of flexible, fully articulating and rotating operating instruments. These instruments include a Flex® Laser Holder, Flex® Monopolar Maryland Dissector and Flex® Fenestrated Grasper for retraction and tissue manipulation, a Flex® Needle Driver for suturing, and a Flex® Monopolar Needle Knife, Flex® Monopolar Spatula, and Flex® Monopolar Scissor to cut tissue. When operating this system, the instruments provide the surgeon with direct tactile feedback.

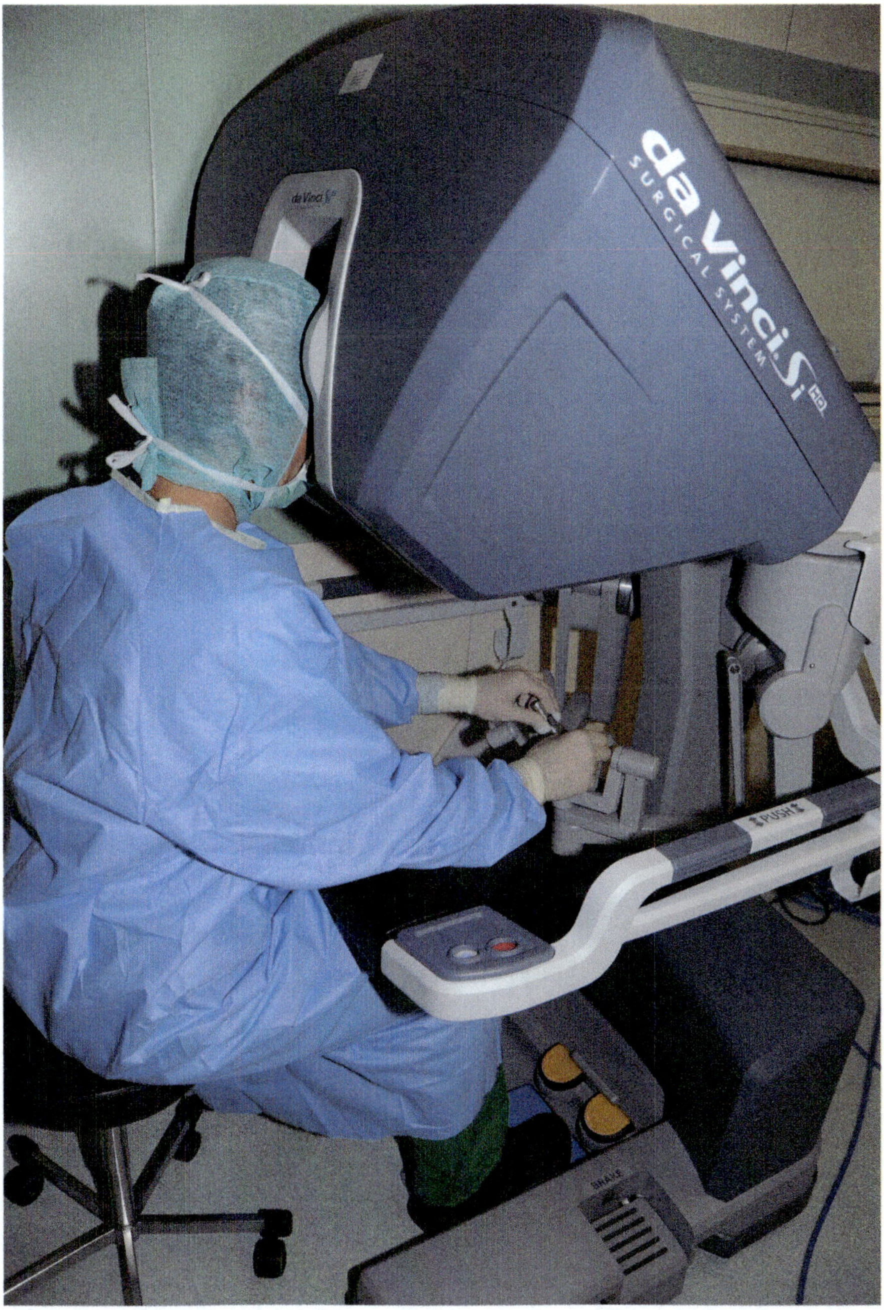

Fig. 1 Da Vinci Si® system

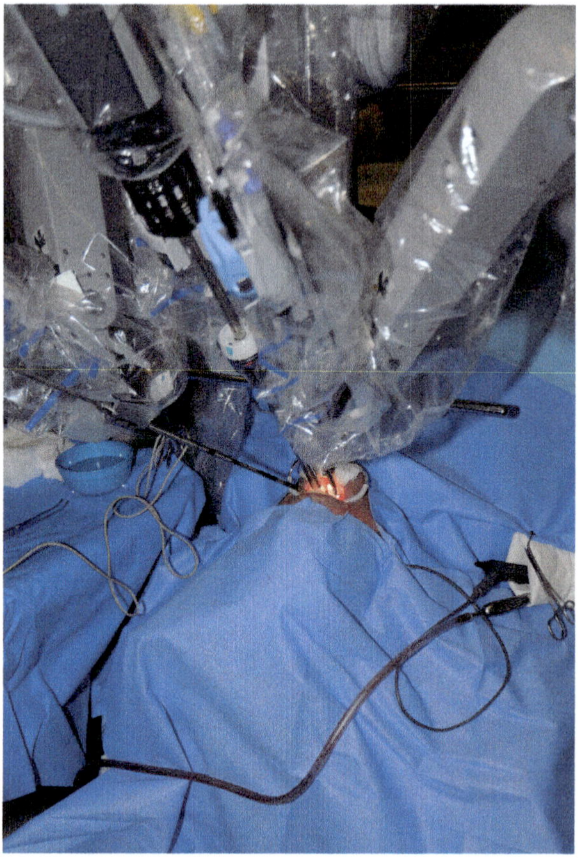

Fig. 2 3D HD endoscope camera

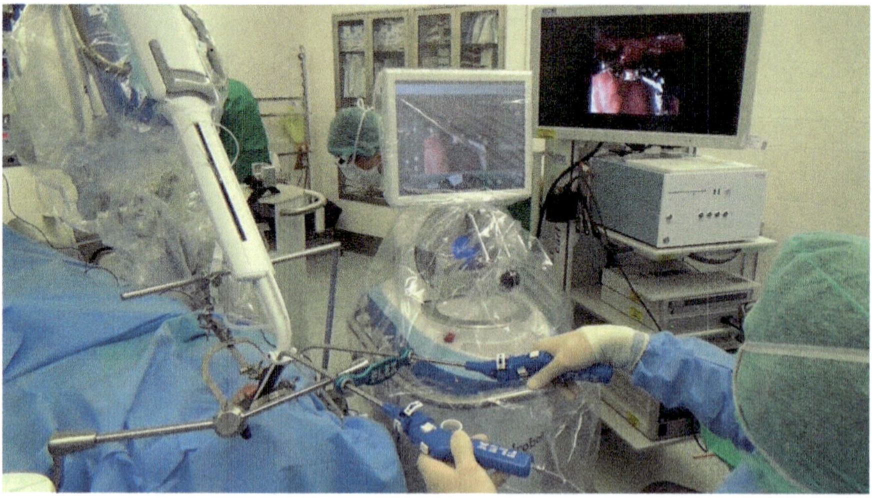

Fig. 3 Three-dimensional movement capacity

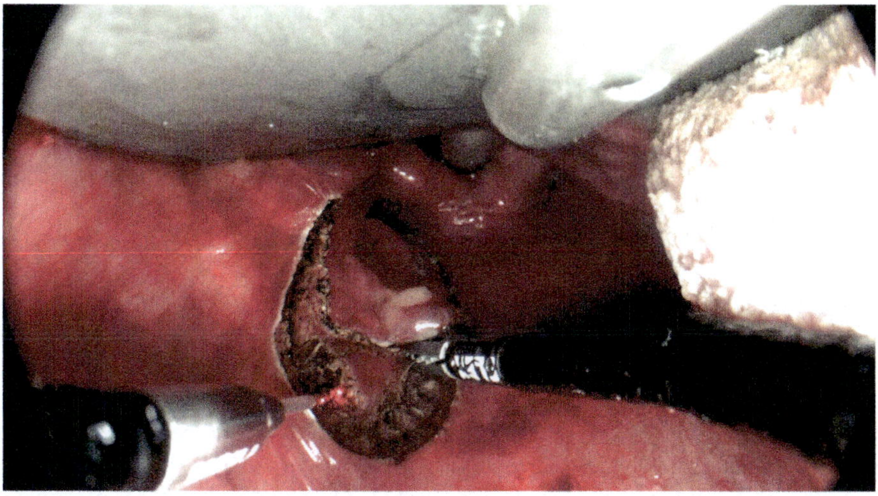

Fig. 4 Self-supporting, stable platform

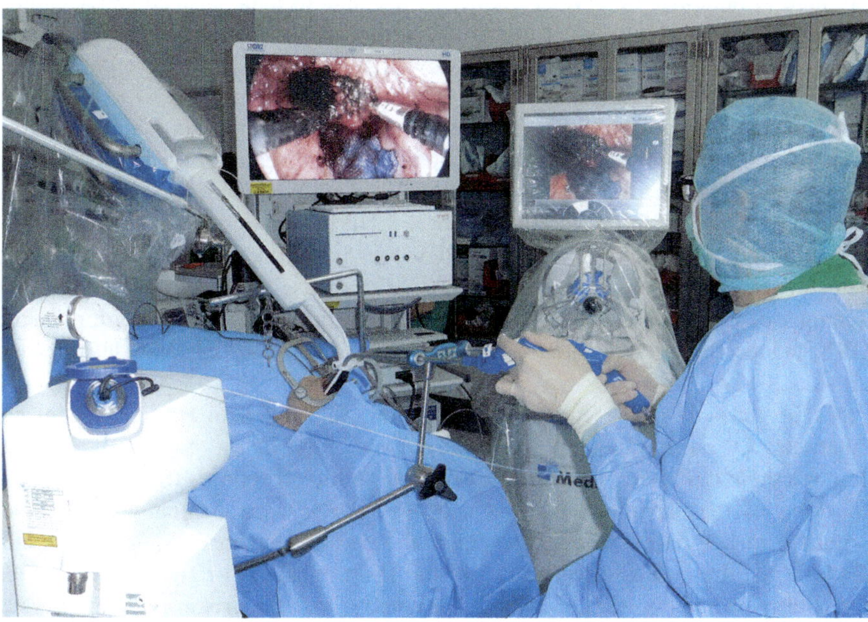

Fig. 5 Flex® Console

5 The Use of TORS in Head and Neck Surgery

The goal of the surgical treatment of HNSCC is complete resection of the cancer with simultaneous preservation of the complex organ functions. Over the past few decades, transoral laser microsurgery (TLM) has been established as an important surgical concept and has become the gold standard for many HNSCC surgeons (Steiner 1994). This was due to comparable oncological outcomes after TLM treatment with reduced comorbidities and loss of function in comparison with classic open surgery techniques. After the introduction of robotic surgery, the systems were investigated with regard to surgical and patient benefits, including length of hospital stay, operating time, quality of surgical resection and quality of life for the patient compared to conventional surgery.

Over the past several years, the development of robotic systems has improved, and therefore, its use in the surgical treatment of HNSCC has become a relevant treatment modality for many patients.

After 2005, indications for TORS started to include the base of tongue (O'Malley et al. 2006), larger tumors of the pharynx (Weinstein et al. 2007) and the parapharyngeal space (O'Malley et al. 2010), tumors of the supraglottic area (Solares and Strome 2007) and the glottis (Desai et al. 2008). Choby and colleagues were able to demonstrate similar quality of life data in patients with OPSCC after TORS in comparison with other transoral surgical approaches and improved results in comparison with open surgery (Choby et al. 2015). Other data indicate an improved swallowing functionality for stage III and IV OPSCC after TORS in comparison with chemoradiotherapy (More et al. 2013). Additionally, different groups suggest the introduction of the TORS-assisted removal of base of tongue tonsil tissue for screening purposes in patients with cancer of unknown primary (CUP) syndrome (Mehta et al. 2013). Since CUP originating from oropharyngeal carcinomas is strongly correlated with HPV positivity, this becomes a particularly interesting aspect in regard to HPV-positive patients (Zengel et al. 2012). For resections of malignant lesions from the supraglottic and epiglottic regions using TORS, a local recurrence rate below 20 % has been reported (Mendelsohn and Remacle 2015).

Despite the enlarged spectrum of indications for TORS in HNSCC, there are limitations: One important factor is the accessibility of the region of interest. Although there have been reports about several glottic procedures (Smith 2014), the exposition of the narrow as well as delicate endolaryngeal structures is limited. Especially in comparison with conventional small endoscopes, the rigid, straight robotic arms, the bulky instruments and the short and broad retractors impair the accessibility (Mattheis et al. 2012). Additionally, in comparison with the crystal clear microscope-based visualization offered by TLM, the current cameras provide lower resolution and lower magnification resulting in reduced visualization of endoluminal structures. With the introduction of the Flex® Robotic System, some of these restrictions have been addressed. The combination with flexible instruments allows for a better accessibility of the relevant structures. Regions of the hypopharynx, especially the pyriform sinus, and regions of the larynx, e.g., the supraglottic region, can be simultaneously visualized, which helps in the assessment of possible infiltration of anatomical structures. The visual resolution remains inferior to the microscope of TLM. Surgeons positively report about the gained tactile feedback. Nevertheless, the system needs prospective clinical trials in order to validate its value and certify improvement in comparison with other established modalities, i.e., TLM.

With the technical advancements over the past few years, many of the early restrictions could be set aside leading to contraindications comparable to those for TLM procedures. Weinstein et al. grouped the contraindications into vascular, functional, oncologic and non-oncologic reasons (Weinstein et al. 2015): Vascular contraindications of TORS for oropharyngeal cancer include close vicinity to important arterial structures such as the carotid artery (e.g., by tumor encasement, or retropharyngeal course of the carotid artery in case of tonsillar cancer) or both lingual arteries (midline tongue base cancer). Functional contraindications include a required resection of more than 50 % of functional relevant structures such as deep tongue base musculature. Oncologic contraindications can result because of size and/or infiltration (T4b, prevertebral fascia), unresectable neck disease or distant metastases and neoplastic-related trismus. Finally, any non-oncologic conditions that prevent either any surgical approach in general or the specific transoral approach such as trismus or cervical spine disease limit the procedure. In our department, we are performing two-thirds base of tongue resections—irrespective of TORS—in selected cases.

Another important factor that potentially limits the use of TORS is the availability of these cost-intensive devices at the surgical centers. One of the main initial critiques of TORS was the high cost. This important factor in modern health care remains an issue. Dombrée and colleagues demonstrated that even in the case of well-trained surgical teams with short surgical times, the costs of the da Vinci system remain higher as compared to conventional surgical strategies in larynx procedures (Dombree et al. 2014). Other sources, however, report shorter periods of hospitalization and treatment-related costs, as well as patient morbidity, partially depending on the tumor location (Richmon et al. 2014; Chung et al. 2015). However, these results are from retrospective studies and their validity may be threatened by biases in areas such as patient selection. In general, additive to the costs of open surgery or TLM, which are mainly determined by personnel, surgical time and hospitalization, the costs of TORS-assisted procedures are also determined by high acquisition costs and the maintenance. This aspect potentially limits the distribution in institutions that are involved in the primary care of HNSCC patients.

6 TORS in HPV-Positive Patients

TORS has demonstrated advantages for a better visualization of the pharynx, especially at the base of tongue. In HPV-related carcinoma, the base of tongue as part of the oropharynx is frequently involved. Surgeons (and therefore patients) potentially benefit from an increased mobility and a better overview in comparison with conventional TLM. In comparison with chemoradiotherapy, TORS has been associated with lower morbidity rates and better functional outcomes. Still, the decision for or against the surgical treatment lies at the end of an interdisciplinary team-based approach including the patient's individual wishes and needs. Therefore, after the decision for surgical treatment has been made, it must then be determined if TORS is indicated. So far, HPV testing is not yet a prognostic predictive marker for a certain established therapeutic alternative and therefore should not change management decisions except in the context of a trial, yet a majority of US physicians report an influence of HPV testing on their treatment approach for OPSCC (Maniakas et al. 2014). As reasons were not given in this survey, one can only speculate that HPV testing may lead to a de-intensification of therapy in the case of HPV-positive test results. To what extent that the TORS procedures will play a role in de-intensification for HPV-positive patients needs to be further evaluated, as the technical development will continue and trials for de-intensification strategies are ongoing.

7 Conclusion

TORS is a valid alternative for surgical transoral procedures in selected cases. Especially for endolaryngeal TORS procedures, additional technical development is mandatory, particularly with respect to visualization and manipulation. The Flex® Robotic System has provided new capabilities that need to be further evaluated. TORS systems are going to improve technical issues and therefore reduce patient morbidity as well as improve surgical handling. The developed systems have to be tested and evaluated in prospective trials in order to be able to identify benefits and disadvantages in patient care. With respect to HPV-related OPSCC, TORS has become a valuable surgical alternative for an increasing number of patients.

References

Best SR, Niparko KJ, Pai SI (2012) Biology of human papillomavirus infection and immune therapy for HPV-related head and neck cancers. Otolaryngol Clin North Am 45:807–822

Choby GW, Kim J, Ling DC, Abberbock S, Mandal R, Kim S, Ferris RL, Duvvuri U (2015) Transoral robotic surgery alone for oropharyngeal cancer: quality-of-life outcomes. JAMA Otolaryngol–Head Neck Surg 141:499–504

Chung TK, Rosenthal EL, Magnuson JS, Carroll WR (2015) Transoral robotic surgery for oropharyngeal and tongue cancer in the United States. The Laryngoscope 125:140–145

Desai SC, Sung CK, Jang DW, Genden EM (2008) Transoral robotic surgery using a carbon dioxide flexible laser for tumors of the upper aerodigestive tract. The Laryngoscope 118: 2187–2189

Dombree M, Crott R, Lawson G, Janne P, Castiaux A, Krug B (2014) Cost comparison of open approach, transoral laser microsurgery and transoral robotic surgery for partial and total laryngectomies. Eur Arch oto-rhino-laryngol (official journal of the European Federation of

Oto-Rhino-Laryngological Societies (EUFOS): affiliated with the German Society for Oto-Rhino-Laryngology—Head and Neck Surgery) 271:2825–2834
Hasskamp P, Lang S, Holtmann L, Stuck BA, Mattheis S (2015) First use of a new retractor in transoral robotic surgery (TORS). Eur Arch oto-rhino-laryngol (official journal of the European Federation of Oto-Rhino-Laryngological Societies (EUFOS): affiliated with the German Society for Oto-Rhino-Laryngology—Head and Neck Surgery)
Haus BM, Kambham N, Le D, Moll FM, Gourin C, Terris DJ (2003) Surgical robotic applications in otolaryngology. The Laryngoscope 113:1139–1144
Himpens J, Leman G, Cadiere GB (1998) Telesurgical laparoscopic cholecystectomy. Surg Endosc 12:1091
Hockstein NG, Nolan J. P, O'Malley WB Jr., Woo YJ (2005) Robotic microlaryngeal surgery: a technical feasibility study using the daVinci surgical robot and an airway mannequin. The Laryngoscope 115:780–785
Kwoh YS, Hou J, Jonckheere EA, Hayati S (1988) A robot with improved absolute positioning accuracy for CT guided stereotactic brain surgery. IEEE Trans Bio-Med Eng 35:153–160
Lawson G, Mendelsohn AH, Van Der Vorst S, Bachy V, Remacle M (2013) Transoral robotic surgery total laryngectomy. The Laryngoscope 123:193–196
Lyford-Pike S, Peng S, Young GD, Taube JM, Westra WH, Akpeng B, Bruno TC, Richmon JD, Wang H, Bishop JA, Chen L, Drake CG, Topalian SL, Pardoll DM, Pai SI (2013) Evidence for a role of the PD-1:PD-L1 pathway in immune resistance of HPV-associated head and neck squamous cell carcinoma. Cancer Res 73:1733–1741
Maniakas A, Moubayed SP, Ayad T, Guertin L, Nguyen-Tan PF, Gologan O, Soulieres D, Christopoulos A (2014) North-American survey on HPV-DNA and p16 testing for head and neck squamous cell carcinoma. Oral Oncol 50:942–946
Mattheis S, Lang S (2015) A new flexible endoscopy-system for the transoral resection of head and neck tumors. Laryngo- rhino- otologie 94:25–28
Mattheis S, Mandapathil M, Rothmeier N, Lang S, Dominas N, Hoffmann TK (2012) Transoral robotic surgery for head and neck tumors: a series of 17 patients. Laryngo- rhino- otologie 91: 768–773
Mattheis S, Kansy B, Hasskamp P, Holtmann L, Lang S (2015) Advances in transoral robotic surgery. Hno 63:752–757
McLeod IK, Melder PC (2005) Da Vinci robot-assisted excision of a vallecular cyst: a case report. Ear Nose Throat J 84:170–172
Mehta V, Johnson P, Tassler A, Kim S, Ferris RL, Nance M, Johnson JT, Duvvuri U (2013) A new paradigm for the diagnosis and management of unknown primary tumors of the head and neck: a role for transoral robotic surgery. The Laryngoscope 123:146–151
Mendelsohn AH, Remacle M (2015) Transoral robotic surgery for laryngeal cancer. Curr Opin Otolaryngol Head Neck Surg 23:148–152
More YI, Tsue TT, Girod DA, Harbison J, Sykes KJ, Williams C, Shnayder Y (2013) Functional swallowing outcomes following transoral robotic surgery vs primary chemoradiotherapy in patients with advanced-stage oropharynx and supraglottis cancers. JAMA Otolaryngol–Head Neck Surg 139:43–48
O'Malley BW Jr, Weinstein GS, Snyder W, Hockstein NG (2006) Transoral robotic surgery (TORS) for base of tongue neoplasms. The Laryngoscope 116:1465–1472
O'Malley BW Jr, Quon H, Leonhardt FD, Chalian AA, Weinstein GS (2010) Transoral robotic surgery for parapharyngeal space tumors. ORL J oto-rhino-laryngol Relat Spec 72:332–336
Pai SI (2013) Adaptive immune resistance in HPV-associated head and neck squamous cell carcinoma. Oncoimmunology 2:e24065
Paul HA, Bargar WL, Mittlestadt B, Musits B, Taylor RH, Kazanzides P, Zuhars J, Williamson B, Hanson W (1992) Development of a surgical robot for cementless total hip arthroplasty. Clin Orthop Relat Res 57–66
Pytynia KB, Dahlstrom KR, Sturgis EM (2014) Epidemiology of HPV-associated oropharyngeal cancer. Oral Oncol 50:380–386

Remacle M, Prasad VMN, Lawson G, Plisson L, Bachy V, Van der Vorst S (2015) Transoral robotic surgery (TORS) with the Medrobotics Flex System: first surgical application on humans. Eur Arch oto-rhino-laryngol (official journal of the European Federation of Oto-Rhino-Laryngological Societies (EUFOS): affiliated with the German Society for Oto-Rhino-Laryngology—Head and Neck Surgery) 272:1451–1455

Richmon JD, Quon H, Gourin CG (2014) The effect of transoral robotic surgery on short-term outcomes and cost of care after oropharyngeal cancer surgery. The Laryngoscope 124:165–171

Smith RV (2014) Transoral robotic surgery for larynx cancer. Otolaryngol Clin North Am 47: 379–395

Solares CA, Strome M (2007) Transoral robot-assisted CO2 laser supraglottic laryngectomy: experimental and clinical data. The Laryngoscope 117:817–820

Steiner W (1994) Therapy of hypopharyngeal cancer. Part III: the concept of minimally invasive therapy of cancers of the upper aerodigestive tract with special reference to hypopharyngeal cancer and trans-oral laser microsurgery. Hno 42:104–112

Tinhofer I, Johrens K, Keilholz U, Kaufmann A, Lehmann A, Weichert W, Stenzinger A, Stromberger C, Klinghammer K, Becker ET, Dommerich S, Stolzel K, Hofmann VM, Hildebrandt B, Moser L, Ervens J, Bottcher A, Albers A, Stabenow R, Reinecke A, Budach V, Hoffmeister B, Raguse JD (2015) Contribution of human papilloma virus to the incidence of squamous cell carcinoma of the head and neck in a European population with high smoking prevalence. Eur J Cancer (Oxford, England: 1990) 51:514–521

Weinstein GS, O'Malley BW Jr., Snyder W, Sherman E, Quon H (2007) Transoral robotic surgery: radical tonsillectomy. Arch Otolaryngol–Head Neck Surg 133:1220–1226

Weinstein GS, O'Malley BW Jr, Rinaldo A, Silver CE, Werner JA, Ferlito A (2015) Understanding contraindications for transoral robotic surgery (TORS) for oropharyngeal cancer. Eur Arch oto-rhino-laryngol (official journal of the European Federation of Oto-Rhino-Laryngological Societies (EUFOS): affiliated with the German Society for Oto-Rhino-Laryngology—Head and Neck Surgery) 272:1551–1552

Zengel P, Assmann G, Mollenhauer M, Jung A, Sotlar K, Kirchner T, Ihrler S (2012) Cancer of unknown primary originating from oropharyngeal carcinomas are strongly correlated to HPV positivity. Virchows Arch: Int J Pathol 461:283–290

Part V
Predictive Factors for Outcome and Quality of Life in HPV Positive and HPV Negative

Risk Groups for Survival in HPV-Positive and HPV-Negative OPSCC

Michelle M. Rietbergen, Ruud H. Brakenhoff and C. René Leemans

Abstract

Over the last three decades, it has become clear that infection with high-risk human papillomavirus (HPV) is etiologically linked to the development of head and neck squamous cell carcinomas, particularly those carcinomas that arise in the oropharyngeal region.

Keywords

De-escalation · Comorbidity · Prognostic model · Biomarkers · Risk groups

1 Introduction

Over the last three decades, it has become clear that infection with high-risk human papillomavirus (HPV) is etiologically linked to the development of head and neck squamous cell carcinomas, particularly those carcinomas that arise in the oropharyngeal region.

Epidemiologic evidence has revealed a rapid increase in the prevalence rates of HPV-induced oropharyngeal squamous cell carcinomas (OPSCCs) in Europe and the rest of the world (Chaturvedi et al. 2011; Nasman et al. 2009; Rietbergen et al. 2013; Shaw and Robinson 2011). HPV-positive oropharyngeal carcinomas are considered to be a different tumor entity, based on biological, epidemiological and clinical differences, compared to the HPV-negative OPSCCs.

M.M. Rietbergen · R.H. Brakenhoff · C. René Leemans (✉)
Department of Otolaryngology/Head and Neck Surgery, VU University Medical Center, Amsterdam, The Netherlands
e-mail: cr.leemans@vumc.nl

W. Golusiński et al. (eds.), *HPV Infection in Head and Neck Cancer*,
Recent Results in Cancer Research 206, DOI 10.1007/978-3-319-43580-0_17

Patients with HPV-positive OPSCC are generally younger by approximately 10 years, male and are less likely to have a history of tobacco or alcohol use compared to patients with HPV-negative OPSCC (Chaturvedi et al. 2011; Gillison et al. 2000, 2008). HPV-positive tumors present mostly at an early primary tumor (T) stage and advanced nodal (N) stage. In general, HPV-associated OPSCCs are TNM stage III and IV disease at presentation. Lymph node metastases are usually cystic and multilevel (Begum and Westra 2008; Hafkamp et al. 2008). Despite the advanced stage, HPV-associated OPSCC has been shown to be more responsive to therapy and has a better outcome than similar HPV-negative tumors (Butz et al. 1996; Lindel et al. 2001; Lindquist et al. 2007). Several retrospective and prospective studies in the USA, Australia and Western Europe have consistently demonstrated that HPV-positive OPSCC is associated with a more favorable prognosis (Ang et al. 2010; Fakhry et al. 2008; Posner et al. 2011; Rischin et al. 2010). One of the first studies to prospectively evaluate in a multicenter clinical trial the association of tumor HPV status with response to treatment and survival in patients (n = 96) with OPSCC was that of Fakhry et al. (2008). Their data confirmed the improved survival outcomes for patients with HPV-positive OPSCC observed in retrospective survival analyses and were consistent with an increased sensitivity of these types of cancers to chemoradiation. Because of the relatively small sample size, however, other favorable prognostic factors also associated with tumor HPV status (e.g., early tumor stage or low comorbidity score) could not be ruled out as an explanation for the observed difference in survival. In 2010, Ang et al. published a study which was performed within a randomized clinical trial conducted by the Radiation Therapy Oncology Group (RTOG; the RTOG 0129 study). This study provided strong evidence that tumor HPV status is an independent prognostic factor for overall survival and progression-free survival among patients (n = 266) with OPSCC. Ang et al. were the first to propose a prognostic model for OPSCC patients, with HPV being the most important prognostic factor. Since then, this model has been validated in other populations, and different prognostic risk models have been developed for OPSCC patients that all include HPV as main prognostic factor (Ang et al. 2010; Dahlstrom et al. 2012).

2 Different Prognostic Models

In the study by Ang et al. (2010), the first recursive partitioning model (RPA) for patients with OPSCC was proposed based on the RTOG 0129 study. In total 266 patients with OPSCC were stratified into three risk groups: patients having a low, intermediate or high risk of death. HPV was tested by p16-immunohistochemistry and in situ hybridization for HPV16. A combination of HPV status, pack years of tobacco smoking and TNM stage could be used to classify patients with OPSCC into these three risk groups (Fig. 1). This is a unique prognostic model that has been validated by others (Granata et al. 2012). However, this model is based on a clinical trial in the USA in which only patients with stage III/IV disease and a good ECOG

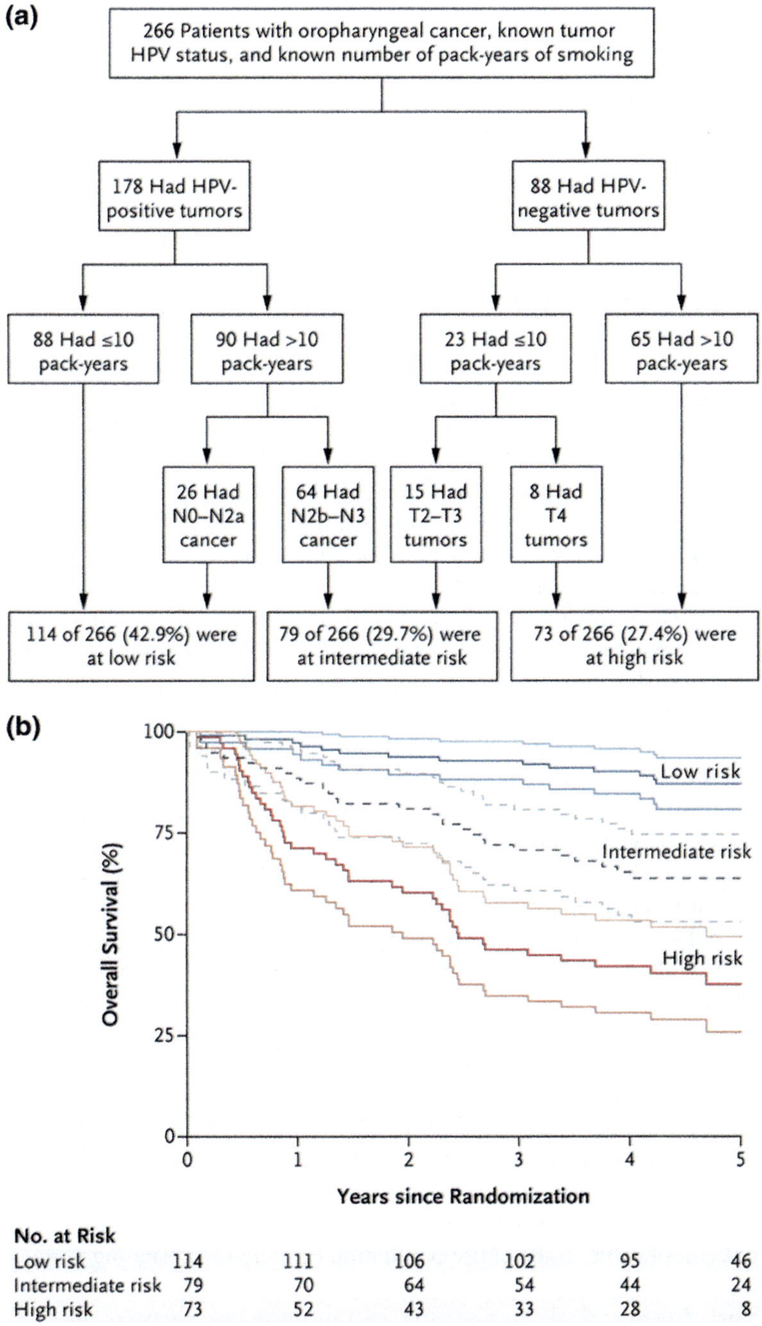

Fig. 1 Classification of risk groups for survival of OPSCC using RPA analysis of 2 RTOG trials by Ang et al.(2010)

performance score (i.e., 0–1) were included. The question therefore arises whether this model would also be applicable for the entire population of patients who present with OPSCC, or if additional prognostic factors need to be considered. Moreover, the HPV-attributable fraction and the smoking behavior in many European countries differ significantly from that in the USA.

In 2013, Rietbergen et al. conducted a study, based on an unselected, consecutive cohort of 723 patients with OPSCC. This study also included patients with stage I/II disease and patients with moderate to severe comorbidity (using the ACE-27 score) (Kallogjeri et al. 2012; Kaplan and Feinstein 1974). HPV status was determined by p16-immunohistochemistry followed by an HPV DNA test on the p16-positive cases. Using this patient group, the prognostic model of the RTOG 0129 study was confirmed (Rietbergen et al. 2013); the 3-year survival rates were similar to those described previously (Ang et al. 2010). However, when analyzing this cohort using the RTOG 0129 prognostic model, the Harrell's C-index was suboptimal. Therefore, an adapted recursive partitioning model was developed, based on this consecutive patient cohort, also including patients with stage I/II disease and patients with moderate to severe comorbidity. This new model confirmed that the major prognostic factor for patients with OPSCC is HPV status. However, comorbidity (instead of smoking) was the most important prognostic factor in HPV-positive patients and the second most important factor in HPV-negative patients after nodal stage (Fig. 2). In HPV-negative patients, nodal stage remained the most important prognostic factor. In HPV-positive patients, nodal stage did not influence the prognosis. The observation that HPV-positive patients have a good prognosis regardless of nodal stage has already been described in several studies (Chaturvedi et al. 2011; Shaw and Robinson 2011; Ang et al. 2010). Interestingly enough, smoking was not a prognostic factor in the prognostic model of Rietbergen et al. Smoking was one of the prognostic determinants of overall survival in the univariate and multivariable analyses. However, in the recursive partitioning analysis, comorbidity was a stronger prognostic factor than smoking. A likely explanation for this observation was that most of the patients in the cohort with a moderate to severe comorbidity were also heavy smokers (83.3 %), and died of smoking-related causes such as cardiovascular disease and lung, esophageal and head and neck cancers. In addition, most of the patients in the cohort smoked more than 10 PY (87.1 %), which is a very high percentage in comparison with other studies (Ang et al. 2010; O'Sullivan et al. 2013).

In 2015, the prognostic model proposed by Rietbergen et al. (2015) was validated with an independent series of patients. Whereas the RTOG 0129 prognostic model focuses on the so-called 'trial population' (i.e., patients with stage III/IV OPSCC having a good ECOG performance score), this new prognostic model seems to be applicable to the entire population of patients presenting with OPSCC. Moreover, this model might be more suitable for a patient population with a high percentage of heavy smokers, as is the case in most European countries. Comorbidity, instead of tobacco smoking, might be a more informative prognostic factor in those populations.

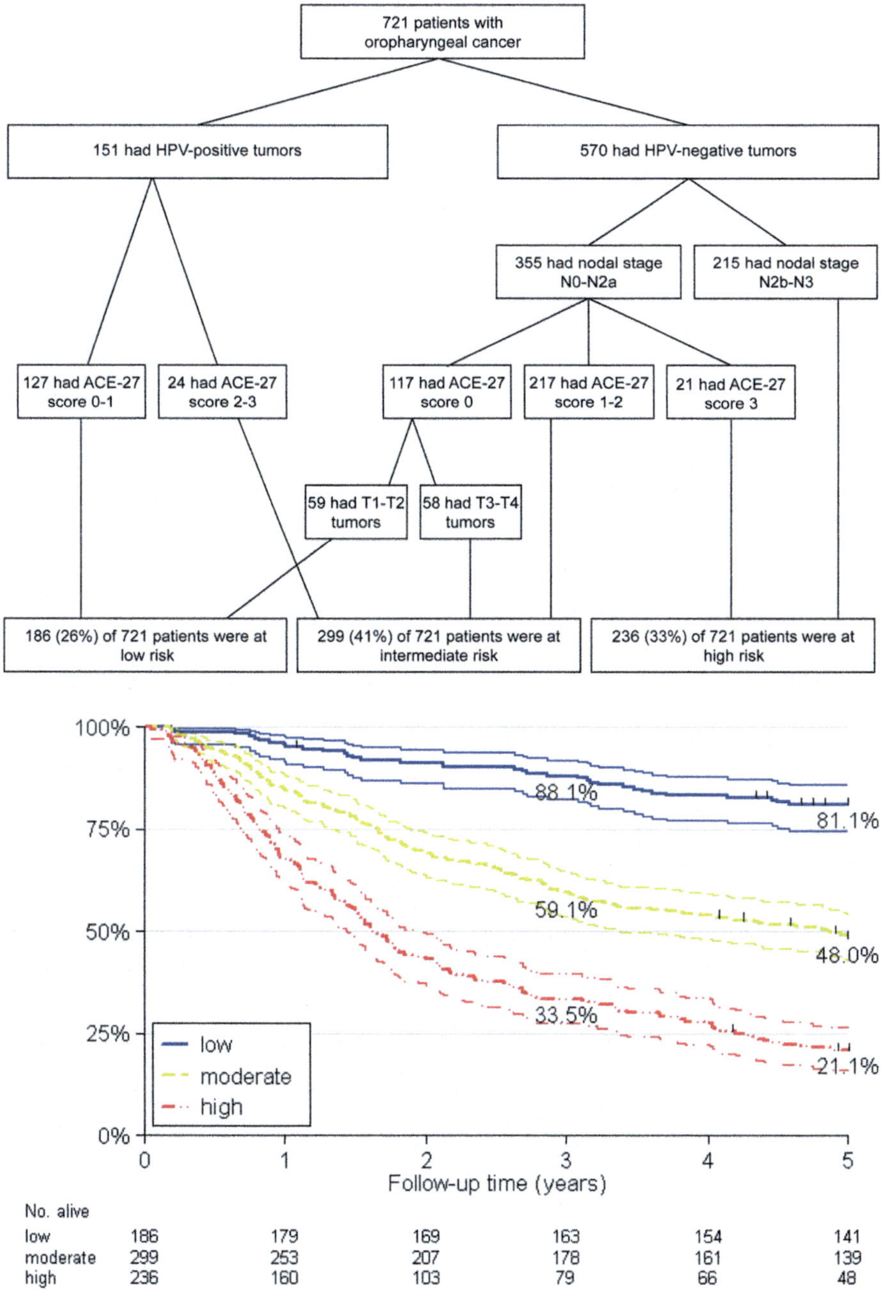

Fig. 2 Classification of risk groups for survival of OPSCC using RPA anlysis of a Netherlands cohort by Rietbergenet al. (2013b)

One of the other remarkable findings in the study of Rietbergen et al. was the fact that survival of patients with p16-positive but HPV DNA-negative OPSCC (16.4 % of p16 positive patients) was significantly different compared to patients with 'truly' HPV-positive OPSCC. The survival curve of this 'discordant' group almost converged the survival curve of patients with an HPV-negative OPSCC. In 2011, Perrone et al. reported similar results; patients in the p16-positive but HPV DNA-negative subgroup showed the same overall survival curves as HPV-negative patients (Perrone et al. 2011). This finding might be important for the inclusion of patients in de-intensification trials. Currently, de-intensification trials are being conducted for which eligibility for randomization only involves positivity on p16-immunohistochemistry. However, this causes the risk to enroll patients with HPV DNA-negative tumors.

Therefore, we encourage to incorporate HPV status into the next (8th) edition of the TNM AJCC/UICC classification. Moreover, we stress the importance of performing reliable HPV DNA testing besides p16-immunohistochemistry to detect a true HPV-related OPSCC.

3 De-intensification of Treatment

As patients with HPV-positive OPSCC have a favorable prognosis, an opportunity now exists to investigate less intense treatment strategies for these patients. These treatment strategies should not compromise survival outcomes but lower the risk of potentially debilitating late effects of treatment. For the most part, patients with HPV-positive OPSCC are younger and generally have a better health status compared to patients with HPV-negative OPSCC. Thus, low treatment-related toxicities and a high level of quality of life after treatment are important considerations in the clinical management of these patients.

In 2010, Ang et al. already suggested, on the basis of their data, that future clinical trials should be designed specifically for patients with HPV-positive OPSCC. Their analysis did not show a significant difference in overall survival between a concomitant-boost accelerated-fractionation regimen of radiotherapy and a standard-fractionation regimen, combined with concurrent, high-dose cisplatin in patients with HPV-positive OPSCC. Therefore, they suggested that either regimen could serve as the comparison for a new therapy being investigated.

Currently, several de-escalation trials are running for patients with HPV-positive OPSCC. The DeESCALATE-HPV trial is a phase III trial that compares radiotherapy plus cetuximab versus chemoradiotherapy in patients with HPV-positive OPSCC. The purpose of this study is to evaluate the application of cetuximab instead of cisplatin, a less toxic alternative for concurrent chemoradiation. A second trial that aims to assess a potential for cetuximab instead of cisplatin, is the (recently closed) RTOG 1016 trial.

Another de-escalation trial is the recently closed ECOG-E1308 phase II trial, for patients with stage III/IV HPV-positive OPSCC. This trial tested whether induction chemotherapy (combination of paclitaxel, cisplatin, and cetuximab followed by concurrent cetuximab and radiotherapy) may allow for safe reduction in radiotherapy dose to the primary site and involved neck nodes. Patients with complete response to induction had modification of the prescribed radiation therapy dose from 69.3 Gy (given for incomplete response) to 54 Gy. Eligibility for randomization in this trial also included HPV16 in situ hybridization besides p16-immunohistochemistry.

The ability to estimate survival probability of OPSCC patients before any type of treatment would be very valuable for decision making, especially for patients who might be enrolled in treatment de-escalation trials. The two prognostic models described above might be used to stratify patients for de-intensification therapy. However, when considering treatment selection, it may also be useful to stratify patients based on their risk of recurrence. Despite the known favorable locoregional and survival outcome of HPV-positive compared with HPV-negative OPSCC, the recent literature shows that distant metastases (DM) rates are the same for both (Ang et al. 2010; O'Sullivan et al. 2012). In addition, DM in HPV-positive patients may occur in unexpected sites and after longer intervals (Huang et al. 2012). DM seems to be the leading cause of death in HPV-positive patients. O'Sullivan et al. (2013) recently demonstrated that HPV-positive patients with nodal stage N2c have a reduced distant control when treated with radiotherapy alone and seem less suited for deintensification strategies that omit chemotherapy. They suggest that deintensification that withholds or reduces chemotherapy intensity should be considered cautiously and might be best deployed in subgroups least likely to develop DM (i.e., T1-3 N0-2c patients).

4 Refinement of Prognostic Models by Other Biomarkers

Besides the main prognostic factors for survival in patients with HPV-positive OPSCC (i.e., smoking, comorbidity, and a high nodal stage), other predictors of survival have recently been suggested. Recent investigations undertaken to improve the staging system for HPV-positive tumors suggest that new biomarkers to complement known risk factors are needed to improve prognostic accuracy (Huang et al. 2012; Rios et al. 2014).

Murphy et al. recently described the relationship between tumor-specific growth rate (TSGR) and oropharyngeal cancer (OPC) outcomes in the HPV-positive patient. TSGR was defined as the primary tumor volume differences between a diagnostic and secondary scan separated >7 days without interval treatment (in percent volume growth/day) (Murphy et al. 2015). This was derived from primary tumor volume doubling time for 85 OPC patients with known p16 status and smoking pack-years managed with (chemo)radiation. TSGR was incorporated into RTOG 0129 risk grouping (0129RG) to assess whether TSGR could improve prognostic accuracy. Incorporation of this radio biomarker into risk stratification with 0129RG improved the predictive quality of the risk groups. It suggests the potential ability of TSGR to improve patient selection for treatment intensification.

Another potential biomarker could be tumor infiltrating lymphocytes (TIL) levels. In 2014, Ward et al. (2014) showed that TIL levels predict for survival in OPSCC patients. In their study, survival in patients with HPV positive, TIL_{low} tumors, was not significantly different than in those with HPV-negative disease. A prognostic model based on low TIL levels, heavy smoking, and late T stage allowed the identification of a group of HPV-positive patients with poor survival.

The prognostic impact of EGFR overexpression remains uncertain. EGFR is abnormally activated in approximately 80 % of head and neck cancers (Thomas et al. 2005). EGFR expression has been associated with prognosis in head and neck cancer, particularly in patients treated with radiotherapy, although some studies have found no relationship between EGFR and treatment response or outcome (Thomas et al. 2005; Putti et al. 2002; Chang et al. 2008; Kong et al. 2009; Fischer et al. 2008).

Hong et al. (2010) examined the prognostic significance of EGFR expression in relation to HPV status in 270 OPSCCs. Their data showed that EGFR and HPV are independent prognostic markers in OPC, although the effect of EGFR was more convincing for locoregional control than for survival. They suggested that use of EGFR in combination with HPV status gives additional prognostic information particularly in terms of locoregional control.

Vainshtein et al. (2014) investigated EGFR overexpression in 184 HPV-positive and 14 HPV-negative patients. EGFR overexpression was related to HPV-negative status and was univariately associated with locoregional (LR) recurrence in the overall population, but was neither retained in the multivariate model after adjustment for HPV status, nor associated with LR recurrence in HPV-positive patients. In HPV-positive patients, only T4- and N3-stages were significant predictors of LR recurrence on multivariate analysis.

In 2015, another potential biomarker was investigated that might influence survival in HPV-positive OPSCC patients; CD98. CD98 has been described as being a novel enrichment marker for cancer stem cells (CSCs) (Martens-de Kemp et al. 2013). CSCs represent a small subpopulation of tumor cells that maintain tumor growth by fuelling the expansion of the malignant cell population infinitely (Bao et al. 2006). CSCs can be distinguished from the bulk of the tumor based on differential expression of protein markers on the cell membrane. Previous studies suggest that treatment failure in head and neck cancer patients might be the consequence of therapy resistance of CSCs (de Jong et al. 2010). Rietbergen et al. (2014) showed that overall survival and progression-free survival was markedly better for HPV-positive patients with a $CD98_{low}$ OPSCC compared to HPV-positive patients with a $CD98_{high}$ OPSCC. Consequently, CD98-expression could be used as an additional prognostic marker for selection of HPV-positive patients in clinical trials. Although a challenging and attractive idea, the use of CD98 as a prognostic marker should first be preceded by a thorough validation phase in prospective clinical trials.

5 Conclusion

Several prognostic models have been proposed in which tumor HPV-status is the most important prognostic factor. These models might be used to stratify patients for de-intensification therapy. Besides tumor HPV status, other prognostic factors such as tobacco smoking, comorbidity, and nodal stage influence the prognosis in OPSCC patients. However, especially when using these models in clinical trial designs, one has to bear in mind that the population on which the prognostic model has been developed should be more or less identical with the population that is enrolled in the clinical (de-escalation) trial. Moreover, we underline the importance of performing reliable HPV DNA testing besides p16-immunohistochemistry to detect a true HPV-related OPSCC and to select patients for de-intensifying trials. To improve prognostic accuracy, radiographic and biological biomarkers may also play a role in the nearby future.

References

Ang KK, Harris J, Wheeler R et al (2010) Human papillomavirus and survival of patients with oropharyngeal cancer. N Engl J Med 363:24–35

Bao S, Wu Q, McLendon RE et al (2006) Glioma stem cells promote radioresistance by preferential activation of the DNA damage response. Nature 444:756–760

Begum S, Westra WH (2008) Basaloid squamous cell carcinoma of the head and neck is a mixed variant that can be further resolved by HPV status. Am J Surg Pathol 32:1044–1050

Butz K, Geisen C, Ullmann A et al (1996) Cellular responses of HPV-positive cancer cells to genotoxic anti-cancer agents: repression of E6/E7-oncogene expression and induction of apoptosis. Int J Cancer 68:506–513

Chang AR, Wu HG, Park CI et al (2008) Expression of epidermal growth factor receptor and cyclin D1 in pretreatment biopsies as a predictive factor of radiotherapy efficacy in early glottic cancer. Head Neck 30:852–857

Chaturvedi AK, Engels EA, Pfeiffer RM et al (2011) Human papillomavirus and rising oropharyngeal cancer incidence in the United States. J Clin Oncol 29:4294–4301

Dahlstrom KR, Calzada G, Hanby JD, et al (2012) An evolution in demographics, treatment, and outcomes of oropharyngeal cancer at a major cancer center: a staging system in need of repair. Cancer

de Jong MC, Pramana J, Van Der Wal JE et al (2010) CD44 expression predicts local recurrence after radiotherapy in larynx cancer. Clin Cancer Res 16:5329–5338

Fakhry C, Westra WH, Li S et al (2008) Improved survival of patients with human papillomavirus-positive head and neck squamous cell carcinoma in a prospective clinical trial. J Natl Cancer Inst 100:261–269

Fischer C, Zlobec I, Stockli E et al (2008) Is immunohistochemical epidermal growth factor receptor expression overestimated as a prognostic factor in head-neck squamous cell carcinoma? A retrospective analysis based on a tissue microarray of 365 carcinomas. Hum Pathol 39:1527–1534

Gillison ML, Koch WM, Capone RB et al (2000) Evidence for a causal association between human papillomavirus and a subset of head and neck cancers. J Natl Cancer Inst 92:709–720

Gillison ML, D'Souza G, Westra W et al (2008) Distinct risk factor profiles for human papillomavirus type 16-positive and human papillomavirus type 16-negative head and neck cancers. J Natl Cancer Inst 100:407–420

Granata R, Miceli R, Orlandi E et al (2012) Tumor stage, human papillomavirus and smoking status affect the survival of patients with oropharyngeal cancer: an Italian validation study. Ann Oncol 23:1832–1837

Hafkamp HC, Manni JJ, Haesevoets A et al (2008) Marked differences in survival rate between smokers and nonsmokers with HPV 16-associated tonsillar carcinomas. Int J Cancer 122:2656–2664

Hong A, Dobbins T, Lee CS et al (2010) Relationships between epidermal growth factor receptor expression and human papillomavirus status as markers of prognosis in oropharyngeal cancer. Eur J Cancer 46:2088–2096

Huang SH, Perez-Ordonez B, Liu FF et al (2012) Atypical clinical behavior of p16-confirmed HPV-related oropharyngeal squamous cell carcinoma treated with radical radiotherapy. Int J Radiat Oncol Biol Phys 82:276–283

Kallogjeri D, Piccirillo JF, Spitznagel EL Jr et al (2012) Comparison of scoring methods for ACE-27: simpler is better. J Geriatr Oncol 3:238–245

Kaplan MH, Feinstein AR (1974) The importance of classifying initial co-morbidity in evaluating the outcome of diabetes mellitus. J Chronic Dis 27:387–404

Kong CS, Narasimhan B, Cao H et al (2009) The relationship between human papillomavirus status and other molecular prognostic markers in head and neck squamous cell carcinomas. Int J Radiat Oncol Biol Phys 74:553–561

Lindel K, Beer KT, Laissue J et al (2001) Human papillomavirus positive squamous cell carcinoma of the oropharynx: a radiosensitive subgroup of head and neck carcinoma. Cancer 92:805–813

Lindquist D, Romanitan M, Hammarstedt L et al (2007) Human papillomavirus is a favourable prognostic factor in tonsillar cancer and its oncogenic role is supported by the expression of E6 and E7. Mol Oncol 1:350–355

Martens-de Kemp SR, Brink A, Stigter-van WM et al (2013) CD98 marks a subpopulation of head and neck squamous cell carcinoma cells with stem cell properties. Stem Cell Res 10:477–488

Murphy CT, Devarajan K, Wang LS et al (2015) Pre-treatment tumor-specific growth rate as a temporal biomarker that predicts treatment failure and improves risk stratification for oropharyngeal cancer. Oral Oncol 51:1034–1040

Nasman A, Attner P, Hammarstedt L et al (2009) Incidence of human papillomavirus (HPV) positive tonsillar carcinoma in Stockholm, Sweden: an epidemic of viral-induced carcinoma? Int J Cancer 125:362–366

O'Sullivan B, Huang SH, Perez-Ordonez B et al (2012) Outcomes of HPV-related oropharyngeal cancer patients treated by radiotherapy alone using altered fractionation. Radiother Oncol 103:49–56

O'Sullivan B, Huang SH, Siu LL et al (2013) Deintensification candidate subgroups in human papillomavirus-related oropharyngeal cancer according to minimal risk of distant metastasis. J Clin Oncol 31:543–550

Perrone F, Gloghini A, Cortelazzi B et al (2011) Isolating p16-positive/HPV-negative oropharyngeal cancer: an effort worth making. Am J Surg Pathol 35:774–777

Posner MR, Lorch JH, Goloubeva O et al (2011) Survival and human papillomavirus in oropharynx cancer in TAX 324: a subset analysis from an international phase III trial. Ann Oncol 22:1071–1077

Putti TC, To KF, Hsu HC et al (2002) Expression of epidermal growth factor receptor in head and neck cancers correlates with clinical progression: a multicentre immunohistochemical study in the Asia-Pacific region. Histopathology 41:144–151

Rietbergen MM, Leemans CR, Bloemena E et al (2013a) Increasing prevalence rates of HPV attributable oropharyngeal squamous cell carcinomas in the Netherlands as assessed by a validated test algorithm. Int J Cancer 132:1565–1571

Rietbergen MM, Brakenhoff RH, Bloemena E et al (2013b) Human papillomavirus detection and comorbidity: critical issues in selection of patients with oropharyngeal cancer for treatment De-escalation trials. Ann Oncol 24:2740–2745

Rietbergen MM, Martens-de Kemp SR, Bloemena E et al (2014) Cancer stem cell enrichment marker CD98: a prognostic factor for survival in patients with human papillomavirus-positive oropharyngeal cancer. Eur J Cancer 50:765–773

Rietbergen MM, Witte BI, Velazquez ER et al (2015) Different prognostic models for different patient populations: validation of a new prognostic model for patients with oropharyngeal cancer in Western Europe. Br J Cancer 112:1733–1736

Rios VE, Hoebers F, Aerts HJ et al (2014) Externally validated HPV-based prognostic nomogram for oropharyngeal carcinoma patients yields more accurate predictions than TNM staging. Radiother Oncol 113:324–330

Rischin D, Young RJ, Fisher R et al (2010) Prognostic significance of p16INK4A and human papillomavirus in patients with oropharyngeal cancer treated on TROG 02.02 phase III trial. J Clin Oncol 28:4142–4148

Shaw R, Robinson M (2011) The increasing clinical relevance of human papillomavirus type 16 (HPV-16) infection in oropharyngeal cancer. Br J Oral Maxillofac Surg 49:423–429

Thomas GR, Nadiminti H, Regalado J (2005) Molecular predictors of clinical outcome in patients with head and neck squamous cell carcinoma. Int J Exp Pathol 86:347–363

Vainshtein JM, Spector ME, McHugh JB et al (2014) Refining risk stratification for locoregional failure after chemoradiotherapy in human papillomavirus-associated oropharyngeal cancer. Oral Oncol 50:513–519

Ward MJ, Thirdborough SM, Mellows T et al (2014) Tumour-infiltrating lymphocytes predict for outcome in HPV-positive oropharyngeal cancer. Br J Cancer 110:489–500

Predictive Factors for Outcome and Quality of Life in HPV-Positive and HPV-Negative HNSCC

Jochen Hess

Abstract

Infection with high-risk types of the human papilloma virus (HPV) is an etiological risk factor for oropharyngeal squamous cell carcinoma (OPSCC) and associated with a better response to therapy and improved survival. A better understanding of the molecular principles underlying the differences in clinical behavior could pave the way to establish more effective and less toxic therapy for HPV-positive OPSCC and their HPV-negative counterparts. Compelling experimental evidence demonstrates that extensive global reprogramming of epigenetic profiles is as important as genetic mutations during neoplastic transformation and malignant progression, including HPV-positive OPSCC. In this chapter, the current knowledge on HPV-related alterations in DNA methylation, histone modification, and chromosome remodeling will be summarized and assessment of cancer-related profiles will be discussed as a valuable tool to gain important diagnostic or prognostic information for therapeutic decision-making and clinical management of HNSCC patients.

Keywords

DNA methylation · Histone modification · Chromosome remodeling · DNMT · HDAC

J. Hess (✉)
Department of Otolaryngology, Head and Neck Surgery,
University Hospital and Research Group Molecular Mechanisms
of Head and Neck Tumors, German Cancer Research Center (DKFZ),
Heidelberg, Germany
e-mail: jochen.hess@med.uni-heidelberg.de

W. Golusiński et al. (eds.), *HPV Infection in Head and Neck Cancer*,
Recent Results in Cancer Research 206, DOI 10.1007/978-3-319-43580-0_18

1 Background and Clinical Relevance

Infection with high-risk types of human papilloma virus (HPV), predominantly type 16, has been identified as important risk factor in an escalating number of patients with head and neck squamous cell carcinoma (HNSCC) (Gillison et al. 2015). HPV-positive tumors arise mainly in the (oropharynx oropharyngeal squamous cell carcinoma (OPSCC)) and display distinct biological and clinical features as opposed to HPV-negative HNSCC (Mehanna et al. 2013; Ndiaye et al. 2014; Hayes et al. 2015; Network 2015). HPV-positive OPSCCs are associated with a better response to therapy and improved survival, justifying the HPV status as one of the most accurate prognostic biomarkers in primary and progressed tumors (Ang et al. 2010; Chaturvedi et al. 2011; Fakhry et al. 2014; Kang et al. 2015). It is foreseen that a better understanding of the molecular principles underlying the differences in clinical behavior could pave the way to establish more effective and less toxic therapy for HPV-positive OPSCC but also their HPV-negative counterparts.

The manifestation of HNSCC is a multifactorial process, which is characterized by the accumulation of genomic events and somatic mutations affecting tumor-relevant signaling and gene regulatory networks. Recent advances in next-generation sequencing provided a valuable tool to unravel the mutational landscape of HNSCC, including differences between HPV-positive and HPV-negative tumors (Hayes et al. 2015; Network 2015). However, most ongoing clinical trials still focus on therapeutic targets that were already known before cancer genomes were mapped. This is mainly due to the fact that our ability to interpret and translate these complex data sets from bench to bedside is hampered by the vast amount of information generated by global sequencing studies (Edwards et al. 2011).

Clinical and experimental studies of the last decades provide compelling evidence that extensive global reprogramming of epigenetic profiles is as important as genetic mutations during neoplastic transformation and malignant progression. Originally, epigenetics was defined as heritable traits that are not linked to changes in the DNA sequence. Nowadays, the term epigenetics is used to describe the mechanisms by which DNA methylation as well as chromatin-associated proteins and their posttranslational modifications regulate gene transcription. Cell-type-specific epigenetic patterning is essential for the establishment and maintenance of cellular integrity during development and tissue homeostasis, and its deregulation has been reported for all human malignancies (Berdasco and Esteller 2010; Baylin and Jones 2011). The most extensively studied epigenetic marker is DNA methylation, and together with posttranslational histone modifications affecting chromatin remodeling and specific miRNA expression signatures, it defines the epigenetic landscape of human cancers, including HNSCC (Kostareli et al. 2012; Koffler et al. 2014; Le et al. 2014; van Kempen et al. 2014; Anayannis et al. 2015). It is well documented that all of the major classes of cancer-causing agents including viruses elicit alterations in epigenetic patterning (Minarovits et al. 2016). This is of particular clinical relevance as many epigenetic modifications persist or increase during disease progression, and assessment of cancer-related profiles provides a valuable tool to gain important diagnostic or prognostic information for therapeutic decision-making and clinical management of HNSCC patients (Koffler et al. 2014; van Kempen et al. 2014). Moreover, the dynamic and reversible nature of epigenetic reprogramming makes key nodes of its regulatory circuits bona fide drug targets for precision medicine (Azad et al. 2013).

2 HPV-Related Alterations in DNA Methylation

DNA methylation is a physiologic epigenetic modification, which occurs primarily on the addition of a methyl group to a CpG dinucleotide in the DNA sequence. CpGs are asymmetrically distributed into poor and dense regions (CpG islands). CpG islands are predominantly located in the promoter regions or first exon of approximately half of all genes (Jones and Baylin 2002). DNA methylation is catalyzed by the enzymatic activity of DNA methyltransferases (DNMTs) of which three variants have been identified in humans: DNMT1, DNMT3A, and DNMT3B (Subramaniam et al. 2014). Aberrant DNA methylation is a hallmark of all human malignancies, including HNSCC, and distinct profiles have been attributed to environmental factors, patient habits (e.g., tobacco and alcohol consumption), and viral infection (Kostareli et al. 2012; van Kempen et al. 2014; Minarovits et al. 2016). The cancer methylome displays a characteristic loss of global DNA methylation in repetitive regions and concomitant accumulation of gene promoter methylation. Although the underlying molecular principles and effect of global DNA hypo-methylation remain elusive, it is thought to contribute to chromosomal instability and activation of proto-oncogene expression (Robertson 2005; Jones and Baylin 2007). It is worth noting that several studies reported a HPV-related difference in hypo-methylation of repetitive LINE-1 elements, indicating a more efficient maintenance of global DNA methylation accompanied by reduced genetic instability in HPV-positive HNSCC (Richards et al. 2009; Poage et al. 2011; Sartor et al. 2011). This assumption is supported by recent studies addressing the quality and quantity of genomic aberrations in HPV-positive and HPV-negative HNSCCs (Klussmann et al. 2009; Wilting et al. 2009; Agrawal et al. 2011; Stransky et al. 2011).

2.1 HPV and Gene Promoter Hyper-Methylation

Gene promoter hyper-methylation often causes reduced transcription of tumor suppressor genes involved in cellular processes of DNA damage repair, detoxification, cell cycle regulation, and apoptosis (Rodriguez-Paredes and Esteller 2011). In cancer, transcriptional silencing by gene promoter methylation may occur even more frequently than structural inactivation of genes by deletion or somatic mutation (Rodriguez-Paredes and Esteller 2011; Azad et al. 2013). Numerous studies have explored HPV-related differences in the profile of gene promoter methylation; however, many reports evaluated only a limited number of selected genes and did not focus solely on OPSCC, which is the most common site for HPV-related tumors in the upper aerodigestive tract (Kostareli et al. 2012; van Kempen et al. 2014). More recent studies focused on global analysis of gene promoter methylation in HPV-positive versus HPV-negative HNSCCs with the aim of gaining a detailed view of clinically relevant alterations and unraveling affected signaling and gene regulatory networks (Koffler et al. 2014). Collectively, these studies reported a trend toward a higher level of gene promoter hyper-methylation in HPV-positive tumors (Sartor et al. 2011; Colacino et al. 2013; Lechner et al. 2013; Lleras et al. 2013). The widespread gain of gene promoter methylation raises the question whether HPV-positive HNSCC resembles a CpG island methylator phenotype (CIMP), which was originally discovered in colorectal cancer (Hughes et al. 2013; Suzuki et al. 2014). Combinatorial ectopic expression of the viral oncogenes E6 and E7 in an HPV-negative cell line partially phenocopied the CIMP signature seen in HPV-positive tumors and established E6 as the main viral effector gene (Lechner et al. 2013). It is worth noting that HPV-related tumors with CIMP had a poor clinical outcome with significantly shorter survival (Lechner et al. 2013). An association of CIMP and poor prognosis was also reported for patients with oral cancer, though CIMP was not an independent factor in predicting prognosis (Jithesh et al. 2013).

2.2 Functional Interaction of Viral Proteins with DNMTs

One molecular mode of action by which HPV might alter profiles of gene promoter methylation is due to direct targeting the expression and enzymatic activity of DNMTs by viral oncoproteins (Minarovits et al. 2016). Increased expression of DNMT1 and DNMT3A was evident in HPV-positive tumor cell lines and primary OPSCCs (Sartor et al. 2011; Lechner et al. 2013; Schlecht et al. 2015). Additionally, viral oncoproteins stimulate DNMT activity in vitro and tumor cell lines, which is at least in part due to a direct physical interaction of E7 and DNMT1 (Burgers et al. 2007; Laurson et al. 2010; D'Costa et al. 2012). Chromatin immunoprecipitation assays further confirmed E7-DNMT1 complex formation at the CCNA1 promoter serving as a model for HPV-related gene promoter methylation (Chalertpet et al. 2015).

2.3 HPV-Related Gene Promoter Methylation Patterns and Signaling Pathways

Distinct HPV-related methylation patterns extrapolated from global gene promoter methylation profiling provide a valuable molecular tool for diagnostic and prognostic assessment of HNSCC patients (Colacino et al. 2013; Kostareli et al. 2013). But, they also facilitate an integrative data analysis to infer clinically relevant differences in signaling and gene regulatory networks taking into account the HPV status (Koffler et al. 2014). This knowledge could pave the way to identify promising new drug targets for a more specific and individualized therapy of HNSCC patients.

As an example, functional annotation of a gene panel with HPV-related promoter methylation indicated differential activity of WNT/β-catenin signaling, PPAR regulation, retinoic acid signaling, c-KIT signaling, and cell–cell or cell–matrix adhesion (Worsham et al. 2013). Differences in retinoic acid metabolism and signaling due to gene promoter methylation and based on the HPV status of OPSCC were also suggested by Kostareli and colleagues (Kostareli et al. 2013). In another study, gene-set enrichment analysis identified several targets of polycomb repressive complex 2 (PRC2) that were affected by HPV-related gene promoter methylation, including multiple members of the cadherin superfamily such as CDH8, CDH15, PCDH8, PCDH9, PCDH10, and PCDHB3 (Lechner et al. 2013). Finally, Fertig and colleagues applied integrative data analysis based on DNA methylation and gene expression patterns to infer biologically significant molecular pathways that may be exploited as therapeutic targets (Fertig et al. 2013). This approach revealed specific gene promoter methylation patterns that regulate gene expression in HPV-negative HNSCC and distinguish it from HPV-positive HNSCC. Analysis of these differentially regulated genes indicated that activation of the Hedgehog pathway was specific for HPV-negative HNSCC, which was confirmed by increased levels of GLI1, the primary Hedgehog target, in HNSCC compared to normal mucosa with the highest GLI1 expression in HPV-negative tumors.

3 HPV-Related Alterations in Chromatin Architecture

Epigenetic regulation of gene expression requires a complex interplay between DNA methylation, histone modifications, and nucleosome remodeling. The most commonly studied covalent modifications of histones are posttranslational acetylation, deacetylation, and methylation at the amino-terminal ends, and key enzymes are histone acetyltransferases (HAT), histone deacetylases (HDAC), and histone methyltransferases (HMT). Moreover, large complexes of nucleosome remodeling factors regulate gene expression by modulation of the chromatin architecture.

Despite compelling evidence that cancer-associated chromatin states are of clinical relevance, our knowledge on HPV-related alterations in histone modification and nucleosome remodeling as well as their functional interaction with DNA methylation profiles remains largely elusive. A recent study on global DNA methylation profiles of HPV-positive and HPV-negative HNSCCs suggested that HPV modulates the cancer epigenome through hyper-methylation of PRC2 target genes, which are implicated in tumor progression and metastasis (Lechner et al. 2013). Sartor and colleagues also reported a distinct promoter hyper-methylation of PRC2 target genes in HPV-positive as compared to HPV-negative HNSCC cell lines (Sartor et al. 2011). PRC2 maintains the transcriptional repression of a large number of genes with key regulatory roles in development and differentiation, and PRC2 proteins are required for normal embryonic development and exhibit a well-established role in stem-cell maintenance (Conway et al. 2015). It is worth noting that cancer-specific promoter hyper-methylation is more likely for PRC2 targets than non-targets (Ohm et al. 2007; Schlesinger et al. 2007).

The enzyme enhancer of zeste homolog 2 (EZH2) is the catalytic component of PRC2 and acts as an HMT at H3K27, resulting in gene silencing via chromatin condensation. Dysregulation of the repressive H3K27 trimethylation (H3K27me3) mark in HNSCC contributes to aberrant squamous differentiation (Gannon et al. 2013), and $p16^{INK4A}$-positive OPSCCs display global elevations of H3K27me3 patterns (Biron et al. 2012). Collectively, these data strongly suggest that viral oncoproteins induce epigenetic regulation of PRC2 target genes during HNSCC pathogenesis by altered expression or activity of HMTs and thereby modulate the chromatin architecture at corresponding gene promoters. Indeed, EZH2 is activated at the transcriptional level in HPV-positive cervical cancer cells by E7-mediated release of E2F from pocket proteins (Holland et al. 2008). In a more recent study, Sharma and colleagues also demonstrated a functional interplay between E7 and HOTAIR, a long noncoding RNA that recruits PRC2 to target gene promoters (Sharma et al. 2015).

4 Conclusion and Perspectives

An increasing body of experimental studies has provided compelling evidence that viral oncoproteins of HPV16 interact with key components of the cellular epigenetic machinery to reprogram the gene expression pattern and thereby alter cellular traits of the infected host cell. Monitoring HPV-related disruption of the epigenetic program represents a powerful tool for diagnosis, prognosis, and treatment decision-making, and due to its reversible nature serves as a bona fide target for a more effective and less toxic treatment of HNSCC patients with HPV-positive tumors. Epigenetic-based therapies for cancer treatment have been approved, and additional inhibitors for key regulators of DNA methylation, histone modification, and chromosome remodeling have shown promise in preclinical trials. Although the biology of epigenetic regulation is complex and our knowledge on the underlying regulatory circuits is incomplete, this new generation of more specific and potent inhibitors will hopefully be available for clinical use in the coming years (Cai et al. 2015). Another promising option for epigenetic-based therapy is its combination with already established or novel treatment regimens. As an example, demethylating drugs improve the efficacy of therapeutic viral DNA vaccines in a variety of HPV-associated malignancies (Lu et al. 2009). However, the lack of reliable molecular biomarkers to predict either clinical activity or resistance of epigenetic-based therapy is a serious problem limiting the translation from bench to bedside (Helin and Dhanak 2013).

References

Agrawal N, Frederick MJ, Pickering CR, Bettegowda C, Chang K, Li RJ, Fakhry C, Xie TX, Zhang J, Wang J, Zhang N, El-Naggar AK, Jasser SA, Weinstein JN, Trevino L, Drummond JA, Muzny DM, Wu Y, Wood LD, Hruban RH, Westra WH, Koch WM, Califano JA, Gibbs RA, Sidransky D, Vogelstein B, Velculescu VE, Papadopoulos N, Wheeler DA, Kinzler KW, Myers JN (2011) Exome sequencing of head and neck squamous cell carcinoma reveals inactivating mutations in NOTCH1. Science 333(6046):1154–1157

Anayannis NV, Schlecht NF, Belbin TJ (2015) Epigenetic mechanisms of human papillomavirus-associated head and neck cancer. Arch Pathol Lab Med 139(11):1373–1378

Ang KK, Harris J, Wheeler R, Weber R, Rosenthal DI, Nguyen-Tan PF, Westra WH, Chung CH, Jordan RC, Lu C, Kim H, Axelrod R, Silverman CC, Redmond KP, Gillison ML (2010) Human papillomavirus and survival of patients with oropharyngeal cancer. N Engl J Med 363 (1):24–35

Azad N, Zahnow CA, Rudin CM, Baylin SB (2013) The future of epigenetic therapy in solid tumours–lessons from the past. Nat Rev Clin Oncol 10(5):256–266

Baylin SB, Jones PA (2011) A decade of exploring the cancer epigenome - biological and translational implications. Nat Rev Cancer 11(10):726–734

Berdasco M, Esteller M (2010) Aberrant epigenetic landscape in cancer: how cellular identity goes awry. Dev Cell 19(5):698–711

Biron VL, Mohamed A, Hendzel MJ, Alan Underhill D, Seikaly H (2012) Epigenetic differences between human papillomavirus-positive and -negative oropharyngeal squamous cell carcinomas. J Otolaryngol Head Neck Surg 41(Suppl 1):S65–S70

Burgers WA, Blanchon L, Pradhan S, de Launoit Y, Kouzarides T, Fuks F (2007) Viral oncoproteins target the DNA methyltransferases. Oncogene 26(11):1650–1655

Cai SF, Chen CW, Armstrong SA (2015) Drugging chromatin in cancer: recent advances and novel approaches. Mol Cell 60(4):561–570

Chalertpet K, Pakdeechaidan W, Patel V, Mutirangura A, Yanatatsaneejit P (2015) Human papillomavirus type 16 E7 oncoprotein mediates CCNA1 promoter methylation. Cancer Sci 106(10):1333–1340

Chaturvedi AK, Engels EA, Pfeiffer RM, Hernandez BY, Xiao W, Kim E, Jiang B, Goodman MT, Sibug-Saber M, Cozen W, Liu L, Lynch CF, Wentzensen N, Jordan RC, Altekruse S, Anderson WF, Rosenberg PS, Gillison ML (2011) Human papillomavirus and rising oropharyngeal cancer incidence in the United States. J Clin Oncol 29(32):4294–4301

Colacino JA, Dolinoy DC, Duffy SA, Sartor MA, Chepeha DB, Bradford CR, McHugh JB, Patel DA, Virani S, Walline HM, Bellile E, Terrell JE, Stoerker JA, Taylor JM, Carey TE, Wolf GT, Rozek LS (2013) Comprehensive analysis of DNA methylation in head and neck squamous cell carcinoma indicates differences by survival and clinicopathologic characteristics. PLoS ONE 8(1):e54742

Conway E, Healy E, Bracken AP (2015) PRC2 mediated H3K27 methylations in cellular identity and cancer. Curr Opin Cell Biol 37:42–48

D'Costa ZJ, Jolly C, Androphy EJ, Mercer A, Matthews CM, Hibma MH (2012) Transcriptional repression of E-cadherin by human papillomavirus type 16 E6. PLoS ONE 7(11):e48954

Edwards AM, Isserlin R, Bader GD, Frye SV, Willson TM, Yu FH (2011) Too many roads not taken. Nature 470(7333):163–165

Fakhry C, Zhang Q, Nguyen-Tan PF, Rosenthal D, El-Naggar A, Garden AS, Soulieres D, Trotti A, Avizonis V, Ridge JA, Harris J, Le QT, Gillison M (2014) Human papillomavirus and overall survival after progression of oropharyngeal squamous cell carcinoma. J Clin Oncol 32 (30):3365–3373

Fertig EJ, Markovic A, Danilova LV, Gaykalova DA, Cope L, Chung CH, Ochs MF, Califano JA (2013) Preferential activation of the hedgehog pathway by epigenetic modulations in HPV negative HNSCC identified with meta-pathway analysis. PLoS ONE 8(11):e78127

Gannon OM, Merida de Long L, Endo-Munoz L, Hazar-Rethinam M, Saunders NA (2013) Dysregulation of the repressive H3K27 trimethylation mark in head and neck squamous cell carcinoma contributes to dysregulated squamous differentiation. Clin Cancer Res 19(2):428–441

Gillison ML, Chaturvedi AK, Anderson WF, Fakhry C (2015) Epidemiology of human papillomavirus-positive head and neck squamous cell carcinoma. J Clin Oncol 33 (29):3235–3242

Hayes DN, Van Waes C, Seiwert TY (2015) Genetic landscape of human papillomavirus-associated head and neck cancer and comparison to tobacco-related tumors. J Clin Oncol 33(29):3227–3234

Helin K, Dhanak D (2013) Chromatin proteins and modifications as drug targets. Nature 502 (7472):480–488

Holland D, Hoppe-Seyler K, Schuller B, Lohrey C, Maroldt J, Durst M, Hoppe-Seyler F (2008) Activation of the enhancer of zeste homologue 2 gene by the human papillomavirus E7 oncoprotein. Cancer Res 68(23):9964–9972

Hughes LA, Melotte V, de Schrijver J, de Maat M, Smit VT, Bovee JV, French PJ, van den Brandt PA, Schouten LJ, de Meyer T, van Criekinge W, Ahuja N, Herman JG, Weijenberg MP, van Engeland M (2013) The CpG island methylator phenotype: what's in a name? Cancer Res 73(19):5858–5868

Jithesh PV, Risk JM, Schache AG, Dhanda J, Lane B, Liloglou T, Shaw RJ (2013) The epigenetic landscape of oral squamous cell carcinoma. Br J Cancer 108(2):370–379

Jones PA, Baylin SB (2002) The fundamental role of epigenetic events in cancer. Nat Rev Genet 3 (6):415–428

Jones PA, Baylin SB (2007) The epigenomics of cancer. Cell 128(4):683–692

Kang H, Kiess A, Chung CH (2015) Emerging biomarkers in head and neck cancer in the era of genomics. Nat Rev Clin Oncol 12(1):11–26

Klussmann JP, Mooren JJ, Lehnen M, Claessen SM, Stenner M, Huebbers CU, Weissenborn SJ, Wedemeyer I, Preuss SF, Straetmans JM, Manni JJ, Hopman AH, Speel EJ (2009) Genetic signatures of HPV-related and unrelated oropharyngeal carcinoma and their prognostic implications. Clin Cancer Res 15(5):1779–1786

Koffler J, Sharma S, Hess J (2014) Predictive value of epigenetic alterations in head and neck squamous cell carcinoma. Mol Cell Oncol 1(2):e954827

Kostareli E, Holzinger D, Bogatyrova O, Hielscher T, Wichmann G, Keck M, Lahrmann B, Grabe N, Flechtenmacher C, Schmidt CR, Seiwert T, Dyckhoff G, Dietz A, Hofler D, Pawlita M, Benner A, Bosch FX, Plinkert P, Plass C, Weichenhan D, Hess J (2013) HPV-related methylation signature predicts survival in oropharyngeal squamous cell carcinomas. J Clin Invest 123(6):2488–2501

Kostareli E, Holzinger D, Hess J (2012) New concepts for translational head and neck oncology: lessons from HPV-related oropharyngeal squamous cell carcinomas. Front Head Neck Cancer 2:1–10

Laurson J, Khan S, Chung R, Cross K, Raj K (2010) Epigenetic repression of E-cadherin by human papillomavirus 16 E7 protein. Carcinogenesis 31(5):918–926

Le JM, Squarize CH, Castilho RM (2014) Histone modifications: targeting head and neck cancer stem cells. World J Stem Cells 6(5):511–525

Lechner M, Fenton T, West J, Wilson G, Feber A, Henderson S, Thirlwell C, Dibra HK, Jay A, Butcher L, Chakravarthy AR, Gratrix F, Patel N, Vaz F, O'Flynn P, Kalavrezos N, Teschendorff AE, Boshoff C, Beck S (2013) Identification and functional validation of HPV-mediated hypermethylation in head and neck squamous cell carcinoma. Genome Med 5 (2):15

Lleras RA, Smith RV, Adrien LR, Schlecht NF, Burk RD, Harris TM, Childs G, Prystowsky MB, Belbin TJ (2013) Unique DNA methylation loci distinguish anatomic site and HPV status in head and neck squamous cell carcinoma. Clin Cancer Res 19(19):5444–5455

Lu D, Hoory T, Monie A, Wu A, Wang MC, Hung CF (2009) Treatment with demethylating agent, 5-aza-2'-deoxycytidine enhances therapeutic HPV DNA vaccine potency. Vaccine 27 (32):4363–4369

Mehanna H, Beech T, Nicholson T, El-Hariry I, McConkey C, Paleri V, Roberts S (2013) Prevalence of human papillomavirus in oropharyngeal and nonoropharyngeal head and neck cancer–systematic review and meta-analysis of trends by time and region. Head Neck 35 (5):747–755

Minarovits J, Demcsak A, Banati F, Niller HH (2016) Epigenetic dysregulation in virus-associated neoplasms. Adv Exp Med Biol 879:71–90

Ndiaye C, Mena M, Alemany L, Arbyn M, Castellsague X, Laporte L, Bosch FX, de Sanjose S, Trottier H (2014) HPV DNA, E6/E7 mRNA, and p16INK4a detection in head and neck cancers: a systematic review and meta-analysis. Lancet Oncol 15(12):1319–1331

Network CGA (2015) Comprehensive genomic characterization of head and neck squamous cell carcinomas. Nature 517(7536):576–582

Ohm JE, McGarvey KM, Yu X, Cheng L, Schuebel KE, Cope L, Mohammad HP, Chen W, Daniel VC, Yu W, Berman DM, Jenuwein T, Pruitt K, Sharkis SJ, Watkins DN, Herman JG, Baylin SB (2007) A stem cell-like chromatin pattern may predispose tumor suppressor genes to DNA hypermethylation and heritable silencing. Nat Genet 39(2):237–242

Poage GM, Houseman EA, Christensen BC, Butler RA, Avissar-Whiting M, McClean MD, Waterboer T, Pawlita M, Marsit CJ, Kelsey KT (2011) Global hypomethylation identifies Loci targeted for hypermethylation in head and neck cancer. Clin Cancer Res 17(11):3579–3589

Richards KL, Zhang B, Baggerly KA, Colella S, Lang JC, Schuller DE, Krahe R (2009) Genome-wide hypomethylation in head and neck cancer is more pronounced in HPV-negative tumors and is associated with genomic instability. PLoS ONE 4(3):e4941

Robertson KD (2005) DNA methylation and human disease. Nat Rev Genet 6(8):597–610

Rodriguez-Paredes M, Esteller M (2011) Cancer epigenetics reaches mainstream oncology. Nat Med 17(3):330–339

Sartor MA, Dolinoy DC, Jones TR, Colacino JA, Prince ME, Carey TE, Rozek LS (2011) Genome-wide methylation and expression differences in HPV(+) and HPV(-) squamous cell carcinoma cell lines are consistent with divergent mechanisms of carcinogenesis. Epigenetics 6 (6):777–787

Schlecht NF, Ben-Dayan M, Anayannis N, Lleras RA, Thomas C, Wang Y, Smith RV, Burk RD, Harris TM, Childs G, Ow TJ, Prystowsky MB, Belbin TJ (2015) Epigenetic changes in the CDKN2A locus are associated with differential expression of P16INK4A and P14ARF in HPV-positive oropharyngeal squamous cell carcinoma. Cancer Med 4(3):342–353

Schlesinger Y, Straussman R, Keshet I, Farkash S, Hecht M, Zimmerman J, Eden E, Yakhini Z, Ben-Shushan E, Reubinoff BE, Bergman Y, Simon I, Cedar H (2007) Polycomb-mediated methylation on Lys27 of histone H3 pre-marks genes for de novo methylation in cancer. Nat Genet 39(2):232–236

Sharma S, Mandal P, Sadhukhan T, Roy Chowdhury R, Ranjan Mondal N, Chakravarty B, Chatterjee T, Roy S, Sengupta S (2015) Bridging links between long noncoding RNA HOTAIR and HPV oncoprotein E7 in cervical cancer pathogenesis. Sci Rep 5:11724

Stransky N, Egloff AM, Tward AD, Kostic AD, Cibulskis K, Sivachenko A, Kryukov GV, Lawrence MS, Sougnez C, McKenna A, Shefler E, Ramos AH, Stojanov P, Carter SL, Voet D, Cortes ML, Auclair D, Berger MF, Saksena G, Guiducci C, Onofrio RC, Parkin M, Romkes M, Weissfeld JL, Seethala RR, Wang L, Rangel-Escareno C, Fernandez-Lopez JC, Hidalgo-Miranda A, Melendez-Zajgla J, Winckler W, Ardlie K, Gabriel SB, Meyerson M, Lander ES, Getz G, Golub TR, Garraway LA, Grandis JR (2011) The mutational landscape of head and neck squamous cell carcinoma. Science 333(6046):1157–1160

Subramaniam D, Thombre R, Dhar A, Anant S (2014) DNA methyltransferases: a novel target for prevention and therapy. Front Oncol 4:80

Suzuki H, Yamamoto E, Maruyama R, Niinuma T, Kai M (2014) Biological significance of the CpG island methylator phenotype. Biochem Biophys Res Commun 455(1–2):35–42 van Kempen PM, Noorlag R, Braunius WW, Stegeman I, Willems SM, Grolman W (2014) Differences in methylation profiles between HPV-positive and HPV-negative oropharynx squamous cell carcinoma: a systematic review. Epigenetics 9(2):194–203

Wilting SM, Smeets SJ, Snijders PJ, van Wieringen WN, van de Wiel MA, Meijer GA, Ylstra B, Leemans CR, Meijer CJ, Brakenhoff RH, Braakhuis BJ, Steenbergen RD (2009) Genomic profiling identifies common HPV-associated chromosomal alterations in squamous cell carcinomas of cervix and head and neck. BMC Med Genomics 2:32

Worsham MJ, Chen KM, Ghanem T, Stephen JK, Divine G (2013) Epigenetic modulation of signal transduction pathways in HPV-associated HNSCC. Otolaryngol Head Neck Surg 149 (3):409–416

Cancer Immunology and HPV

Barbara Wollenberg

Abstract

HNSCC is a heterogeneous group of tumors located in the oral cavity, oropharynx, hypopharynx and larynx. Originally, tobacco and alcohol exposures were the main risk factors for HNSCC. In the last two decades, HPV infections have been identified as a risk factor for HNSCC, especially for oropharyngeal tumors. Whereas the HPV-induced oropharyngeal carcinomas predominantly express the HPV16 related E6 and E7 oncoproteins, the HPV-negative HNSCC are associated with an overexpression of p53. However, if the therapy successes for HPV-negative and HPV-positive HNSCCs are compared, there are significantly higher total survival rates for HPV-positive oropharyngeal tumors compared to HPV-negative tumors. It is important to understand this phenomenon in order to improve and adapt therapy concepts.

Keywords

Immunology · Immune cell infiltration · Microenvironment · Immunotherapy

1 Cancer Immunology and HPV

HNSCC is a heterogeneous group of tumors located in the oral cavity, oropharynx, hypopharynx and larynx. Originally, tobacco and alcohol exposures were the main risk factors for HNSCC. In the last two decades, HPV infections have been identified as a risk factor for HNSCC, especially for oropharyngeal tumors, with the

B. Wollenberg (✉)
Department of Otorhinolaryngology, University of Schleswig-Holstein Campus Lübeck, Ratzeburger Allee 160, 23538 Lübeck, Germany
e-mail: Barbara.Wollenberg@uksh.de

W. Golusiński et al. (eds.), *HPV Infection in Head and Neck Cancer*,
Recent Results in Cancer Research 206, DOI 10.1007/978-3-319-43580-0_19

tonsil area being the most commonly affected area with 45–70 % HPV-positive cases (Mellin et al. 2002; Ritta et al. 2013).

More than 180 papilloma viruses have been identified to date, with approximately 120 genotypes isolated from humans. Whereas the HPV-induced oropharyngeal carcinomas predominantly express the HPV16 related E6 and E7 oncoproteins, the HPV-negative HNSCC are associated with an overexpression of p53 (Bernard et al. 2010).

However, if the therapy successes for HPV-negative and HPV-positive HNSCCs are compared, there are significantly higher total survival rates for HPV-positive oropharyngeal tumors compared to HPV-negative tumors (Gillison 2008; Ragin and Taioli 2007). It is important to understand this phenomenon in order to improve and adapt therapy concepts.

2 Immune Cell Infiltrations

Human solid tumor tissues are known to be infiltrated by various kinds of immune cells which are modulated within the tumor microenvironment (Hartmann et al. 2003; Heimdal et al. 2000; Pries and Wollenberg 2006; Veltri et al. 1986).

Several HPV-related immunologic features have been described in HNSCC.

In general, HPV-positive tumors have been shown to possess characteristic immune cell infiltrates compared to HPV-negative HNSCC. Recently, Partlova et al. 2015 have shown that HPV-positive tumors were infiltrated by significantly higher numbers of IFNgC CD8C T lymphocytes, IL-17C CD8C T lymphocytes, myeloid dendritic cells and proinflammatory chemokines. Furthermore, HPV-positive tumors had significantly lower expression of COX2 mRNA and higher expression of PD1 mRNA (Partlova et al.).

Spanos et al. 2009 have shown, for human and murine HPV-transformed cell lines, that neither radiation nor cisplatin therapy cured immune-incompetent mice, whereas in vivo, HPV-positive tumors were more sensitive to radiation and cisplatin treatment. Surprisingly, adoptive transfer of wild-type immune cells into immune-incompetent mice restored HPV-positive tumor clearance with cisplatin therapy. These data suggest that HPV-positive tumors are not more curable because of an increased epithelial sensitivity to cisplatin or radiation therapy, but because of an HPV-related immunity (Spanos et al. 2009).

These implications of a HPV-related immunity were corroborated by a study with an unselected group of 50 patients with HNSCC, where T lymphocytes were isolated from tumors and lymph nodes. Comprehensive investigations of the HPV16-specific T cell responses revealed a broad repertoire of CD41 T helper type 1 and type 2 cells, CD41 regulatory T cells and CD81 T cells reactive to HPV16. Heusinkveld et al. identified circulating HPV16-specific T cells in 63.6 % of the HPV-positive HNSCC, but only in 24.1 % of the HPV-negative HNSCC (Heusinkveld et al. 2012).

Similarly, Albers et al. found increased levels of T cells toward HPV16 E7 in HPV-positive HNSCC patients (Albers et al. 2005).

The local presence of HPV16-specific T cell immunity in HPV16-induced HNSCC was underlined by an additional study, which demonstrated increased infiltrations of CD3+ and FoxP3+ T cells in correlation with higher HPV16 copy numbers in solid HNSCC (Ritta et al. 2013).

Correspondingly, it has been shown that targeting CD137, which is an inducible receptor on activated T lymphocytes, synergizes with cisplatin and radiation therapy in HPV-positive HNSCC (Lucido et al. 2014).

Furthermore, increased amounts of effector memory and effector T cells were found in patients with human HPV-positive oropharyngeal squamous cell carcinomas, suggesting a virus-induced T cell activation (Turksma et al. 2013).

In addition, increased numbers of different types of antigen presenting cells such as myeloid dendritic cells (mDC), plasmacytoid dendritic cells (pDC), macrophages and monocytes have been found in HPV-associated HNSCC (Levovitz et al.). Comprehensive immune profiling using qRT-PCR and immunohistochemistry identified a significantly increased infiltration of HPV-positive HNSCC by CD20 + B cells, as well as by invasive margin FoxP3+ Treg (Russell et al. 2013).

Similar findings have recently been demonstrated for HPV-related cervical cancers, where the HPV infection was associated with macrophage differentiation, a compromised cellular immune response, an abnormal imbalance between type 1 T–helper cells (Th1) and Th2 cells, regulatory T cell infiltration, and downregulated DC activation and maturation (Song et al. 2015).

3 Microenvironment Modulation

All these different types of immune cells are known to release numerous cytokines and inflammatory mediators with proangiogenic and prometastatic effects, and the potential to drive tumor progression.

For example, IL-1 is produced by monocytes, macrophages, dendritic cells and various other cells, and in HNSCC IL-1α and IL-1β have also been demonstrated to modestly induce the production of gelatines, which are family members of the matrix metalloproteinases (MMPs) and contribute to tumor invasion and metastasis (Mann et al. 1995).

IL-1α was furthermore identified to promote the transcriptional activator NF-κB which is known to participate in various aspects of cancer induction and maintenance (Wolf et al. 2001).

TGFβ is known to inhibit the proliferation and function of T and B lymphocytes as well as the function of macrophages (Chen et al. 1999; Mann et al. 1992).

Levovitz et al. (2014) have shown an overexpression of TGFßR1 in HPV-related oropharyngeal cancer and cervical cancer, which implicates TGFβR1/TGFβ signaling in the development of both cancer types (Levovitz et al. 2014).

In addition, HNSCC cell lines have recently been demonstrated to express IL-18 which is a proinflammatory cytokine that plays an important role in NK cell activation and Th1 cell response (Martone et al. 2004).

For HPV-positive tumors, the critical parameter to escape from efficient immune responses is the interference of HPV with the expression of interferons (IFNs), which are produced by virus-infected cells and reveal immuno-stimulatory properties. Furthermore, HPV interacts with antigen presentation to reduce adaptive immune responses and to downregulate HLA class I (Ferris 2015).

Thus, the cancer immunology has a huge impact on the tumor progression and its therapy response, and has to be distinguished between HPV-positive and HPV-negative HNSCCs.

In addition to the mentioned HPV-specific T cell profiles, the Warburg phenomenon has been discussed concerning its effect on antitumoral immune responses, since the accumulation of tumor-derived lactate inhibits cytotoxic T cells. An immunohistochemical analysis of oropharyngeal carcinomas showed an enhanced antitumoral immune response (CD8/CD4 ratio) together with increased levels of proteins involved in transmembranous metabolite transportation (GLUT1 and CD147) and respiratory metabolism (COX5B) in HPV-positive HNSCC (Krupar et al. 2014).

Concerning the incurrence of HPV-related HNSCC, several publications discussed HPV-specific humoral immune responses. Indeed, the presence of antibodies to HPV proteins E6 and/or E7 has been shown to be associated with a significant increased risk for oropharyngeal cancer. Antibodies to HPV16 have been detected in some patients more than 15 years before their cancer diagnosis (Gillison et al. 2012).

4 Immunotherapeutic Approaches

Generally, immune therapy provides active and passive as well as specific and unspecific forms of antitumoral activity. The currently closest approach to clinical application is different HPV-related vaccination approaches. Several approaches are under development in HNSCC, using specific peptide vaccines such as melanoma antigen A3/HPV-16 peptide (NCT00257738), HPV-16 E7 *Listeria* vaccine (Sewell et al. 2004) or vaccinia-based E6/E7 vaccine (Davidson et al. 2004).

Furthermore, adoptive T cell transfer is currently evaluated for HNSCC immunotherapy, where T cells are first removed from the patient before they get reintroduced after specific modifications in order to enhance their activity against HPV-associated head and neck cancer (NCT01585428) (Ferris 2015).

In summary, the current state of knowledge suggests that the presence of HPV may induce an increased immune response and may be responsible for a more favorable prognosis of HPV-positive HNSCC.

References

Albers A, Abe K, Hunt J, Wang J, Lopez-Albaitero A, Schaefer C, Gooding W, Whiteside TL, Ferrone S, DeLeo A, Ferris RL (2005) Antitumor activity of human papillomavirus type 16 E7-specific T cells against virally infected squamous cell carcinoma of the head and neck. Cancer Res 65:11146–11155

Bernard HU, Burk RD, Chen Z, van Doorslaer K, zur Hausen H, de Villiers EM (2010) Classification of papilloma viruses (PVs) based on 189 PV types and proposal of taxonomic amendments. Virology 401:70–79

Chen Z, Malhotra PS, Thomas GR, Ondrey FG, Duffey DC, Smith CW, Enamorado I, Yeh NT, Kroog GS, Rudy S, McCullagh L, Mousa S, Quezado M, Herscher LL, Van Waes C (1999) Expression of proinflammatory and proangiogenic cytokines in patients with head and neck cancer. Clin Cancer Res 5:1369–1379

Davidson EJ, Faulkner RL, Sehr P, Pawlita M, Smyth LJ, Burt DJ, Tomlinson AE, Hickling J, Kitchener HC, Stern PL (2004) Effect of TA-CIN (HPV 16 L2E6E7) booster immunisation in vulval intraepithelial neoplasia patients previously vaccinated with TA-HPV (vaccinia virus encoding HPV 16/18 E6E7). Vaccine 22:2722–2729

Ferris RL (2015) Immunology and Immunotherapy of head and neck cancer. J Clin Oncol 33:3293–3304

Gillison ML (2008) Human papillomavirus-related diseases: oropharynx cancers and potential implications for adolescent HPV vaccination. J Adolesc Health 43:S52–S60

Gillison ML, Alemany L, Snijders PJ, Chaturvedi A, Steinberg BM, Schwartz S, Castellsague X (2012) Human papillomavirus and diseases of the upper airway: head and neck cancer and respiratory papillomatosis. Vaccine 30(5):F34–F54

Hartmann E, Wollenberg B, Rothenfusser S, Wagner M, Wellisch D, Mack B, Giese T, Gires O, Endres S, Hartmann G (2003) Identification and functional analysis of tumor-infiltrating plasmacytoid dendritic cells in head and neck cancer. Cancer Res 63:6478–6487

Heimdal JH, Aarstad HJ, Olofsson J (2000) Peripheral blood T-lymphocyte and monocyte function and survival in patients with head and neck carcinoma. Laryngoscope 110:402–407

Heusinkveld M, Goedemans R, Briet RJ, Gelderblom H, Nortier JW, Gorter A, Smit VT, Langeveld AP, Jansen JC, van der Burg SH (2012) Systemic and local human papillomavirus 16-specific T-cell immunity in patients with head and neck cancer. Int J Cancer 131:E74–E85

Krupar R, Robold K, Gaag D, Spanier G, Kreutz M, Renner K, Hellerbrand C, Hofstaedter F, Bosserhoff AK (2014) Immunologic and metabolic characteristics of HPV-negative and HPV-positive head and neck squamous cell carcinomas are strikingly different. Virchows Arch 465:299–312

Levovitz C, Chen D, Ivansson E, Gyllensten U, Finnigan JP, Alshawish S, Zhang W, Schadt EE, Posner MR, Genden EM, Boffetta P, Sikora AG (2014) TGFbeta receptor 1: an immune susceptibility gene in HPV-associated cancer. Cancer Res 74:6833–6844

Lucido CT, Vermeer PD, Wieking BG, Vermeer DW, Lee JH (2014) CD137 enhancement of HPV positive head and neck squamous cell carcinoma tumor clearance. Vaccines (Basel) 2:841–853

Mann EA, Spiro JD, Chen LL, Kreutzer DL (1992) Cytokine expression by head and neck squamous cell carcinomas. Am J Surg 164:567–573

Mann EA, Hibbs MS, Spiro JD, Bowik C, Wang XZ, Clawson M, Chen LL (1995) Cytokine regulation of gelatinase production by head and neck squamous cell carcinoma: the role of tumor necrosis factor-alpha. Ann Otol Rhinol Laryngol 104:203–209

Martone T, Bellone G, Pagano M, Beatrice F, Palonta F, Emanuelli G, Cortesina G (2004) Constitutive expression of interleukin-18 in head and neck squamous carcinoma cells. Head Neck 26:494–503

Mellin H, Dahlgren L, Munck-Wikland E, Lindholm J, Rabbani H, Kalantari M, Dalianis T (2002) Human papillomavirus type 16 is episomal and a high viral load may be correlated to better prognosis in tonsillar cancer. Int J Cancer 102:152–158

Partlova S, Boucek J, Kloudova K, Lukesova E, Zabrodsky M, Grega M, Fucikova J, Truxova I, Tachezy R, Spisek R, Fialova A (2015) Distinct patterns of intratumoral immune cell infiltrates in patients with HPV-associated compared to non-virally induced head and neck squamous cell carcinoma. Oncoimmunology 4:e965570
Pries R, Wollenberg B (2006) Cytokines in head and neck cancer. Cytokine Growth Factor Rev 17:141–146
Ragin CC, Taioli E (2007) Survival of squamous cell carcinoma of the head and neck in relation to human papillomavirus infection: review and meta-analysis. Int J Cancer 121:1813–1820
Ritta M, Landolfo V, Mazibrada J, De Andrea M, Dell'Oste V, Caneparo V, Peretti A, Giordano C, Pecorari G, Garzaro M, Landolfo S (2013) Human papillomavirus tumor-infiltrating T-regulatory lymphocytes and P53 codon 72 polymorphisms correlate with clinical staging and prognosis of oropharyngeal cancer. New Microbiol 36:133–144
Russell S, Angell T, Lechner M, Liebertz D, Correa A, Sinha U, Kokot N, Epstein A (2013) Immune cell infiltration patterns and survival in head and neck squamous cell carcinoma. Head Neck Oncol 5:24
Sewell DA, Shahabi V, Gunn GR 3rd, Pan ZK, Dominiecki ME, Paterson Y (2004) Recombinant Listeria vaccines containing PEST sequences are potent immune adjuvants for the tumor-associated antigen human papillomavirus-16 E7. Cancer Res 64:8821–8825
Song D, Li H, Dai J (2015) Effect of human papillomavirus infection on the immune system and its role in the course of cervical cancer. Oncol Lett 10:600–606
Spanos WC, Nowicki P, Lee DW, Hoover A, Hostager B, Gupta A, Anderson ME, Lee JH (2009) Immune response during therapy with cisplatin or radiation for human papillomavirus-related head and neck cancer. Arch Otolaryngol Head Neck Surg 135:1137–1146
Turksma AW, Bontkes HJ, van den Heuvel H, de Gruijl TD, von Blomberg BM, Braakhuis BJ, Leemans CR, Bloemena E, Meijer CJ, Hooijberg E (2013) Effector memory T-cell frequencies in relation to tumour stage, location and HPV status in HNSCC patients. Oral Dis 19:577–584
Veltri RW, Rodman SM, Maxim PE, Baseler MW, Sprinkle PM (1986) Immune complexes, serum proteins, cell-mediated immunity, and immune regulation in patients with squamous cell carcinoma of the head and neck. Cancer 57:2295–2308
Wolf JS, Chen Z, Dong G, Sunwoo JB, Bancroft CC, Capo DE, Yeh NT, Mukaida N, Van Waes C (2001) IL (interleukin)-1alpha promotes nuclear factor-kappaB and AP-1-induced IL-8 expression, cell survival, and proliferation in head and neck squamous cell carcinomas. Clin Cancer Res 7:1812–1820

Part VI
HPV - Prevention Vaccination, Ongoing Trials

Update on De-intensification and Intensification Studies in HPV

Hisham Mehanna

Abstract

In this chapter, we discuss de-esclation of treatment for patients with HPV-positive disease. We discuss the rationale for de-escalation (why de-escalate?), patient selection criteria (who to de-esclate?) and what the treatment options for de-esclation are and the studies that are currently being run in those areas (how to de-escalate?). We stress the importance of clinicians NOT changing the management of oropharyngeal cancer patients outside clinical trials, and encourage them to recruit to the ongoing studies.

Keywords

De-escalation of HPV · Epidemiology of HPV · Head and neck cancer · Molecular biology of HPV · Testing of HPV · Treatment of HPV

As we have seen in previous chapters, the seminal paper by Ang et al. (2010) demonstrated that there were several prognostic groups within oropharyngeal cancer. This prognostic classifier has been validated in other cohorts. There are other prognostic classifiers that have also been developed that show similar findings with some variations. However, they consistently demonstrate that HPV-positive disease has better outcomes than HPV-negative disease (Huang et al. 2015). In addition, it would appear that HPV positivity maintains its prognostic effect regardless of the type of treatment (Haughey and Sinha 2012). As a consequence of

H. Mehanna (✉)
Chair of Head and Neck Surgery, School of Cancer Sciences,
University of Birmingham, Birmingham, England, UK
e-mail: h.mehanna@bham.ac.uk

H. Mehanna
Institute of Head and Neck Studies and Education,
University of Birmingham, Birmingham, England, UK

W. Golusiński et al. (eds.), *HPV Infection in Head and Neck Cancer*,
Recent Results in Cancer Research 206, DOI 10.1007/978-3-319-43580-0_20

the improved prognosis of HPV-positive patients, many clinicians and researchers around the world have considered and are considering de-intensification of treatment for HPV-positive disease. There are several studies that have been completed or are being currently run for this indication. In this article, we will discuss the following aspects:

- Why should we de-intensify treatment?
- Who should we de-intensify treatment for?
- How should we de-intensify treatment?

1 Why Should We De-intensify Treatment?

As can be seen from the prognostic classifiers, the low-risk HPV-positive patients have excellent survival. These patients tend to be younger than the traditional head and neck cancer patient. This means that as they have a higher chance of cure, they will live longer with the substantial effects of treatment. Indeed, we know that chemoradiotherapy results in considerable early and late toxicities (Trotti et al. 2007), and that late toxicity is cumulative (Machtay et al. 2008). Therefore, it would seem reasonable to try to reduce the toxicity profile in these patients who have excellent long-term survival to improve their overall quality of life and reduce the long-term burden of treatment.

In addition, it would appear that patients are supportive of de-intensification of chemoradiotherapy regimens for HPV-positive low-risk disease. However, the majority of them are supportive only if there is little or no chance of detriment to their overall survival. Furthermore, it should be noted that over a quarter do not want de-intensification. In addition, the majority of those who are in favour of de-intensification would reduce the chemotherapy part of the treatment, and only 20 % would wish to reduce radiotherapy (Brotherston et al. 2013).

2 Who Should We De-intensify Treatment for?

The overall principle guiding treatment is *primum non nocere—first do no harm.* These patients have excellent survival, and are in the main, cured of their disease. Many studies, including the one quoted above by Brotherstone, show that patients' most important aim for treatment is cure followed by prolonged survival. Therefore, in all our discussions on de-intensification the maintenance of the very high cure rates for patients should be paramount.

When considering what the causes of treatment failure are in patients with high-risk disease, one identifies that they most often fail locoregionally. This was apparent in the RTOG 0129 study by Ang et al. (2010). In that study, distant metastatic failure did not differ significantly between HPV-positive and HPV-negative disease. Other studies e.g. by O'Sullivan et al. (2013) have shown that HPV-positive disease and HPV-negative disease have similar distant control rates. Work by the same group in Toronto has shown that the risk of distant metastasis in HPV-positive patients is highest in those who were treated with radiotherapy alone [with N2b disease and who are heavy smokers, or who have N2c or N3 disease]. Distant metastasis is also high in patients who have HPV-positive T4 disease. Therefore, we should be aware of de-intensifying treatment, especially by removing chemotherapy, in these patients who in the main constitute the intermediate HPV-positive risk category.

3 What Are the Options for De-intensification?

There are several options for de-intensification: using less toxic chemotherapy regimens, removing chemotherapy, reducing the radiotherapy dose, and incorporating surgery and reducing post-operative chemoradiotherapy regimens. Fortunately, there has been a strong emphasis on ensuring that these de-intensification options are tested within clinical trials, and that clinicians do **NOT** change the management of HPV-positive patients outside of clinical trials. In this next section, we will discuss the different options for de-intensification and the ongoing trials within that area.

3.1 Primary Non-Surgical Therapies

3.1.1 Less Toxic Chemoradiotherapy Regimens

Several trials have explored the use of biological therapies instead of chemotherapy to reduce the burden of toxicity. In particular, cetuximab has been found to be effective in head and neck cancer (Bonner et al. 2006) and more recently found to be particularly effective in HPV-positive patients (Rosenthal—look at most recent JCO publication). In addition, cetuximab is thought to have less toxicity than platinum-based regimens (Bonner et al. 2006). Three large trials are therefore exploring the use of cetuximab and radiotherapy compared to cisplatin and radiotherapy.

The RTOG 1016 study includes all HPV-positive patients (low risk and intermediate risk). The primary outcome is overall survival. It has recruited $\sim$1000 patients and is currently in follow-up and is due to report in 2019.

The De-ESCALaTE study, run by our group at InHANSE, has also very recently completed recruitment of 304 patients. The primary outcome is overall (acute and late) toxicity and cost-effectiveness. It is also due to report in 2019.

The TROG group also have a similar study aiming to recruit 200 patients. Its primary outcome is swallowing and is also looking at the weekly toxicity profile of both treatments. Both De-ESCALaTE and TROG studies limit eligibility to low-risk HPV-positive patients only.

3.1.2 Removal of Chemotherapy—(Radiotherapy Alone)

Based on data from Toronto, it was identified that the lowest risk HPV-positive patients were those who were non-smokers and did not have N3 or T4 disease. In those lowest risk patients, the addition of chemotherapy to radiotherapy did not seem to significantly increase overall survival benefit. This suggested that chemotherapy may be omitted completely in this very low-risk group of patients.

The NRG 002 study looks to recruit HPV-positive, non-smokers, but excludes T4 and N3 disease. It is randomising patients to chemoradiotherapy of 60 Gy in six weeks with weekly cisplatin of 40 mg/m^2 versus slightly accelerated radiotherapy of 60 Gy in five weeks with 6 fractions per week. This phase 2 trial is currently ongoing.

3.1.3 Reduction of Radiotherapy Dose

Incremental radiotherapy doses result in considerably higher overall toxicity. Therefore, by reducing the overall radiotherapy dose, a reduction in overall long-term toxicity may occur. Groups have hypothesised that by increasing chemotherapy, especially in an induction format, there may be a possibility of reducing the overall radiotherapy dose.

The ECOG 1308 (Cmelak et al. 2014), a phase II trial, recruited patients to three cycles of induction cisplatin, cetuximab and paclitaxel. Those patients who showed complete response were then given cetuximab and a reduced radiotherapy dose (54 Gy in 27 fractions). Those that did not show complete response were given cetuximab plus the standard radiotherapy dose of 69 Gy in 33 fractions. This study did not meet its own minimum threshold for overall two-year disease-free survival. However, patients who were deemed to have the best prognosis (T1 to T3 N1, to N1 N2b with less than 10 pack years of smoking) did very well, showing an overall two-year survival of 97 % despite having the low dose of radiotherapy. However, for the higher-risk patients who received full-dose intensity-modulated radiotherapy, the overall survival was 87 % and the 2-year progression-free survival was 65 %. The results suggest that the low-risk patients could be given less radiotherapy and still achieve excellent survival. Therefore, a phase III study, the Quarterback study, has been initiated. In this trial, patients are given induction TPF. Those who then achieve complete or partial response are randomised to either carboplatin plus standard radiotherapy of 70 Gy or to carboplatin plus reduced radiotherapy of 56 Gy. Patients who do not achieve partial or complete response receive 70 Gy of radiotherapy. This study is currently ongoing.

3.1.4 Post-operative Surgical Patients

In the surgically treated, post-operative patients, there is good evidence to suggest that adjuvant treatment post-operatively is highly protective (Haughey and Sinha 2012; Sinha et al. 2012). Additionally, some studies have shown that there may be no difference in overall survival between patients who receive post-operative radiotherapy alone and those who receive post-operative chemoradiotherapy. However, the numbers included in these subgroup analyses were very small and therefore highly prone to type 2 errors. Some studies have shown that extracapsular spread may not have as much significance in HPV-positive patients who are treated with post-operative adjuvant therapy as in HPV-negative patients. This is especially true for minimal extracapsular spread of <1 mm (Haughey and Sinha 2012; Sinha et al. 2012). However, these studies have yet to be validated prospectively in large studies. These data have been used to generate hypotheses regarding the reduction of radiotherapy or chemoradiotherapy doses post-operatively after transoral and transrobotic surgery.

The ECOG 1311 recruits HPV-positive patients who have had transoral robotic or transoral laser robotic surgery and who require post-operative radiotherapy or chemoradiotherapy. This study limits recruitment to HPV-positive patients with T1—T3, N1—N2b disease. Patients who are at low risk and require no adjuvant treatment are observed. Those patients who are high risk and have positive margins or extracapsular spread of >1 mm or 4 or more lymph nodes receive standard chemoradiotherapy. Those patients who have intermediate disease with clear margins, <1-mm extracapsular spread or 2–3 metastatic lymph nodes, perineural invasion or lymphovascular invasion are randomised to standard IMRT radiotherapy of 60 Gy in 30 fractions or reduced IMRT radiotherapy of 50 Gy in 25 fractions. The primary endpoint is 2-year progression-free survival. This study has now completed recruitment and is in follow-up.

The PATHOS trial run by the Cardiff Clinical Trials Unit in the UK has taken this a step further. They also randomise the high-risk patients to cisplatin plus radiotherapy (60 Gy in 30 fractions) or radiotherapy alone (60 Gy in 30 fractions) with no cisplatin. The endpoint of this phase II study is swallowing function. If an improvement in swallowing function is demonstrated compared to control, then a larger phase III study will be undertaken.

The ADEPT study run by the University of Washington is randomising 496 patients of T1–T4a HPV-positive disease undergoing transoral resection who have extracapsular extension of nodes and negative margins to standard chemoradiotherapy with IMRT 60 Gy and weekly cisplatin versus the experimental arm of radiotherapy alone (IMRT 60 Gy). The endpoints are disease-free survival and progression-free survival.

3.1.5 Escalation Trials

It should also be noted that whilst there is a lot of interest in de-escalation, many groups are now turning their thoughts to the intermediate-risk HPV-positive group and HPV-positive patients with T4 or N3 disease. In this group, the overall survival is approximately 70 % at three years. Many have noted that this outcome is not comparable to that of low-risk patients, especially when considering that these are younger patients. Therefore, some groups have considered escalating treatment for this particular higher-risk group of patients.

In the UK, the COMPARE trial, run by our group at InHANSE, is randomising patients to standard chemoradiotherapy (70 Gy in 35 fractions), compared to three experimental arms: TPF plus chemoradiotherapy; cisplatin plus dose-escalated radiotherapy; and surgery plus chemoradiotherapy. The outcome is overall survival.

Recruitment has just started to this 650 patient trial, which uses the efficient multiarm, multimodal trial design. Other groups are also considering other forms of escalation including the use of immunotherapy in combination with chemoradiotherapy.

4 Conclusion

It is clear that there are several possible ways to achieve de-escalation and indeed escalation of treatment in HPV-positive patients. The coming few years will reveal the results of many interesting trials which will help direct our management of these groups of patients. We again would encourage clinicians to not change the management of HPV-positive patients, but to continue to treat them as they would treat other oropharyngeal cancer patients, and that they strongly consider recruiting these patients into the relevant clinical trials to ensure that we find out quickly the best way to treat these patients.

References

Ang KK, Harris J, Wheeler R et al (2010) Human papillomavirus and survival of patients with oropharyngeal cancer. N Engl J Med 363(1):24–35

Bonner JA, Harari PM, Giralt J et al (2006) Radiotherapy plus cetuximab for squamous-cell carcinoma of the head and neck. N Engl J Med 354(6):567–578

Brotherston DC, Poon I, Le T et al (2013) Patient preferences for oropharyngeal cancer treatment de-escalation. Head Neck 35(2):151–159

Cmelak A, Li S, Marur S, et al (2014) E1308: reduced-dose IMRT in human papilloma virus (HPV)-associated resectable oropharyngeal squamous carcinomas (OPSCC) after clinical complete response (cCR) to induction chemotherapy (IC). In: ASCO annual meeting proceedings 2014, p LBA6006

Haughey BH, Sinha P (2012) Prognostic factors and survival unique to surgically treated p16+ oropharyngeal cancer. Laryngoscope 122(Suppl 2):S13–S33

Huang SH, Xu W, Waldron J et al (2015) Refining American joint committee on cancer/union for international cancer control TNM stage and prognostic groups for human papillomavirus-related oropharyngeal carcinomas. J Clin Oncol 33(8):836–845

Machtay M, Moughan J, Trotti A et al (2008) Factors associated with severe late toxicity after concurrent chemoradiation for locally advanced head and neck cancer: an RTOG analysis. J Clin Oncol 26(21):3582–3589

O'Sullivan B, Huang SH, Siu LL et al (2013) Deintensification candidate subgroups in human papillomavirus-related oropharyngeal cancer according to minimal risk of distant metastasis. J Clin Oncol 31(5):543–550

Sinha P, Lewis JS, Piccirillo JF, Kallogjeri D, Haughey BH (2012) Extracapsular spread and adjuvant therapy in human papillomavirus-related, p16-positive oropharyngeal carcinoma. Cancer 118(14):3519–3530

Trotti A, Pajak TF, Gwede CK et al (2007) TAME: development of a new method for summarising adverse events of cancer treatment by the radiation therapy oncology group. Lancet Oncol 8(7):613–624

Vaccination Expectations in HNSCC

Stina Syrjänen and Jaana Rautava

Abstract

HPV-associated head and neck squamous cell carcinoma (HNSCC), more specifically the incidence of oropharyngeal cancer, is dramatically increasing in industrialized countries. According to what has been learned from anogenital vaccination programs, there are reasons to believe that current human papillomavirus (HPV) vaccinations may be potentially effective also against HNSCC. However, before specific results on HNSCC are available, one must keep in mind that carcinogenesis in the head and neck region may differ from that of the anogenital tract. Furthermore, the current evidence supports the view that HPV infection is much more complex than simply a sexually transmitted disease. HPV is present in the semen, placenta and in the newborns, and these infections of the newborns create cell-mediated immunity (CMI) against HPV, including the T memory cells. Acquisition of HPV infection in early life will rise new series of questions in the field of HPV vaccination.

Keywords

Human papillomavirus (HPV) · Head and neck squamous cell carcinoma (HNSCC) · Vaccination

S. Syrjänen (✉) · J. Rautava
Department of Oral Pathology, Faculty of Medicine, Turku University Hospital, Institute of Dentistry, University of Turku, Lemminkäisenkatu 2, 20520 Turku, Finland
e-mail: stina.syrjanen@utu.fi

W. Golusiński et al. (eds.), *HPV Infection in Head and Neck Cancer*,
Recent Results in Cancer Research 206, DOI 10.1007/978-3-319-43580-0_21

1 HPV Vaccines

In 1992, Kirnbauer and his associates descried a novel technique how to make human papillomavirus-like particles (VLP) in vitro (1992) by expressing the L1 major capsid proteins of HPV16 in insect cells using a baculovirus vector. In this system, the L1 proteins were expressed at high levels and, surprisingly, assembled into structures that closely resembled PV virions (Kirnbauer et al. 1992) with immunogenicity similar to that of infectious virions. This novel L1 VLP preparation was immediately recognized as a potential candidate for serological tests to measure antibodies to conformational virion epitopes, as well as for a vaccine to prevent HPV infections (Kirnbauer et al. 1992). Subsequent studies on these lines have resulted in the development of the first-generation prophylactic vaccines against HPV6, 11, 16, 18 (Gardasil®, Merck Sharp & Dohme Corp., Whitehouse Station, NJ, USA) or against HPV16 and HPV18 (Cervarix®, GlaxoSmithKline Biologicals, Rixensart, Belgium). In 2015, The U.S. Food and Drug Administration approved a new nonavalent HPV vaccine Gardasil 9® (HPV6, 11, 16, 18, 31, 33, 45, 52 and 58) with promising preliminary results (for review Fruscalzo et al. 2016). Table 1 summarizes the characteristics of the current HPV VLP vaccines and their indications for use.

Table 1 Characteristics of Cervarix®, Gardasil® and Gardasil 9® vaccines

	Cervarix	Gardasil	Gardasil 9
HPV coverage	16, 18	6, 11, 16, 18	6, 11, 16, 18, 31, 33, 45, 52, 58
Manufacturer	GlaxoSmithKline	Merck	Merck
Producing cells	Trichoplusia ni (Hi 5) insect cell line infected with L1 recombinant baculovirus	Saccharomyces cerevisiae (baker's yeast) expressing L1	Saccharomyces cerevisiae (baker's yeast) expressing L1
Adjuvant	Aluminum hydroxyl-phosphate sulfate	Aluminum hydroxide, 3-O-deacylated-4'-monophosphoryl lipid A	Aluminum hydroxide, 3-O-deacylated-4'-monophosphoryl lipid A
Administration	Intramuscular	Intramuscular	Intramuscular
Injection schedule	0, 1, 6 months	0, 2, 6 months	0, 1–2, 6 months
Indications for use (HPV-associated diseases)	Cervical cancer and precancer and adenocarcinoma in situ	Women 9–26 years: cervical, vulvar, vaginal, anal cancer and precancer; genital warts. Men 9–26 years: anal cancer and precancer; genital warts	Women 9–26 years: cervical, vulvar, vaginal, anal cancer and precancer; genital warts. Men 9–26 years: anal cancer and precancer; genital warts

Both of the first-generation prophylactic vaccines have exhibited excellent safety and effectiveness. However, neither of the vaccines has shown efficacy against a prevalent infection (Schiller et al. 2012). There has been no standard assay for assessing immunogenicity in HPV VLP vaccine trials, making direct comparisons difficult. However, regardless of the assays used, studies have demonstrated antibody responses that are strong and durable up to 6–8 years (Brotherton et al. 2016; Einstein et al. 2014; Roteli-Martins et al. 2012; Olsson et al. 2007).

One of the key issues in HPV vaccination is the most optimal timing for the HPV vaccines to provide maximal protection of HPV-naïve individuals (Malagon et al. 2012). Recent studies have confirmed that HPV is present in the semen, placenta and in the newborns (Rintala et al. 2004, 2005; Sarkola et al. 2008; Laprise et al. 2014; Skoczynski et al. 2015; Chisanga et al. 2015). Data from our Finnish Family HPV cohort indicate that persistent oral HPV infections among newborn are predicted by mother's placental HPV positivity (Koskimaa et al. 2012). This implicates that the timing of HPV vaccination needs to be re-evaluated. In already infected women, HPV vaccination will not alter the course of their genital tract infection although it induces higher HPV IgG antibody titers. During pregnancy, there might be more efficient transplacental transfer of maternal HPV antibodies to prevent the newborn to contract HPV infection during delivery. The natural history of the first HPV exposure is not elucidated yet, but there is a possibility that the first site of HPV entry is the oral mucosa (Syrjänen et al. submitted; Rintala et al. 2005).

2 Natural History of HPV in Head and Neck Region

The prevalence and natural history of HPV infection in the head and neck region has not been well established yet. Our prospective Finnish Family HPV cohort on HPV dynamics among family members has shown that HPV infection can be acquired vertically by the newborn before, during and after delivery, and HPV can be found both in the oral and genital mucosa (Sarkola et al. 2008; Rintala et al. 2004, 2005; Syrjänen et al. submitted). The site of the first HPV infection may be through oral mucosa more likely than the genital mucosa. These infections of the newborns create cell-mediated immunity (CMI) against HPV, including the T memory cells (Koskimaa et al. 2014, 2015). In adult life, HPV prevalence seems to be lower in oral mucosa than in the genital region (Chung et al. 2013). Studies using mouth rinses/gargles have found HPV prevalence ranging between 0.9 and 7.5 % (Edelstein et al. 2012; Gillison et al. 2012; Pickard et al. 2012; Smith et al. 2007; Summersgill et al. 2001). With mucosal swab samples and using more sensitive HPV detection methods, HPV prevalence is considerably higher (Kero et al. 2012, 2014; Rautava et al. 2012a, b).

Understanding the natural history of HPV infection in its whole, and the events leading to head and neck infection and cancer in particular, is the critical questions to be solved before conclusions can be drawn whether the current HPV vaccine strategies of adolescents also protect against HNSCC.

3 HPV Antibodies in Saliva

Oral cavity has its own specific environment including saliva. Saliva has secretory immunoglobulin A (sIgA) which is important in the control of infectious agents on oral mucosal surfaces. A study showed that low levels of sIgA could make the individual more susceptible to oral HPV infection (Gonçalves et al. 2006). Saliva could be a noninvasive testing alternative to serum testing for HPV antibodies (Cameron et al. 2003). Women with cervical neoplasia showed significantly more sIgA for HPV16 than women with no cervical neoplasia (Marais et al. 2006). However, opposite results were reported from Costa Rican women by Kemp and co-workers (2012). Immunoglobulin levels could be more site specific than compartmental between mucosal sites (Passmore et al. 2007). Women with a persistent oral HPV infection showed higher levels of salivary IgG and lysozyme than women with no oral HPV infection (Haukioja et al. 2014). In this study, smoking was a risk of persistent oral HPV infection. Prophylactic HPV vaccination has also been shown to induce neutralizing antibodies in saliva (Handisurya et al. 2016). An approach of mucosal HPV immunization has also been explored, because mucosal surfaces are the site of HPV infection (Kichaev et al. 2013). In Sweden, it was shown that after gradual introduction of public HPV vaccination during 2007–2012, between 2013 and 2014, when 73 % of the women were HPV vaccinated, but not necessarily before their sexual debut, oral HPV prevalence had dropped to 1.4 % as compared with 9.3 % in 2009–2011 ($p < 0.00001$) (Grun et al. 2015).

4 Prevention of HPV-Associated Head and Neck Cancer with Vaccination

HPV-associated HNSCC, more specifically the incidence of oropharyngeal cancer, is dramatically increasing in industrialized countries (Gooi et al. 2016; Marur and Forastiere 2016), but there are no data on vaccine efficacy against oropharyngeal HPV infections (Chaturvedi et al. 2011). Table 2 summarizes the prevalence of HPV in HNSCCs derived from systematic reviews including meta-analyses. Because the most common oncogenic HPV genotypes (HPV16 and HPV18) found in the head and neck malignancies are the same as in cervical cancer, the question is: do prophylactic HPV vaccines effectively prevent HPV-related head and neck pathologies (Beachler et al. 2015; Herrero et al. 2013). However, HNSCCs may also harbor HPV genotypes that are not so common in genital malignancies (Rautava et al. 2012a, b). Moreover, Gardasil has demonstrated protection against genital warts and penile/vulvar/vaginal/anal neoplasia in addition to cervical cancer (Schiller et al. 2012; Garland and Smith 2010; Goldstone et al. 2013). Vaccination efficacy is lower when the subjects have already an ongoing HPV infection (Lu et al. 2011). These data suggest that vaccinating the males protects them also against most vaccine HPV-type-related anogenital diseases, which has led to registration and use of these vaccines for males in some countries (Palefsky et al. 2011;

Table 2 Systematic reviews including meta-analysis of head and neck cancers

Reference	Sample size	Cancer	HPV positivity	Population
Gama et al. (2016)	7347	Laryngeal SCC	1830 (25 %)	Global
Shaikh et al. (2015)	7280	Head and neck carcinoma	36 %	Asian Pacific region
Zhang et al. (2014)	3429	Esophageal cancer	HPV16 prevalence 0.381 (95 % CI: 0.283, 0.479)	China
Aboqunrin et al. (2014)	3649	Head and neck cancers	40 %	European
Hardefeldt et al. (2014)	132 studies	Esophageal SCC	24.8 %	Global
Syrjänen and Syrjänen (2013)	492	Sinonasal SCC	133 (27.0 %)	Global
Syrjänen (2013)	10,234	Esophageal SCC	3135 (30.6 %)	Global
Mehanna et al. (2013)	19,368 (5396 oroph, 13,972 non-oroph)	Oropharyngeal/non-oropharyngeal SCC	Oroph 47.7 % Non-oroph 21.8 %	Global
Termine et al. (2008)	4852	Head and neck SCC/oral SCC	34.5 %/38.1 %	Global

Giuliano et al. 2011). For men, immunization through the oral mucosa might be even more important than for women, because the largest mucosal area of men is in the oral cavity (Marais et al. 2006). Quadrivalent vaccination also induces neutralizing antibodies in oral mucosal fluids (Handisurya et al. 2016). Cost-effectiveness analysis has shown that HPV vaccination for boys aged 12 years could be a cost-effective strategy for the prevention of oropharyngeal carcinoma (Graham et al. 2015).

Today, there is no knowledge of the preceding lesions in the continuum of oropharyngeal carcinogenesis. However, it has been shown that HPV16 E6 antibodies are detectable 10 years prior to the detection of oropharyngeal cancer (Lang Kuhs et al. 2016; Anderson et al. 2015; Kreimer et al. 2013).

5 Therapeutic HPV Vaccines and HNSCC

Therapeutic HPV vaccines could eliminate preexisting lesions and infected cells. Before using HPV vaccine in the treatment of a certain patient, there should be established HPV status and histological results. However, today there is no agreed standard method for HPV testing. Most therapeutic vaccines have been developed with HPV16, against its oncoproteins. Targets for therapeutic intervention are HPV

E6 and E7 oncoproteins since they are expressed at all levels of the HPV-infected epithelium and play a role in the induction and maintenance of HPV-related cancer.

There are trials ongoing with several different molecular targets. A phase I dose escalation trial of MAGE-A3- and HPV16-specific peptide immunomodulatory vaccines GL-0810 and GL-0817 showed T cell and antibody responses in a majority of HNSCC patients (*n* = 16) (Zandberg et al. 2015). One consequence of E6/E7 over-expression in HPV-associated oropharyngeal cancer is a strong expression of the cellular protein $p16^{INK4a}$ (Reuschenbach et al. 2016). A recent report of phase 1/2a first-in-human trial on HPV DNA vaccine against cyclin-dependent kinase inhibitor $p16^{INK4a}$ showed induction of cellular and humoral immune responses in advanced tumors without severe toxicities (Reuschenbach et al. 2016). This study with 26 patients included seven HNSCCs. With a mouse model, local irradiation and Shiga Toxin B-based HPV vaccination for treatment of HNSCC have shown promising results and are approaching early-phase clinical trials (Mondini et al. 2015). In another study with mice, intradermal DNA vaccines forming E7 recombinant retroviral virus-like particles (pVLP-E7) cured mice with already established tumors when combined with toll-like receptor (TLR) 7 and TLR 9 agonists (Lescaille et al. 2013). Also the PD-1:PD-L1 pathway has shown a possibility of therapeutic blockade analyzing tissue samples from tonsillar carcinoma patients (Lyford-Pike et al. 2013). For comparison, quadrivalent vaccination effectiveness in low-risk HPV-induced respiratory papillomatosis has either shown no effect in children (Hermann and Weckx 2016) or prolonged the intervals between the surgical interventions (Hocevar-Boltezar et al. 2014).

6 Conclusions

How to prevent the transmission and expression of oncogenic HPV of the head and neck region is an open question. Or is the early HPV infection part of the normal natural history and more focus should be on understanding what makes an HPV infection prone to malignant transformation? The answer may be found from the individual's immunological status. According to what has been learned from anogenital vaccination programs, there are reasons to believe that vaccinations might be potentially effective also against head and neck neoplasia (Takes et al. 2015). However, before specific results on HNSCC are available, one must keep in mind that carcinogenesis in the head and neck region may differ from that of the anogenital tract. Furthermore, the current evidence supports the view that HPV infection is much more complex than simply a sexually transmitted disease. Acquisition of HPV infection in early life will rise new series of questions in the field of HPV vaccination.

References

Aboqunrin S, Di Tanna GL, Keeping S, Carroll S, Iheanacho I (2014) Prevalence of human papillomavirus in head and neck cancers in European populations: a meta-analysis. BMC Cancer 14:968

Anderson KS, Gerber JE, D'Souza G, Pai SI, Cheng JN, Alam R, Kesiraju S, Chowell D, Gross ND, Haddad R, Gillison ML, Posner M (2015) Biologic predictors of serologic responses to HPV in oropharyngeal cancer: the HOTSPOT study. Oral Oncol 51(8):751–758

Beachler DC, Kreimer AR, Schiffman M, Herrero R, Wacholder R, Rodriguez AC, Lowy DR, Porras C, Schiller JT, Quint Q, Jimenez S, Safaeian M, Struijk L, Schussler J, HIlderheim A, Gonzalez P, Costa Rica HPV Vaccine Trial (CVT) Group (2015) Multisite HPV16/18 vaccine efficacy against cervical, anal and oral HPV infection. J Natl Cancer Inst 108(1)

Brotherton M, Jit M, Gravitt PE, Brisson M, Kreimer AR, Pai SI, Fakhry C, Monsonego J, Franceschi S. (2016) Eurogin roadmap 2015: how has HPV knowledge changed our practice: vaccines. Int J Cancer (Epub ahead of print)

Cameron JE, Snowhite IV, Chaturvedi AK, Hagensee ME (2003) Human papillomavirus-specific antibody status in oral fluids modestly reflects serum status in human immunodeficiency virus-positive individuals. Clin Diagn Lab Immunol 10(3):431–438

Chaturvedi AK, Engels EA, Pfeiffer RM, Hernandez BY, Xiao W, Kim E, Jiang B, Goodman MT, Sibug-Saber M, Cozen W, Liu L, Lynch CF, Wentzensen N, Jordan RC, Alterkruse S, Anderson WF, Rosenberg PS, Gillison ML (2011) Human papillomavirus and rising oropharyngeal cancer incidence in the United States. J Clin Oncol 29:4294–4301

Chisanga C, Eggert D, Mitchell CD, Wood C, Angeletti PC (2015) Evidence for placental HPV infection in both HIV positive and negative women. J Cancer Ther 6(15):1276–1289

Chung CH, Bagheri A, D'Souza G (2013) Epidemiology of oral human papillomavirus infection. Oral Oncol S1368-8375(13):00685-4

Edelstein ZR, Schwartz SM, Hawes S, Hughes JP, Feng Q, Stern ME et al (2012) Rates and determinants of oral human papillomavirus infection in young men. Sex Trans Dis 39:860–867

Einstein MH, Takacs P, Chatterjee A, Sperling RS, Chakhtoura N, Blatter MM, Lalezari J, David MP, Lin L, Struyf F, Dubin G; HPV-101 Study Group (2014) Comparison of long-term immunogenicity and safety of human papillomavirus (HPV)-16/18 AS04-adjuvanted vaccine and HPV-6/11/16/18 vaccine in healthy women aged 18–45 years: end-of-study analysis of a phase III randomized trial. Human Vaccin Immunother 10(12):3435–3445

Fruscalzo A, Londero AP, Bertozzi S, Lelle RJ (2016) Second-generation prophylactic HPV vaccines: current options and future strategies for vaccines development. Minerva Med 107:26–38

Gama RR, Carvalho AL, Filho AL, Scorsato AP, Lopez RV, Rautava J, Syrjänen S, Syrjänen K (2016) Detection of human papillomavirus in laryngeal squamous cell carcinoma: systematic review and meta-analysis. Laryngoscope 126(4):885–893

Garland SM, Smith JS (2010) Human papillomavirus vaccines: current status and future prospects. Drugs 70:1079–1098

Gillison ML, Broutian T, Pickard RK, Tong ZY, Xiao W, Kahle L, Graubard BI, Chaturvedi AK (2012) Prevalence of oral HPV infection in the United States, 2009–2010. JAMA 307:693–703

Giuliano AR, Palefsky JM, Goldstone S, Moreira ED Jr, Penny ME, Aranda C, Vardas E, Moi H, Jessen H, Hillman R, Chang YH, Ferris D, Rouleau D, Bryan J, Marshall JB, Vuocolo S, Barr E, Radley D, Haupt RM, Guris D (2011) Efficacy of quadrivalent HPV vaccine against HPV infection and disease in males. N Engl J Med 364(5):401–411

Goldstone SE, Jessen H, Palefsky JM, Giuliano AR, Moreira ED Jr, Vardas E, Aranda C, Hillman RJ, Ferris DG, Coutlee F, Marshall JB, Vuocolo S, Haupt RM, Guris D, Garner E (2013) Quadrivalent HPV vaccine efficacy against disease related to vaccine and non-vaccine HPV types in males. Vaccine 31:3849–3855

Gonçalves AK1, Giraldo P, Barros-Mazon S, Gondo ML, Amaral RL, Jacyntho C (2006) Secretory immunoglobulin A in saliva of women with oral and genital HPV infection. Eur J Obstet Gynecol Reprod Biol 124(2):227–231
Gooi Z, Chan JY, Fakhry C (2016) The epidemiology of the human papillomavirus related to oropharyngeal head and neck cancer. Laryngoscope 126(4):894–900
Graham DM, Isaranuwatchai W, Habbous S, de Oliveira C, Liu G, Siu LL, Hoch JS (2015) A cost-effectiveness analysis of human papillomavirus vaccination of boys for the prevention of oropharyngeal cancer. Cancer 121:1785–1792
Grun N, Åhrlund-Richter A, Franzen J, Mirzaie L, Marions L, Ramqvist T, Dalianis T (2015) Oral human papillomavirus (HPV) prevalence in youth and cervical HPV prevalence in women attending a youth clinic in Sweden, a follow up-study 2013-2014 after gradual introduction of public HPV vaccination. Infect Dis 47(1):57–61
Handisurya A, Schellenbacher C, Haitel A, Senger T, Kirnbauer R (2016) Human papillomavirus vaccination induces neutralizing antibodies in oral mucosal fluids. Br J Cancer 114:409–416
Hardefeldt HA, Cox MR, Eslick GD (2014) Association between human papillomavirus (HPV) and oesophageal squamous cell carcinoma: a meta-analysis. Epidemiol Infect 124 (6):1119–1137
Haukioja A, Asunta M, Söderling E, Syrjänen S (2014) Persistent oral human papillomavirus infection is associated with smoking and elevated salivary immunoglobulin G concentration. J Clin Virol 61(1):101–106
Hermann JS, Weckx LY, Monteiro NJ, Santor GF Jr, Campos PAC, Nagata PSS (2016) Effectiveness of the human papillomavirus (types 6, 11, 16 and 18) vaccine in the treatment of children with recurrent respiratory papillomatosis. Int J Pediatr Otorhinolaryngol 83:94–98
Herrero R, Quint W, HIldesheim A, Gonzalez P, Struijk L, Katki HA, Porras C, Schiffman M, Rodriguez AC, Solomon D, Jimenez S, Schiller JT, Lowy DR, van Doorn LJ, Wacholder S, Kreimer AR, CVT Vaccine Group (2013) Reduced prevalence of oral human papillomavirus (HPV) 4 years after bivalent HPV vaccination in a randomized clinical trial in Costa Rica. PLoS ONE 8(7):e68329
Hocevar-Boltezar I, Maticic M, Sereq-Bahar M, Gale N, Poljak M, Kocjan B, Zargi M (2014) Human papilloma virus vaccination in patients with an aggressive course of recurrent respiratory papillomatosis. Eur Arch Otorhinolaryngol 271:3255–3262
Kemp TJ, Safaeian M, Miner S, Williams MC, Rodrigues AC, Herrero R, Hildesheim A, Pinto AL (2012) Oral immunoglobulin levels are not a good surrogate for cervical immunoglobulin levels. Front Oncol 2:61
Kero K, Rautava J, Syrjänen K, Grenman S, Syrjänen S (2012) Oral mucosa as a reservoir of human papillomavirus: point prevalence, genotype distribution, and incident infections among males in a 7-year prospective study. Eur Urol 62(6):1063–1070
Kero K, Rautava J, Syrjänen K, Willberg J, Grenman S, Syrjänen S (2014) Smoking increases oral HPV persistence among men: 7-year follow-up study. Eur J Clin Microbiol Infect Dis 33 (1):123–133
Kichaev G, Mendoza JM, Amante D, Smith TR, McCoy JR, Sardesai NY, Broderick KE (2013) Electroporation mediated DNA vaccination directly to a mucosal surface results in improved immune responses. Hum Vaccin Immunother 9(10):2014–2018
Kirnbauer R, Booy F, Cheng N, Lowy DR, Schiller JT (1992) Papillomavirus L1 major capsid protein self-assembles into virus-like particles that are highly immunogenic. Proc Natl Acad Sci USA 89(24):12180–12184
Koskimaa HM, Waterboer T, Pawlita M, Grenman S, Syrjänen K, Syrjänen S (2012) Human papillomavirus genotypes present in the oral mucosa of newborns and their concordance with maternal cervical human papillomavirus genotypes. J Pediatr 160(5):837–843
Koskimaa HM, Paaso AE, Welters MJ, Grenman SE, Syrjänen KJ, van der Burg SH, Syrjänen SM (2014) J Transl Med 12:44
Koskimaa HM, Paaso A, Welters MJ, Grenman S, Syrjänen K, van der Burg SH, Syrjänen S (2015) Human papillomavirus 16-specific cell-mediated immunity in children born to mothers

with incident cervical intraepithelial neoplasia (CIN) and to those constantly HPV negative. J Transl Med 13:370

Kreimer AR, Johansson M, Waterboer T, Kaaks R, Chang-Claude J, Drogen D, Tjonneland A, Overvad K, Quiros JR, Gonzalez CA, Sanchez MJ, Larranaga N, Navarro C, Barricarte A, Travis RC, Khaw KT, Wareham N, Trichopoulos A, Lagiou P, Trichopoulos D, Peeters PH, Panico S, Masala G, Grioni S, Tumino R, Vineis P, Bueno-de-Mesquita HB, Laurell G, Hallmans G, Manjer J, Ekström J, Skele G, Lund E, Weiderpass E, Ferrari P, Byrnes G, Romineu I, Riboli E, Hildesheim A, Boeing H, Pawlita M, Brennan P (2013) Evaluation of human papillomavirus antibodies and risk of subsequent head and neck cancer. J Clin Oncol 31 (21):2708–2715

Lang Kuhs KA, Pawlita M, Gibson SP, Schmitt NC, Trivedi S, Argiris A, Kreimer AR, Ferris RL, Waterboer T (2016) Characterization of human papillomavirus antibodies in individuals with head and neck cancer. Cancer Epidemiol 42:46–52

Laprise C, Trottier H, Monnier P, Coutlee F, Mayrand MH (2014) Prevalence of human papillomavirus in semen: a systematic review and meta-analysis. Hum Reprod 29(4):640–651

Lescaille G, Pitoiset F, Macedo R, Baillou C, Huret C, Klatzmann D et al (2013) Efficacy of DNA vaccines forming E7 recombinant retroviral virus-like particles for the treatment of human papillomavirus-induced cancers. Hum Gen Ther 24:533–544

Lu B, Viscidi RP, Lee JH, Wu Y, Villa LL, Lazcano-Ponce E, da Silva RJ, Baggio ML, Quiterio M, Salmeron J, Smith DC, Abrahamsen M, Papenfuss M, Stockwell HG, Giuliano AR (2011) Human papillomavirus (HPV) 6, 11, 16 and 18 seroprevalence is associated with sexual practice and age: results from the multinational HPV infection in men study (HIM study). Cancer Epidemiol Biomark Prev 20:990–1002

Lyford-Pike S, Peng S, Young GD, Taube JM, Westra WH, Akpeng B, Bruno TC, Richmon JD, Wang H, Bishop JA, Chen L, Drake CG, Topallan SL, Pardoll DM, Pai SI (2013) Evidence for a role of the PD-1: PD-L1 pathway in immune resistance of HPV-associated head and neck squamous cell carcinoma. Cancer Res 73(6):1733–1741

Malagon T, Drolet M, Bolly MC, Franco EL, Jit M, Brisson J, Brisson M (2012) Cross-protective efficacy of two human papillomavirus vaccines: a systematic review and meta-analysis. Lancer Infect Dis 12(10):781–789

Marais DJ, Sampson C, Jeftha A, Dhaya D, Passmore JA, Denny L, Rybicki EP, Van Der Walt E, Stephen LX, Williamson AL (2006) More men than women make mucosal IgA antibodies to Human papillomavirus type 16 (HPV-16) and HPV-18: a study of oral HPV and oral HPV antibodies in a normal healthy population. BMC Infect Dis 6:95

Marur S, Forastiere AA (2016) Head and neck squamous cell carcinoma: update on epidemiology, diagnosis, and treatment. Mayo Clin Proc 91(3):386–396

Mehanna H, Beech T, Nicholson T, El-Hariry I, McConkey C, Paleri V, Roberts S (2013) Head Neck 35(5):747–755

Mondini M, Nizard M, Tran T, Mauge L, Loi M, Clemenson C, Dugue D, Maroun P, Louvet E, Adam J, Badoual C, Helley D, Dransart E, Johannes L, Vozenin MC, Perfettini JL, Tartour E, Deutsch E (2015) Synergy of radiotherapy and a cancer vaccine for the treatment of HPV-associated head and neck cancer. Mol Cancer Ther 14:1336–1345

Olsson SE, Villa LL, Costa RL, Petta CA, Andrade RP, Malm C, Iversen OE, Hoye J, Steinwall M, Riis-Johannssen G, Andersson-Ellstrom A, Elfgren K, von Krogh G, Lehtinen M, Paavonen J, Tamms GM, Giacoletti K, Lupinacci L, Esser MT, Vuocolo SC, Saah AJ, Barr E (2007) Induction of immune memory following administration of a prophylactic quadrivalent human papillomavirus (HPV) types 6/11/16/18 virus-like particle (VLP) vaccine. Vaccine 21 (25):4931–4939

Palefsky JM, Giuliano AR, Goldstone S, Moreira ED Jr, Aranda C, Jessen H, Hillman R, Ferris D, Coutlee F, Stoler MH, Marshall JB, Radley D, Vuocolo S, Haupt RM, Guris D, Garner EI (2011) HPV vaccine against anal HPV infection and anal intraepithelial neoplasia. N Engl J Med 365(17):1576–1585

Passmore JA, Marais DJ, Sampson C, Allan B, Parker N, Milner M, Denny L, Williamson AL (2007) Cervicovaginal, oral, and serum IgG and IgA responses to human papillomavirus type 16 in women with cervical intraepithelial neoplasia. J Med Virol 79:1375–1380
Pickard RK, Xiao W, Broutian TR, He X, Gillison ML (2012) The prevalence and incidence of oral human papillomavirus infection among young men and women, aged 18-30 years. Sex Transm Dis 39:559–566
Rautava J, Willberg J, Louvanto K, Wideman L, Syrjänen K, Grenman S, Syrjänen S (2012a) Prevalence, genotype distribution and persistence of human papillomavirus in oral mucosa of women: a six-year follow-up study. PLoS ONE 7(8):e42171
Rautava J, Kuuskoski J, Syrjänen K, Grenman R, Syrjänen S (2012b) HPV genotypes and their prognostic significance in head and neck squamous cell carcinomas. J Clin Virol 53:116–120
Reuschenbach M, Pauligk C, Karbach J, Rafiyan MR, Kloor M, Prigge ES, Sauer M, Al-Batran SE, Kaufmann AM, Schneider A, Jäger E, von Knebel Doeberitz M (2016) A phase 1/2a study to test the safety and immunogenicity of a p 16^{INK4a} peptide vaccine in patients with advanced human papillomavirus-associated cancers. Cancer 112(9):1425–1433
Rintala MA, Grenman SE, Pöllänen PP, Suominen JJ, Syrjänen SM (2004) Detection of high-risk HPV DNA in semen and its association with the quality of semen. Int J STD AIDS 15 (11):740–743
Rintala MA, Grenman SE, Järvenkylä ME, Syrjänen KJ, Syrjänen SM (2005) High-risk types of human papillomavirus (HPV) DNA in oral and genital mucosa of infants during their first 3 years of life: experience from the Finnish HPV Family Study. Clin Infect Dis 41(12):1728–1733
Roteli-Martins C, NAud P, De Borba P, Teixeira J, De Carvalho N, Zahaf T et al (2012) Sustained immunogenicity and efficacy of the HPV-16/18 As04-adjuvant vaccine: up to 8.4 years of follow-up. Hum Vaccin Immunother 8(3):1
Sarkola ME, Grenman SE, Rintala MA, Syrjänen KJ, Syrjänen SM (2008) Human papillomavirus in the placenta and umbilical cord blood. Acta Obstet Gynecol Scand 87(11):1181–1188
Schiller JT, Castellsague X, Garland SM (2012) A review of clinical trials of human papillomavirus prophylactic vaccines. Vaccine 20(30):5
Shaikh MH, McMillan NA, Johnson NW (2015) HPV-associated head and neck cancers in the Asia Pacific: a critical literature review and meta-analysis. Cancer Epidemiol 39(6):923–938
Skoczynski M, Gozdzicka-Jozefiak A, Kwasniewska A (2015) The prevalence of human papillomavirus between the neonates and their mothers. Biomed Res Int 2015:126417
Smith EM, Swarnavel S, Ritchie JM, Wang D, Haugen TH, Turek LR (2007) Prevalence of human papillomavirus in the oral cavity/oropharynx in large population of children and adolescents. Pediatr Infect Dis J 26:836–840
Summersgill KF, Smith EM, Levy BT, Allen JM, Haugen TH, Turek LP (2001) Human papillomavirus in the oral cavities of children and adolescents. Oral Sug Oral Med Oral Pathol Oral Radiol Endod 91:62–69
Syrjänen K (2013) Geographic origin is a significant determinant of human papillomavirus prevalence in oesophageal squamous cell carcinoma: systematic review and meta-analysis. Scand J Infect Dis 45:1–18
Syrjänen K, Syrjänen S (2013) Detection of human papillomavirus (HPV) in sinonasal carcinoma: systematic review and meta-analysis. Hum Pathol 44:983–991
Syrjänen S, Rintala M, Willberg J, Rautava J, Koskimaa H, Paaso A, Kero K, Louvanto K, Syrjänen K, Grenman S. Oral HPV infections in nonsexually active children six-year incidence, clearance and persistence. Submitted
Takes RP, Wierzbicka M, D'Souza G, Jackowska J, Silver CE, Rodrigo JP, Dikkers FG, Olsen KD, Rinaldo A, Brakenhoff RH, Ferlito A (2015) HPV vaccination to prevent oropharyngeal carcinoma: What can be learned from anogenital vaccination programs? Oral Oncol 51(21):1057–1060
Termine N, Panzarella V, Falaschini S, Russo A, Matranga D, Lo Muzio L, Campisi G (2008) HPV in oral squamous cell carcinoma vs head and neck squamous cell carcinoma biopsies: a meta-analysis (1988–2007). Ann Oncol 19(10):1681–1690

Zandberg DP, Rollins S, Goloubeva O, Morales RE, Tan M, Taylor R, Wolf JS, Schumaker LM, Cullen KJ, Zimrin A, Ord R, Lubek JE, Suntharalingam M (2015) A phase I dose escalation trial of MAGE-A3- and HPV16-specific peptide immunomodulatory vaccines in patients with recurrent/metastatic (RM) squamous cell carcinoma of the head and neck (SCCHN). Cancer Immunol Immunother 64:367–379

Zhang SK, Guo LW, Chen Q, Zhang M, Liu SZ, Quan PL, Lu JB, Sun XB (2014) Prevalence of human papillomavirus 16 in esophageal cancer among the Chinese population: a systematic review and meta-analysis. Asian Pac J Cancer Prev 15(23):10143–10149

Printed by Printforce, the Netherlands